MENTAL STATUS EXAMINATION

52 CHALLENGING CASES, MODEL DSM-5 AND ICD-10 INTERVIEWS, QUESTIONNAIRES, AND COGNITIVE TESTS FOR DIAGNOSIS AND TREATMENT

VOLUME 1 OF THE MENTAL STATUS EXAMINATION SERIES

BY

WES BURGESS, M.D., PH.D.

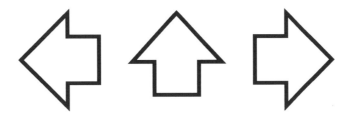

For Amber, with all our love.

Mental Status Examination: 52 Challenging Cases, Model DSM-5 and ICD-10 Interviews, Questionnaires and Cognitive Tests for Diagnosis and Treatment
Volume 1 of the Mental Status Examination Series

Third Edition, Copyright © 2013 by Wes Burgess
Second Edition, Copyright © 2013 by Wes Burgess
First Edition, Copyright © 2011 by Wes Burgess

Figures copyright © 2011 by Wes Burgess
Photo of the author by Cheryl Rizzo
All rights reserved. No part of this book may be reproduced, scanned, or distributed in any print or electronic form without written permission from the author except in the case of brief quotations embodied in articles or reviews. However, *original* purchasers of the book are entitled to use, reproduce, and modify the clinical evaluation forms in Appendices I-VII for their own personal clinical use, as long as correct credit is given.

ISBN-13: 9781482552959
ISBN-10: 1482552957

Diagnoses that are unchanged from the *Diagnostic and Statistical Manual of Mental Disorders,* Fourth Edition, Text Revision (Copyright © 2000) are reprinted with permission from American Psychiatric Association.

Library of Congress Cataloging-In-Publication Data

Burgess, Wes
Mental Status Examination / 52 Challenging Cases, Model DSM-5 and ICD-10 Interviews, Questionnaires and Cognitive Tests for Diagnosis and Treatment / Wes Burgess

pp; cm
Includes bibliographical references (pp 177-178)
1. Mental Health, 2. Medical School, 3. Psychiatry, 4. Psychology, 5. Social Work, 6. Counseling, 7. Nursing, 8. Hospital, 9. Emergency Room

TABLE OF CONTENTS

Introduction 5
Chapter 1. The Diagnostic Examination 6
The Reason for the Consultation. History: Medical, Psychiatric, Developmental, and Social. Observing and Listening to Your Patient. DSM-5 and ICD-10. Administering and Interpreting the Diagnostic Interview and Questionnaire. Panic Disorder. Generalized Anxiety Disorder. Somatic Symptom Disorder. Illness Anxiety Disorder. Conversion Disorder. Factitious Disorder. Malingering. Attention-Deficit/Hyperactivity Disorder. Major Depressive Disorder. Melancholic Depression. Persistent Depressive Disorder. Atypical Depression. Bipolar I Disorder. Bipolar II Disorder. Cyclothymic Disorder. Psychosis. Schizophrenia. Schizophreniform Disorder. Brief Psychotic Disorder. Delusional Disorder. Schizotypal Disorder. Schizoaffective Disorder. Social Anxiety Disorder. Anorexia Nervosa. Bulimia Nervosa. Obsessive-Compulsive Disorder. Acute Stress Disorder. Posttraumatic Stress Disorder. Adjustment Disorders. Suicidality and Violence. Sleep-Wake Disorders. Substance Use Disorders: Alcohol; Opioids; Cannabis: Sedatives, Hypnotics, or Anxiolytics; Cocaine; Amphetamine-Type Stimulants; Hallucinogens; Phencyclidine; Tobacco; Inhalants. Personality Disorders.

Chapter 2. The Cognitive Examination 21
The Cognitive Examination Test Battery. Why Measure Cognition? Standardized Test Batteries. Monitoring Patients' Progress. Psychobiology of the Cognitive Examination. Attention. Language and Aphasias. Memory. Abstract Thinking. Sequential Thinking. Nonverbal Tests of Abstract and Sequential Thinking. The Luria Figure Drawing Test of Sequential Thinking. Administering and Interpreting the Cognitive Interview and Questionnaire. The Cognitive Interview. The Cognitive Questionnaire. Interpreting Patterns of Response to the Cognitive Examination. Tailoring the Cognitive Examination to Your Patient. Delirium. Mild Neurocognitive Disorder. Major Neurocognitive Disorder. Alzheimer's Disease. Traumatic Brain Injury. Frontotemporal Disease. Prion Disease. Human Immunodeficiency Virus (HIV) Infection. Parkinson's Disease. Lewy Body Disease. Huntington's Disease. Vascular Disease. Substance-Induced Neurocognitive Disorders.

Chapter 3. The Mental Status Examination in the Emergency Room 34
Case 1. The Woman Who Was Struck by the Wrath of God 34
Case 2. Mrs. Black Is Too Nervous 47
Case 3. Where Is Roberto? 40
Case 4. Mr. Smith Has Voodoo Worms! 42
Case 5. Jane and the Night Visitors 44
Case 6. Sam and Dave Make a Pact 46
Case 7. Roger Goes through the Roof 50
Case 8. Little Judi Screams in Terror 52
Case 9. Dr. Frank Studies Asian Medicine 54
Case 10. Johnnie Wants to Kill His Friends 57
Case 11. Zebra Boy 61

Chapter 4. The Mental Status Examination in the Hospital 63
Case 12. Keep Kenneth off Our Unit! 63
Case 13. Dr. Ralph Has the Worst Trip of His Life 66
Case 14. Mrs. Tempe Sucks Her Spoon 70
Case 15. "Rule Out Psych" 72
Case 16. Multicolored Dancing Golf Balls 74
Case 17. Carl Falls Down and Feels Better 77
Case 18. Missy Barely Moves 79
Case 19. Marty Is a TV Star 82
Case 20. A Famous Apartment Manager 85

Case 21. George and Anna Can't Move and Lucy Can't Stop 88
Case 22. They're Killing All the Cats! 92
Case 23. Gloria's Friends 95
Case 24. Suzie Moves Out 98

Chapter 5. The Mental Status Examination in the Clinic.. **101**
    Case 25. Is Father Losing His Mind?.. 101
    Case 26. Pat's Problems Come Back... 104
    Case 27. What Happened to Sarah?... 107
    Case 28. Jim's Roommate Dies.. 110
    Case 29. Mr. Snow Has Bad Luck... 113
    Case 30. Maudie Smiles... 117
    Case 31. Laura Itches... 119
    Case 32. Anne's Beautiful Long, Red Hair.. 123
    Case 33. Terry Worries about His Game... 125
    Case 34. Is June Demented?.. 128
Chapter 6. The Mental Status Examination in Private Practice.. **130**
    Case 35. Ted Doesn't Like Emotions... 130
    Case 36. Marilyn Makes a Comeback... 133
    Case 37. Help! I Can't Tell You what's Wrong... 135
    Case 38. Miss Zelda Tumbles.. 137
    Case 39. Tony has a Perfect Plan... 140
    Case 40. Louise's Party Surprise.. 143
    Case 41. Anita Is Not the Woman I Married... 146
    Case 42. I'll be Your Easiest Patient.. 149
    Case 43. Alice Factory Smells Feathers.. 152
    Case 44. Mary Gets a Bite.. 157
    Case 45. Bobbie the Terror... 153
    Case 46. Julie's Nocturnal Adventure.. 161
    Case 47. Freddi Hangs Out at the Fair... 163
    Case 48. Harry has a Hang-Up... 166
Chapter 7. The Mental Status Examination in Legal and Forensic Settings..................................... **168**
    Case 49. Richard Runs in Fear... 168
    Case 50. Don's Curious Crime... 171
    Case 51. Jack Sees Red.. 174
    Case 52. Me and My Uncle.. 178
Chapter 8. Resources.. **181**
Appendix I. The Diagnostic Interview... **183**
Appendix II. The Diagnostic Questionnaire.. **186**
Appendix III. The Cognitive Interview.. **189**
Appendix IV. The Cognitive Questionnaire... **196**
Appendix V. The Cognitive Questionnaire Score Sheet... **200**
Appendix VI. The Nonverbal Tests of Abstract and Sequential Thinking.. **203**
Appendix VII. The Luria Figure Drawing Test... **205**
The Author... **206**
Also from this Author.. **206**
Disclaimer.. **206**

INTRODUCTION

Mental Status Examination is for clinical students, interns, residents, and practicing professionals who want to painlessly perfect their evaluation skills. This book explains how to perform and interpret a complete DSM-5 and ICD-10 mental status examination and a cognitive battery that has been validated in refereed professional journals like the *American Journal of Psychiatry, Psychiatry Research, Biological Psychiatry, Psychiatric Services,* and *Psychological Reports.*

You are introduced to 52 challenging, real-life patients who tell you their stories just as if you were their personal clinician. All patients were given the same examinations described above. With this information, you must discover the correct diagnosis and the clinical treatment that solves each patient's problem. Then the correct clinical solution is revealed and confirmed by the patient's successful treatment response and follow-up. Every step of the diagnostic thinking process is explained so that when you see a similar patient in the Emergency Room, hospital, clinic, private office, or forensic setting, you will know just what to do. By the end of the book, you will have mastered the clinical tools you need to unlock the mystery of your patients' problems.

Mental Status Examination gives you the opportunity to diagnose patients with conditions of Major Depressive Disorder; Attention-Deficit/Hyperactivity Disorder; Bipolar I and II Disorders; Panic Disorder; Generalized Anxiety Disorder; Social Anxiety Disorder; Acute and Posttraumatic Stress Disorders; Schizophrenia; Intoxication, Abuse, and Dependence on pharmaceuticals, alcohol, street drugs, and supplements; Borderline Personality Disorder; Antisocial Personality Disorder; and Psychopathic Personality.

You will diagnose patients suffering from Delusional Disorder, Sleep Terrors, Intellectual Disability, Catatonia, Conversion Disorder, Trichotillomania, and Formication, as well as cultural and religious practices that complicate patients' evaluations, including coining, Santeria, *folie á deux,* and suicide pacts. We explain medical conditions that masquerade as mental disorders, such as aphasias, drug side effects, brain trauma, hypotension, stroke, Creutzfeldt-Jakob disease, multiple sclerosis, *herpes zoster*, Parkinsonism, epilepsy, and cancer.

Mental Status Examination explains how to use a model Diagnostic Examination employing DSM-5 and ICD-10 criteria and a Cognitive Examination battery that measures attention, language, memory, abstract thinking, and sequential thinking (executive function). Both are supplied in both an interview version that you can adapt or read *verbatim* and a questionnaire version that your patients can fill out in advance. The book ends with a Resources chapter with sources you will use.

Time is precious for clinicians—we care for our patients, meet with their families, attack mountains of paperwork, and complete the requirements of our ongoing education. Diagnostic skill is essential for our success. Let's get started now!

CHAPTER 1
THE DIAGNOSTIC EXAMINATION

A mental status examination consists of a diagnostic evaluation and cognitive testing. The examination given in this book will give you the information you need to make an accurate diagnosis. In Appendix I, you will find a complete script for the Diagnostic Interview. If you wish, you can simply read the script to your patients and check off their responses, or you can adapt the wording to suit your individual style. It is worth studying this script because it contains the most important criteria from the American Psychiatric Association's *Diagnostic and Statistical Manual of Mental Disorders* (DSM-5) and the *International Statistical Classification of Diseases and Related Health Problems 10th Revision* (ICD-10) referenced in Chapter 8.

In Appendix II, you will find the Diagnostic Questionnaire. This contains every question from the Diagnostic Interview script arranged so that your patients can complete their answers by themselves. You may hand out this Questionnaire to your new patients in advance of their evaluation to collect information necessary for diagnosis. Then you will be free to use the rest of the interview time to focus on other important clinical issues.

Both versions help organize your diagnostic information and provide a permanent record for the chart. *Original* purchasers of this book are permitted to use, reproduce, and modify the Diagnostic Interview and Diagnostic Questionnaire, as long as proper credit is given.

The Reason for the Consultation

The first step of every interview is to ask patients why they have come for evaluation. Beginning with this question helps get the interviewer and interviewee working together. It is very important that patients believe they can express their chief complaints clearly and that you are listening to what they say. In addition, patients' stated problems often convey useful information about their condition. A patient hospitalized with a huge head wound who says he is only in the hospital for an ingrown toenail may be confused or in denial. A patient with hallucinations and delusions who says he is only being evaluated because he "wants to get to know you," may be guarded or possess impaired insight. Try to get patients to condense their problem into a short statement, so you both can understand it clearly. I open evaluations by saying, "Why are we here today?" or simply, "Tell me your story."

History: Medical, Psychiatric, Developmental, and Social

Sometime during the evaluation, you must take your patient's history, including previous medical and psychiatric problems, past diagnoses, hospitalizations, and treatments (including psychotherapy, prescription medications, and over-the-counter drugs). Developmental history includes information on family members' health and the patient's childhood, developmental milestones, and stressors. A social history can include information about the use of tobacco, coffee, alcohol, and drugs of abuse; school, work, and home situation; as well as current and past relationships. Note that you must base your diagnosis on your patient's current clinical problem, Diagnostic Examination, and Cognitive Examination—diagnoses should never be based on previous diagnoses or the presumptive effects of past stressors.

Observing and Listening to Your Patient

You will learn much by observing your patient during the evaluation. Key times to look at your patient are the moment she meets you, while she is telling you her story, and as you perform your Diagnostic Examination. Is your patient's appearance odd, drab, disheveled, too formal or casual, unkempt, or fragrant with perfume? Is her posture straight or slumped? Does she sit or lean close to you, touch you, or stay as far away as possible? Is her level of activity high? Does she gesture broadly, fidget, cry, wring her hands, or cross her legs and arms? Does she demonstrate any tremors, habits (like biting her fingernails or pulling hair), tics, or stereotypies (purposeful movements out of context, like flicking her fingers in the air)?

Does your patient appear overly warm, friendly, and chummy; or cold, aloof, and distant? Does he act submissive, obsequious, conspiratorial, dramatic, seductive, argumentative, or aggressive? Is he cooperative or uncooperative with the evaluation process?

Is his facial expression and body language (affect) ecstatic, sad, worried, fearful, or angry? Are his expressed emotions appropriate to the situation—for example, does he laugh as he tells you a sad story? Are his expressions *restricted* to just one or two emotions? Is his affect *constricted,* showing a full range of different emotions that are never very strong? Is his affect *flat*, devoid of expression, with emotions that appear to be absent or unreadable? All these aspects of appearance will be valuable in determining your diagnosis.

If you have enough time, you should let your patients explain their situation spontaneously without interruption, asking only broad, open-ended questions when necessary to elicit essential information. This helps patients understand that you care about them and that you are interested in their problem. While your patients are speaking, you may use the Diagnostic Interview or Questionnaire to keep track of their answers and to make sure that you have not omitted anything from your Diagnostic Examination. There is no need to repeat questions that your patient has answered in his or her story.

Remember that a patient needs more than the required symptoms of mental illness for you to give them a diagnosis of mental illness—you must establish that the patient's symptoms are causing clinically significant impairment in school, work, home, social life, or other important areas of living.

DSM-5 AND ICD-10

The Diagnostic and Statistical Manual of Mental Disorders (DSM-5) of the American Psychiatric Association and the *International Statistical Classification of Diseases and Related Health Problems 10th Revision* (ICD-10) of the World Health Organization are research-based publications that define what mental illnesses exist and how to recognize them. DSM-5 and ICD-10 provide official diagnostic criteria that have been accepted throughout the United States and much of the world. DSM-5 is more specific than ICD-10, although both systems generally agree. By using these official diagnostic criteria, trained clinicians with different backgrounds and different credentials can agree on the same diagnosis whether they are general practitioners, psychiatrists, professional psychologists, counselors, nurses, or social workers.

Please note that the names of the DSM-5 and ICD-10 disorders are not the same as the disorders themselves. Unipolar Major Depressive Disorder is responsible for the biggest confusion—many people who claim to feel "depressed" do not meet the largely physical diagnostic criteria and do not have unipolar Major Depressive Disorder. You will also see anhedonic patients that do have unipolar Major Depressive Disorder but deny feeling sadness or depressed mood.

Similarly, many people who claim to have feelings of panic or anxiety do not meet the physiological criteria for Panic Disorder or Generalized Anxiety Disorder and should not receive either diagnosis. Alternatively, you will have patients for whom emotions of fear or anxiety are not the presenting complaint, who nonetheless meet the diagnostic criteria for Panic Disorder or Generalized Anxiety Disorder.

A patient can experience a Manic Episode without any mood elevation if he is angry or expansive, and many individuals with Bipolar I Disorder will never have a manic episode or cycle while you are their caretaker. A patient with Schizophrenia who shows sadness or other strong emotion does not necessarily have Schizoaffective Disorder. Individuals with Obsessive-Compulsive Personality do not exhibit the obsessive thoughts and compulsive behaviors seen in Obsessive-Compulsive Disorder. Individuals with Borderline and Antisocial Personalities are usually quite pleasant when you first meet them in person.

A standardized set of diagnoses is essential for guiding medical, psychotherapeutic, and social treatment; gauging patients' recovery process; billing purposes; and other paperwork. However, there are always individuals who chafe when forced into any external system of categorization and yearn to approach assessment on their own terms with their own labels or lack of them. You will hear from too many medical doctors, mental health clinicians, teachers, and administrators who make "snap diagnoses" on first sight of the patient, without feeling the need to learn or apply official DSM-5 or ICD-10 criteria. I have heard many psychotherapists remark, "It doesn't matter what the diagnosis is—my treatment will be the same." Unfortunately, this approach invariably leads to misdiagnosis and mistreatment.

The diagnostic criteria in this book are a synthesis designed to be both understandable and consistent with both DSM-5 and ICD-10. Some diagnostic criteria are in DSM-5 are unchanged from DSM-IV. Have a copy of the DSM-5 or ICD-10 available during your practice so you can be sure of the *exact* diagnostic criteria that apply to your patient (see Chapter 8).

ADMINISTERING AND INTERPRETING THE DIAGNOSTIC INTERVIEW AND QUESTIONNAIRE

The first step in performing the Diagnostic Examination is to choose the form you wish to use for your patient. The one-on-one Diagnostic Interview is personal and easy to use at the bedside. Try to ask your questions in an unhurried conversational tone that will put your patients at ease. Alternatively, using the Diagnostic Questionnaire will speed the evaluation, especially if your patient completes it in the waiting room before his scheduled appointment. This will free valuable time to discuss your patient's personal problems and to formulate your diagnosis and treatment plan.

The Diagnostic Examination questions are organized around DSM-5 and ICD-10 diagnoses to make scoring and interpretation faster and easier. The numbers below refer to sections of the Diagnostic Interview and Diagnostic Questionnaire (see Appendices I and II).

SECTION 1. CYCLIC ACTIVITY PATTERNS

Many diagnostic criteria consist of physical processes such as sleep duration, time of sleep onset, midcycle waking, early waking, and sleeplessness, as well as the patient's exercise activity, nutrition, appetite, and weight. For example, Generalized Anxiety Disorder can be associated with difficulty falling asleep or midcycle waking. Patients with melancholic unipolar Major Depressive Disorder typically exhibit weight loss and early morning wakening. Major Depressive Disorder with Atypical Features is characterized by weight gain and oversleeping in the morning. Bipolar Manic Episodes are associated with decreased sleeping and advancing sleep cycle—watch for increased goal-directed activity that keeps the patient up late at night.

SECTION 2. PHYSICAL ANXIETY:

Panic Disorder (DSM-5 300.01, ICD-10 F41.0)

Your patient may be having a Panic Attack if she endorses having four of the following symptoms that peaked within minutes: pounding or racing heart; excessive sweating; trembling or shaking; shortness of breath; choking; chest pain; nausea or stomachache; dizziness, lightheadedness, or unsteadiness; chills or hot flushes; numbness and tingling in the fingers or face (paresthesias); a feeling of detachment from self (depersonalization) or the environment (derealization); fear of losing control or going crazy; or fear of dying. These attacks must be followed by one month of worry about additional Panic Attacks and/or maladaptive attempts to avoid having attacks.

Do not routinely give the diagnosis of Panic Disorder solely because patients complain of nervous, anxious, panicky, or fearful emotions—the criteria for Panic Disorder are mainly physical symptoms that are also associated with increased blood levels of adrenaline (epinephrine), lactic acid, and increased blood pH. Even the "psychological" symptoms of derealization, depersonalization, and fears of dying, losing control, and going crazy can be reproduced by artificially altering blood adrenaline levels and acid/base balance. For this reason, you cannot diagnose Panic Disorder if substance intoxication, substance withdrawal, or any other medical disorder causes the symptoms.

If you suspect another medical cause, consider a physiological stress reaction with elevated levels of stress neurotransmitters (like adrenaline) and steroid stress hormones (like cortisol). These can be ameliorated with stress-reduction exercises and meditation (such as those in my book *Calm Your Mind*, see Chapter 8). If the patient endorses dizziness or lightheadedness, chest pain, pounding heart, excessive sweating, or shortness of breath, consider consultation with a cardiac specialist or pulmonologist. If the patient endorses tingling fingers or face, dizziness, and chest pain, consider hyperventilation, which makes blood alkaline, constricts cerebral blood vessels, and decreases the amount of oxygen available to the brain and central nervous system. Lactic acid in the blood following exercise or fear can also precipitate hyperventilation and symptoms of Panic Attacks. In women, chills or hot flushes can indicate menopausal symptoms. Persistent stomach pain can be indicative of stomach ulcer, with concurrent pain and weakness due to bleeding (ask about alcohol and aspirin consumption).

Anxiety in unipolar Major Depressive Disorder, overwhelmed feelings in bipolar depression, agitation in bipolar mania, and tension in Schizophrenia are often misdiagnosed as Panic Attacks. You cannot make a diagnosis of Panic Disorder if another anxiety disorder such as Social Anxiety Disorder, Obsessive-Compulsive Disorder, Posttraumatic Stress Disorder, or Separation Anxiety better accounts for the symptoms.

The chronic anxiety, emotional instability, and emptiness of Personality Disorders are sometimes mistaken for panic symptoms (see *Mental Status Examination for Personality Disorders*, Chapter 8). Such patients may describe Panic Attacks lasting hours or days, whereas the usual Panic Attack lasts between seconds and minutes. Other patients may claim they are in the middle of a Panic Attack as they calmly describe their symptoms. Many clinicians ask their patients the date and time of their first Panic Attack, which individuals with true Panic Disorder can often recall.

SECTION 3. GENERAL ANXIETY:

Generalized Anxiety Disorder (DSM-5 300.02, ICD-10 F41.1)

Patients may qualify for the diagnosis of Generalized Anxiety Disorder if they have uncontrollable worried thoughts about activities or events such as school or work performance that occur most days for at least six months, and endorse at least three of the following symptoms: feeling restless, keyed-up, or edgy; being easily fatigued; having difficulty concentrating or feeling their mind going blank; irritability; muscle tension; or sleep disturbance, such as difficulty falling or staying asleep or restless, unsatisfying sleep. These symptoms must cause distress and impairment in school, work, home, or social functioning.

Do not routinely give patients the diagnosis of Generalized Anxiety Disorder solely because they complain of anxiety or nervousness, without worried thoughts and physical symptoms.

When patients complain of anxiety in the Diagnostic Examination, it is necessary to ascertain what they really mean. For example, patients with intellectual (worried thoughts), emotional (meaningless, floating dread), and physical (agitation and edginess) symptoms may all call their condition "anxiety," despite obvious differences in their experiences. Some patients mislabel other emotions as anxiety. For example, when parents and teachers send me children described as nervous or anxious, the children often describe angry (not anxious) emotions during their Diagnostic Examinations. Many patients, particularly those with Bipolar Disorder, indiscriminately label a variety of concurrent emotions as either "anxious," "fearful," or "depressed," without clearly discriminating between the three states. It is helpful to ask patients specific questions to see what they are really experiencing.

When fatigue is extreme despite efforts to exercise, always consider covert cancer, hypothyroidism, stimulant abuse, or other metabolic disorders. Note that obsessive worries, muscle tension, irritability, edginess, insomnia, and poor focus overlap the symptoms of bipolar mania. Leaden fatigue, irritability, hypersomnia with restless sleep, poor focus, and empty mentation frequently indicate depression with Atypical Features or bipolar depression. You cannot make a diagnosis of Generalized Anxiety Disorder if the symptoms can be accounted for by Bipolar Disorder, unipolar Major Depressive Disorder, Schizoaffective Disorder, Schizophrenia, organic brain problems, or substance-related problems.

In children, fatigue, irritability, agitation, poor sleep, and poor attention in school are final common pathways for many problems, and do not necessarily represent Generalized Anxiety Disorder.

SECTION 4. OTHER PHYSICAL SYMPTOMS:

Somatic Symptom Disorder (DSM-5 300.82, ICD-10 F45.1)

Illness Anxiety Disorder (Hypochondriasis) (DSM-5 300.7, ICD-10 F45.21)

Conversion Disorder (Functional Neurological Symptom Disorder) (DSM-5 300.11, ICD-10 F44)

Factitious Disorder (DSM-5 300.19, ICD-10 F68.1),

Malingering (DSM-5 V65.2, ICD-10 Z76.5)

Headache, neckache, back pain, joint pain, abdominal pain, diarrhea, urinary frequency, low sexual drive, and anorgasmia are among the most common physical problems mentioned by patients. These can all be duplicated in normal individuals by the administration of adrenaline, the major component of the physical stress response. Adrenaline levels also rise with hormonal cycles of menstruation, pregnancy, and menopause, as well as with the use of (and/or withdrawal from) alcohol, narcotics, tobacco, caffeine, amphetamine, cocaine, and other stimulants. These physical symptoms are *not* diagnostic for Panic Disorder or Generalized Anxiety Disorder but they often appear during and in between episodes of unipolar Major Depressive Disorder and Bipolar Disorder. When one of these symptoms is prominent, you should consider an internal medicine workup. If there seems to be no medical basis for the symptoms, they may represent somatic disorders.

Consider Somatic Symptom Disorder when patients' somatic symptoms are distressing or disrupt their daily life and their expression of their symptoms and health concerns are 1) disproportionate to the seriousness of the complaints, 2) expressed with persistently high anxiety, and/or 3) take up excessive time and energy. Although somatic symptoms may change, the state of being symptomatic is persistent, typically lasting more than six months.

Consider Illness Anxiety Disorder (Hypochondriasis) if the patient is excessively preoccupied with the notion that he has a specific serious disease, is anxious and easily alarmed about health issues, and is excessive or avoidant about health-care. Again, although the specific illness that is feared may change, the preoccupation is persistent, typically lasting more than six months.

When a patient experiences problems in voluntary motor control or sensation that are incompatible with neurological or medical diagnoses, warrant medical evaluation and/or cause significant distress or impairment in school, work, home, or social function, consider Conversion Disorder. Conversion Disorder appeared to be more common in the heyday of classical psychodynamic theory, where it was explained as a physical reaction to psychological conflict, but it is sometimes seen today.

Consider Factitious Disorder when patients intentionally fake the symptoms of a physical or mental disorder with the intention of assuming the rôle of patient or invalid. Beware of Factitious Disorder Imposed on Another, where individuals manufacture symptoms to place others (often children or the elderly) in the rôle of patients.

When the intentional faking of physical or mental symptoms is motivated by external incentives, such as obtaining money, avoiding work, obtaining drugs, or evading criminal prosecution, consider Malingering.

SECTION 5. FOCUS PROBLEMS: ATTENTION-DEFICIT/HYPERACTIVITY DISORDER

ADHD, Predominantly Inattentive (DSM-5 314.00, ICD-10 90.0)

You may give your patient the diagnosis of Attention-Deficit/Hyperactivity Disorder, Predominantly Inattentive Presentation if he or she satisfies six of the following symptoms: poor attention to details; difficulty sustaining attention; problems listening to others; failure to finish projects because of poor task persistence; difficulty organizing tasks and activities (including difficulty managing *sequential thinking* tasks); dislike or reluctance to do assigned tasks that require sustained mental effort; losing things necessary for tasks or activities; distractibility; or forgetfulness in daily activities. These symptoms must have been present for at least six months and must interfere with school, work, home, or social life. Some of the symptoms must have been present before 12 years of age and some must be present in at least two settings. If you suspect Attention-Deficit/Hyperactivity Disorder, Primarily Inattentive Presentation, it is best to follow up with a continuous performance behavioral task (CPT) to measure actual inattention.

SECTION 6. ACTIVITY SYMPTOMS:

ADHD, Predominantly Hyperactive-Impulsive (DSM-5 314.01, ICD-10 90.1)

You may give your patient the diagnosis of Attention-Deficit/Hyperactivity Disorder, Predominantly Hyperactive-Impulsive Presentation, if he or she satisfies any six of the following symptoms: fidgeting or squirming, difficulty sitting in one place, restless feelings or behavior, difficulty quieting down during leisure activities, appearing to be "on the go" or "driven like a motor," talking excessively, blurting out answers before questions have been completed, problems waiting one's turn to speak or act, and interrupting others' speech or actions. These symptoms must have been present for at least six months and must interfere with school, work, family, or social life. Some of the symptoms must have been present before 12 years of age and some must be present in at least two settings.

If your patient qualifies for both Inattentive (Section 5) *and* Hyperactive-Impulsive (Section 6) Presentations, you may give him or her the diagnosis of Attention-Deficit/Hyperactivity Disorder, Combined Presentation (DSM-5 314.01, ICD-10 F90.2).

Do Not Diagnose ADHD when the Symptoms Are Explained by another Disorder

Bear in mind that any disorder that causes inattention, impulsivity, or hyperactivity can mimic the symptoms of Attention-Deficit/Hyperactivity Disorder (See Chapter 2). Therefore, you cannot diagnose Attention-Deficit/Hyperactivity Disorder during the course of Schizophrenia or if your patient also meets the criteria for unipolar Major Depressive Disorder, Bipolar Disorder, Dissociative Disorder, Personality Disorder, Autistic Spectrum Disorder, medication or substance use effects, or any other condition that can explain the inattentive, impulsive, or hyperactive symptoms.

For example, the diagnostic criteria for a bipolar Manic Episode include distractibility (which causes difficulty sustaining attention, problems listening to others, poor task persistence, difficulty organizing tasks and activities, reluctance to do tasks that require sustained mental effort, a tendency to lose things necessary for tasks or activities, and forgetfulness in daily activities). By themselves, these criteria would lead to an erroneous diagnosis of Attention-Deficit/Hyperactivity Disorder, Predominantly Inattentive Presentation.

Similarly, the diagnostic criteria for a bipolar Manic Episode include excessive talking and pressured speech (where individuals have problems listening to others, blurt out answers, have difficulty waiting their turn to speak, and interrupt others' speech) and psychomotor agitation (where individuals fidget and squirm, have difficulty sitting in one place, exhibit restless feelings and behavior, have difficulty quieting down during leisure activities, and appear to be "on the go" or "driven like a motor"). By themselves, these criteria would lead to an erroneous diagnosis of Attention-Deficit/Hyperactivity Disorder, Predominantly Hyperactive-Impulsive Presentation. You must look at the pattern of *all* your patient's symptoms and find the diagnosis that best accounts for them all.

SECTION 7. ACUTE AND CHRONIC EMOTIONS

Acute emotions may be defined as those emotions that have been present at least once in the last two weeks. Emotions such as sadness, hopelessness, anxiety, irritability, and anger can be pathological, especially if they are uncontrollable or extreme.

"On top of the world!" is a nonperjorative inquiry about mood elevation (euphoria or elation), a diagnostic criterion for bipolar Manic Episodes that is frequently endorsed by bipolar patients. Occasionally patients will endorse "on top of the world!" if they desire to minimize their pathology or exaggerate their good feelings. Patients can also experience euphoria during intoxication, brain injury, or metabolic imbalances.

Schizophrenic patients and individuals suffering from Personality Disorders often report strong emotions without showing them in facial expressions, postures, or gestures. Many patients with Bipolar Disorder do not clearly discriminate between types of emotions and will endorse many negative or positive emotions simultaneously. When they feel several negative emotions as one, bipolar patients may call their condition "depression" or "anxiety" interchangeably, to the chagrin of their interviewer.

Chronic emotions are present nearly every day over a period of at least two years. Most people do not experience chronic emotions and they are usually pathological. Chronic depression, with unremitting sadness, loneliness, and emptiness is often seen in Persistent Depressive Disorder and the depression of Personality Disorders. For example, patients with Borderline Personality Disorder frequently endorse strong, chronic feelings of sadness and emptiness. Some patients with Bipolar Disorder will cycle through mild-to-severe depression without any remission, resulting in chronic emotions of sadness, irritability, and anger (see *Mental Status Examination for Personality Disorders*).

SECTION 8. LOW FEELINGS:

Major Depressive Episode

Patients may qualify for the diagnosis of a Major Depressive Episode if they endorse at least five of the following symptoms nearly every day for at least two weeks: a sad, depressed mood; a loss of interest or pleasure in most activities (anhedonia); a significant change in appetite or weight; insomnia or hypersomnia; psychomotor depression or agitation; fatigue or low energy; thoughts of guilt or worthlessness; difficulty concentrating or making decisions; or recurrent thoughts of death, suicide, or a suicidal attempt or plan. The symptoms must cause a significant impairment in school, work, home, or social life; and they must include either depressed mood or anhedonia.

Note that a loss of interest and pleasure in life is enough for a diagnosis of Major Depressive Episode—the presence of sadness, hopelessness, or depressed mood is not necessary.

Most of the diagnostic criteria for a Major Depressive Episode reflect physical body states (activity, sleep, fatigue, appetite, weight) and brain states (problems concentrating, making decisions, and obsessive thoughts about worthlessness and death), emphasizing the strong physiological and genetic underpinnings of the disorder. Because patients have widely varying interpretations of "depressed feelings," focusing on your patients' physical symptoms will help you make accurate diagnoses of Major Depressive Episode.

Major Depressive Disorder, Single Episode (DSM-5 296.2, ICD-10 F32).

Major Depressive Disorder, Recurrent (DSM-5 296.3, ICD-10 F33).

If this is the first Major Depressive Episode, you may diagnose Major Depressive Disorder, Single Episode. If there have been prior Major Depressive Episodes, you may diagnose Major Depressive Disorder, Recurrent. You can code the severity of your patient's depression with an additional decimal (e.g., 296.33). For DSM-5, mild=1, moderate=2, severe=3, and with psychosis=4. For ICD-10, mild=0, moderate=1, severe=2, and with psychosis=3.

Major Depressive Disorder cannot be diagnosed if a patient has ever had a Manic or Hypomanic Episode. If there is evidence of a prior Manic Episode (see Section 10), diagnose Bipolar I Disorder, Most Recent Episode Depressed (DSM-5 296.5, ICD-10 F31). Manic symptoms often occur together with major depressive symptoms in Bipolar I Disorder.

Depression with Melancholic Features

Unfortunately, the criteria for a Major Depressive Episode alone do not discriminate between unipolar depression and the distinctively different disorder of bipolar depression. Many clinicians associate the Melancholic Features of depression with *unipolar* Major Depressive Disorder. Patients qualify for Melancholic Features if they endorse either anhedonia or they cannot feel better, even temporarily, when something good happens, and they also endorse at least three of the following symptoms: despondent, morose, despair, or empty mood; early morning depression; depression worse in the morning;, psychomotor depression; anorexia; and excessive guilt. Give these patients the diagnosis of Major Depressive Disorder with Melancholic Features.

Bereavement

In addition to generating feelings of loss, emptiness, and longing for the loved one, death can also trigger or exacerbate unipolar and bipolar Major Depression. When physiological symptoms such as changes in appetite or weight; insomnia or hypersomnia; psychomotor depression or agitation; fatigue or low energy; or difficulty concentrating are prominent, or grief symptoms do not attenuate within 2-6 months, grieving patients should be evaluated for therapeutic treatment of unipolar or bipolar depression. Appropriate focused psychotherapy and either antidepressants for unipolar Major Depressive Disorder, or lithium and anticonvulsants for depressed Bipolar Disorder can help depressed individuals resume their normal lives more quickly.

Persistent Depressive Disorder (DSM-5 300.4, ICD-10 F34.1).

Patients who do not meet the full criteria for Major Depressive Disorder may meet the criteria for Persistent Depressive Disorder (Dysthymia), if they have a chronically depressed mood (see Section 7) for most of the day, more days than not, for at least two years without a break of more than two months. Patients must also confirm that at least two of the following symptoms have been present for at least two years without a break of more than two months: poor appetite or overeating, insomnia or hypersomnia, low energy or fatigue, low self-esteem, poor concentration or difficulty making decisions, or feelings of hopelessness. Persistent Depressive Disorder cannot be diagnosed if a patient has ever had a Manic or Hypomanic Episode or Cyclothymic Disorder. If there is evidence of a prior Manic Episode, diagnose Bipolar I Disorder, Most Recent Episode Depressed (DSM-5 296.5, ICD-10 F31).

SECTION 9. ATYPICAL LOW FEELINGS:

Depression with Atypical Features

Patients qualify for Atypical Features if they endorse mood reactivity ("good news is cheering") and at least two of the following symptoms: significant increase in appetite or weight gain; hypersomnia; leaden paralysis—a heavy, leaden fatigue; and sensitivity to rejection.

Patients with mood reactivity ("good news is cheering") can experience a brightening of depressed mood temporarily in response to good news. If a patient is not sure whether their dysphoria would brighten after positive events, you may ask, "Would you feel better, even for a few minutes, if you found out that you had won a million dollars?" Hypersomnia (sleeping too much) usually refers to a pattern of sleeping 10 hours or more per day but it can also denote strong feelings of sleepiness during the day if the patient is forced to keep a daytime work schedule. Patients describe leaden paralysis as a peculiar sense of being "paralyzed," "unable to function," "unable to cope," or "unable to get motivated to do anything." Sensitivity to rejection refers to a long-standing pattern of easily hurt feelings that may be present even between episodes.

Clinicians have described Atypical Features since the early days of psychiatry, when they were called Hysteroid Dysphoria. Many clinicians believe that depression with Atypical Features is more likely to be *bipolar* depression.

If the patient endorses criteria for Sections 8 and 9, you may diagnose unipolar Major Depressive Disorder with Atypical Features. If the patient has ever had a Manic Episode (see Section 10), you must diagnose Bipolar I Disorder, Most Recent Episode Depressed (DSM-5 296.5, ICD-10 F31). If you are convinced from your evaluation that your patient has Bipolar Disorder but you cannot demonstrate a prior Manic Episode, you may make the diagnosis of Major Depressive Episode with Atypical Features, rule out Bipolar I Disorder, Most Recent Episode Depressed.

Unipolar versus Bipolar Depression

Many studies of pharmacology, physiology, and neuroanatomy confirm that unipolar depression and bipolar depression are distinct disorders, localized in different parts of the brain, and optimally treated with different types of medicine and psychotherapy. However, there is rampant confusion of the two. Misdiagnosis can cause unipolar and bipolar depressed patients to receive inappropriate psychotherapy or medications that prolong their illnesses and subject them to needless suffering. For example, when patients with unipolar Major Depressive Disorder are treated for Bipolar Disorder, they can receive lithium salts and anticonvulsants that may not provide effective treatment and may produce unnecessary side effects.

Currently, the history of a Manic Episode is necessary to diagnose Bipolar Disorder. However, most bipolar sufferers experience mainly depressive symptoms during their lifetimes and many bipolar patients do not have their first Manic Episode until 10-20 years after their first depressed symptoms. Studies show that more than 50% of depressed Bipolar Disorder patients receive the incorrect diagnosis of unipolar Major Depressive Disorder. When depressed patients with Bipolar Disorder receive only psychotherapy treatment, their symptoms will not remit and their illness may become irreversibly more severe. When depressed Bipolar I Disorder patients receive antidepressants, they can have the following reactions: 1) the antidepressants may be partially or completely ineffective; 2) the antidepressants may worsen the bipolar depression symptoms; 3) the antidepressants may trigger or worsen Manic Episodes; 4) the antidepressants may trigger Psychotic Episodes, suicide, and violence; and 5) the antidepressants may cause the lifetime course of Bipolar Disorder to become irreversibly more severe and less responsive to appropriate lithium or anticonvulsant medications.

Clinicians use the presence of Atypical Features, a family history of Bipolar Disorder, psychomotor agitation, cyclic recurrent depression, grandiose symptoms, postpartum psychosis, and a poor response to antidepressants as markers for bipolar depression. If you have reasons to suspect depressed Bipolar Disorder but you can find no history of a prior Manic or Mixed Episode, you may make the diagnosis of Major Depressive Disorder, rule out Bipolar I Disorder, Most Recent Episode Depressed, and plan your treatment accordingly.

SECTION 10. ACTIVATED CONDITIONS:

Manic Episode Criterion A

Patients who experience a distinct period of increased goal-directed activity or energy, and abnormal and persistent elevated, expansive, or irritable mood nearly every day lasting at least one week (or any duration if hospitalization is necessary), satisfy the first criterion for a bipolar Manic Episode. Patients have increased goal-directed activity when they are engaged in tasks (particularly at night)—they need not feel that the tasks are productive or valuable. Elevated mood or euphoria is often characterized as "feeling super good." Expansive moods are characterized by exaggerated emotional expression, overoptimism, and an infectious, "bigger than life" persona.

Note that patients need *never* have been euphoric or expansive to receive the diagnosis of a Manic Episode if they have a week-long episode of significant irritability. In fact, most clinicians find that high-functioning bipolar outpatients present with angry emotions far more frequently than with euphoric or expansive emotions.

If the patient satisfies these criteria, go on to Criterion B.

Manic Episode Criterion B

To diagnose a Manic Episode, in addition to mood symptoms, the patient must also endorse three of the following symptoms (four if the mood is only irritable): inflated self-esteem or grandiosity ("feeling like you could lick the world"), a decreased need for sleep, talking more than usual or interrupting others (pressured speech), rapid or racing thoughts, distractibility, increased goal-directed activity or psychomotor agitation, and excessive involvement in activities that have a high potential for painful consequences (costly or risky impulsive actions). These symptoms must be severe enough to cause a significant impairment in school, work, home, or social activity, necessitate hospitalization, or be accompanied by psychotic symptoms.

If your patient endorses overfocussed activities, ask separately about inordinate time, energy, and money spent on socializing, sexual activities, or projects at school, work, home, or place of worship. If your patient endorses impulsive actions, ask separately about specific acts like impulsive sex, buying sprees (shopping binges), taking sudden trips, speeding, reckless driving, foolish business investments, or other poor life decisions.

Hypomania

A Hypomanic Episode is the same as a Manic Episode except that Criterion A symptoms need only be present for four days, and there is not a "marked impairment in social or occupational functioning," but only an "unequivocal change in functioning that is uncharacteristic of the individual." For a diagnosis of hypomania, the symptoms must *not* cause a significant impairment in school, work, home, or social activities; necessitate hospitalization; or be accompanied by any psychotic symptoms.

In practice, most patients who come to see clinicians are experiencing a significant impairment in school, work, home, or social function as a result of their disease, and are having Manic Episodes. Even if the patient's bipolar symptoms appear mild, the clinician must make sure that there has never been a Manic Episode where the patient's functioning has been impaired, the patient was hospitalized, or any psychotic symptoms were present.

Bipolar I Disorder, Most Recent Episode Manic (DSM-5 296.4, ICD-10 F31).

Bipolar I Disorder, Most Recent Episode Hypomanic (DSM-5 296.40, ICD-10 F31.0).

Bipolar I Disorder, Most Recent Episode Depressed (DSM-5 296.5, ICD-10 F31)

Only one Manic Episode during the lifetime is necessary to diagnose Bipolar I Disorder. If the most recent episode is manic, diagnose Bipolar I Disorder, Most Recent Episode Manic. If the most recent episode is hypomanic, diagnose Bipolar I Disorder, Most Recent Episode Hypomanic. If the most recent episode is depressed, diagnose Bipolar I Disorder, Most Recent Episode Depressed. If both manic and depressed features are present, add the descriptor, with Mixed Features.

You can code the severity of your patient's bipolar episode with additional decimals (e.g., 296.43). For DSM-5, mild=1, moderate=2, severe=3, and with psychosis=4. For ICD-10, the codes distinguish manic and depressed symptoms: mania=1 (mild mania=11, moderate mania=12, severe mania=13), mania with psychosis=2, mild-moderate depression=3, severe depression=4, depression with psychosis=5, mixed mania and depression=6.

Bipolar II Disorder (DSM-5 296.89, ICD-10 F31.81)

Cyclothymic Disorder (DSM-5 301.13, ICD-10 F34.0)

Patients who have only had Hypomanic Episodes and Major Depressive Episodes may be given the diagnosis of Bipolar II Disorder. Patients who have had numerous periods with hypomanic symptoms that do not meet full criteria for a Hypomanic Episode and numerous periods with depressed symptoms that do not meet full criteria for a Major Depressive Episode may be given the diagnosis of Cyclothymic Disorder. In my experience, these criteria may net a mixed and unstable population—some patients who meet these criteria will develop Bipolar I Disorder, while others suffer personality disorders, organic brain disorders, and other problems.

Other Activated Conditions

Note that patients with both manic and depressed Bipolar Disorder often feel a strong physical agitation combined with intrusive thoughts that they describe as "anxiety" or "panic." They may describe such symptoms as a feeling of tremendous energy, overactive thoughts, morning panic, or feeling overwhelmed. They may describe feelings like "jumping out of my skin" or "not feeling right in my body." Secondary symptoms include a need for constant distraction, prolonged insomnia, working >12 hours daily, and difficulty finishing projects. In addition to bipolar Manic Episodes, these symptoms occur in organic brain disorder, stimulant drug abuse, steroid abuse, hyperthyroidism, Cushing's Syndrome, congenital adrenal hyperplasia, and pheochromocytoma.

SECTION 11. ADULT EXPERIENCES: FORMAL THOUGHT DISORDER AND HALLUCINATIONS

Several normal experiences can be mistaken for psychosis. For example, ringing in the ears (tinnitus) is sometimes mistaken for auditory hallucinations. Patients who endorse "knowing others' thoughts" may be thinking of normal phenomena such as guessing what close friends or family are going to say or do ("I always know when Marline is going to call").

Alternately, "knowing others' thoughts" may indicate a formal thought disorder. Amnesia episodes and a sense of leaving the body suggest dissociative disorders. Visions and "hearing noises or voices" usually point to the presence of hallucinations. Whenever you are in doubt, ask the patient to describe his experience in more detail.

Formal thought disorder and hallucinations are most likely to be associated with Schizophrenia, psychotic Bipolar Disorder, or psychotic unipolar Major Depressive Disorder, especially if hallucinations occur with delusions. However, transient hallucinations and sensory illusions may also be present in patients with Substance Intoxication and Withdrawal; Borderline, Histrionic, Narcissistic, Schizoid, and Schizotypal Personality Disorders; stroke; brain trauma; and general nervous system insults including metabolic and hormonal imbalances, hypoxia, uremia, hepatic encephalopathy, poisoning, and other toxic states.

Psychosis

Psychosis is a patient's inability to assess his or her internal and external environment accurately, sometimes called "poor reality testing." In principle, most people define psychosis as the presence of hallucinations or delusions. Psychotic patients may also exhibit blunted affect and disorganized speech and behavior.

Hallucinations are sensory experiences that are not supported by fact or evident to other people. Patients can experience hallucinations in visual, auditory, somatic, olfactory, or gustatory modalities. Common hallucinations include hearing voices that represent themselves as God, Satan or one of their minions (hyperreligious hallucinations) or voices that tell the patient to do things (command hallucinations). Other common auditory hallucinations include a voice describing or keeping up a running commentary on the patient's thoughts or actions, voices that argue with the patient, or two or more voices conversing with each other. Hallucinations in other sensory modalities include seeing visions, smelling perfume or burning feathers, or feeling things crawling on or below the skin.

Some nomenclature is useful in discussing hallucinations. Primary hallucinations are also called sensory illusions—they usually involve the assignment of meaning to a sensation naturally occurring in the environment. For example, the face of a clock may look like a human face, a spot on the skin may look like an insect, or the sound of an air conditioner may seem like whirring cameras in the walls. Primary hallucinations are most often found in organic brain dysfunction resulting from intoxication, toxicity, trauma, stroke, or cancer.

Secondary hallucinations are internally produced sensations, usually associated with a meaning, that the patient acknowledges but sometimes realizes exist only in his head. The obsessions of Obsessive-Compulsive Disorder may fall into this category—the patient realizes that the images she sees are unreasonable, yet she acts as if they are real.

Clinicians are most familiar with tertiary hallucinations, which patients believe to be real despite all evidence to the contrary. Tertiary hallucinations can seem to originate inside your patient's head or in the outside environment. For example, a patient may perceive visions of God, sounds of music, her deceased mother speaking to her, or the feeling of cancer eating through her body. The patient usually assigns meaning to these hallucinations, which are reflected in delusions.

Delusions are the belief in events and conditions that are not supported by fact or evident to other people. Common delusions can be persecutory (a belief that others have malevolent intent), nihilistic (a conviction of imminent doom), erotomanic (a belief that others are in love with the patient), somatic (a belief in undiagnosed physical illnesses), or grandiose (a belief in inflated power, status, or relationship to powerful people or deities).

The psychotic symptoms from many disorders look alike. You can find hallucinations, delusions, blunted affect, disordered speech, and disorganized behavior in patients suffering from Schizophrenia, psychotic Bipolar Disorder, psychotic unipolar Major Depressive Disorder, severe Obsessive-Compulsive Disorder, Delirium, Major Neurocognitive Disorders, epilepsy, and many other medical conditions. Under stress, individuals with Intellectual Disability and personality disorders can experience both hallucinations and delusions. Under the right conditions, antidepressants, sedatives, hypnotics, anxiolytics, steroid hormones, stimulants, narcotic analgesics, hallucinogens, and other substances can trigger or exacerbate psychotic symptoms.

Hallucinations and delusions tend to mimic the mood and egocentricity of the illness—thus schizophrenic hallucinations and delusions may be unemotional, solitary, and dissociated from the individual. Bipolar hallucinations and delusions are likely to reflect strong emotions and personalized, social, religious, and grandiose themes.

Depressed hallucinations and delusions involve guilty, self-deprecating themes. Depressed hallucinations often take the form of critical comments, barely intelligible voices fighting, or incomprehensible noise. In severe depressed hallucinations, the depressed patient may see himself disappearing bit by bit. In depressed delusions, the patient believes that he is responsible for the death of loved ones; that he has failed himself, his family, and his career; and that he has been forsaken by God and society. He may be convinced that his life has been ruined or truncated by an unspeakable personal flaw, an abhorrent physical deficit, or an incurable disease.

Formal Thought Disorder is a form of psychosis characterized by perceived changes in the patient's thoughts and internal environment. Thought broadcasting is the sense that surrounding people can hear the patient's thoughts. Thought insertion is the perception that a foreign thought has been placed into the patient's mind. Thought deletion is the sense that one of the patient's thoughts has been removed from his mind. Thought control is the perception that the patient's thoughts are being directed by some external source. Thought echo is the sense that a patient's thoughts are being spoken aloud (echoed) by a hallucinatory voice.

Ideas of Reference contain meaningful content originating in the surrounding environment. The most common idea of reference is the sense that others are talking about the patient behind her back. Sometimes external messages border on normal experience, like listening to a song on the radio and perceiving a vague, personal message, such as "that love song means I should get back together with my ex-boyfriend." Alternatively, the patient may hear her name spoken in a song or the song's words may form an explicit message. Similarly, a patient may see a billboard that carries her name and a personal message, like "God is watching you" or "don't trust anybody." One of my patients was watching a television soap opera when she saw the main character turn and speak directly to her before resuming his written dialog.

Occasionally, a patient will hear a nearby person making a personal or offensive remark to them. For example, an Emergency Room patient once turned to me and asked, "Did you just say I was an asshole?" I replied, "No, I didn't say that and I'm not thinking it, either. But I'm glad that you asked me so we could clear that up. Please feel free to ask me about anything like that in the future."

SCHIZOPHRENIA SPECTRUM AND OTHER PSYCHOTIC DISORDERS

Schizophrenia (DSM-5 295.90, ICD-10 F20.9)

The diagnosis of Schizophrenia is partly based on symptoms and partly based on the course of the illness. At least two of the following must be usually present during a one-month period: hallucinations, delusions, disorganized speech (with frequent stopping, derailment or incoherence), disorganized behavior, or so-called negative symptoms—diminished expression of emotion (flat affect), diminished words or content in speech (alogia), or failure to engage or persist in activities (avolition). At least one of these must be either hallucinations, delusions or disorganized speech. Continuous signs of the illness must persist for at least six months. During this time, two symptoms may be milder or only negative symptoms may be present. There must be significant impairment in self-care, school, work, home, or social function since the onset of the disturbance.

Unfortunately, Schizophrenia is largely a diagnosis of exclusion because many mental disorders and other medical conditions cause psychosis that duplicate these schizophrenic symptoms. You cannot not diagnose Schizophrenia if there has been a Manic or Depressive Episode; if you can diagnose Bipolar I Disorder, Bipolar II Disorder, or unipolar Major Depressive Disorder; or if the patient's symptoms may result from drug intoxication or withdrawal, medication side effects, or another medical or mental disorder.

Schizophreniform Disorder (DSM-5 295.40, ICD-10 F20.81)

If a schizophrenic episode lasts at least 1 month but less than 6 months, diagnose Schizophreniform Disorder.

Brief Psychotic Disorder (DSM-5 298.8, ICD-10 F23)

If a patient exhibits hallucinations, delusions, disorganized speech, or disorganized behavior for less than one month, with full return to the previous level of functioning, and there is no evidence of psychosis from any other condition, consider Brief Psychotic Disorder.

Delusional Disorder (DSM-5 297.1, ICD-10 F22.0)

When delusions are present for at least one month, without any other diagnosable illness or functional impairment, and behavior is not odd or bizarre, consider the diagnosis of Delusional Disorder.

Schizotypal Personality Disorder (DSM-5 301.22, ICD-10 F21)

Patients with Schizotypal Personality Disorder exhibit at least five of the following criteria which begin early and continue throughout life: social anxiety, avoidance of closeness or intimacy, odd appearance and behavior, inappropriate and flat affect, odd thought and speech patterns, suspicious and paranoid ideas, odd beliefs or magical thinking, ideas of reference, or sensory illusions. Not all clinicians agree that personality disorders share mechanisms or demographics with Schizophrenia. For more details, see *Mental Status Examination for Personality Disorders*.

Schizoaffective Disorder (DSM-5 295.70, ICD-10 F25)

Schizoaffective Disorder can be diagnosed when the full diagnostic symptoms of a Manic Episode or Major Depressive Episode coexist with Schizophrenia for the majority of the duration of the illness and there has been a period of at least two weeks when hallucinations or delusions were present without mood symptoms. However, these criteria are rarely met and I discourage the use of this diagnosis. Most patients who have come to me with this diagnosis have turned out to have psychotic Bipolar Disorder or unipolar Major Depressive Disorder. Patients with psychosis look alike—if your patient is too psychotic to evaluate, it may be best to delay final diagnosis or reassess the patient after the psychotic symptoms have waned, as treatment for one condition may worsen the course of another.

SECTION 12. SOCIAL ANXIETY:

Social Anxiety Disorder (DSM-5 300.23, ICD-10 F40.10)

Patients with Social Anxiety Disorder have excessive fear and avoidance of social situations where they might be humiliated, embarrassed, or rejected because of their anxiety symptoms. This fear typically lasts for six months or more and causes clinically significant distress or impairment in school, work, home, or social function. You may ask patients how they feel around groups of strangers or when speaking in public, which are often the loci of Social Anxiety symptoms.

SECTION 13. PAST BEHAVIORS:

Anorexia Nervosa (DSM-5 307.1, ICD-10 F50.0)

Bulimia Nervosa (DSM-5 307.51, ICD-10 F50.2)

Suicide History

When patients restrict food and/or purge (resulting in a significantly low body weight), exhibit an intense fear of gaining weight, and a disturbance in the perception of body weight and shape, consider Anorexia Nervosa.

When patients binge at least once a week and fast, purge, or abuse medications or exercise to prevent weight gain, consider the diagnosis of Bulimia Nervosa.

Past suicide attempts may predict future suicidality. If endorsed, you should discuss them further with your patient.

SECTION 14. THOUGHTS AND BEHAVIORS:

Obsessive-Compulsive Disorder (DSM-5 300.3, ICD-10 F42)

Obsessive-Compulsive Disorder is defined by the presence of obsessions, compulsions, or both. Obsessions are recurrent and persistent thoughts, impulses, or images that patients experience as intrusive and try to ignore, suppress, or neutralize with another thought or action. Obsessions are not just exaggerated worries about daily life or mental illness symptoms. Compulsions are repetitive behaviors or mental acts that patients feel driven to perform in response to obsessions or rigid rules. Patients perform Compulsions in order to reduce the stress response or avoid some disastrous consequence, but they are excessive and serve no real protective function. Patients may not realize that their obsessions are unreasonable or their compulsions are excessive, and their lack of touch with reality often reaches psychotic proportions. These thoughts and behaviors occupy at least one hour per day and/or cause significant distress or impairment in school, work, home, or social function.

Obsessions are also present in the ruminative thoughts of unipolar Major Depressive Disorder, the recursive thoughts of Bipolar Disorder, the excessive worried thoughts of Generalized Anxiety Disorder, and the preoccupation with food in eating disorders. Compulsive behavior often occurs in psychotic disorders, mood disorders, impulse control disorders, and substance-related disorders. Obsessions and compulsions can appear transiently when individuals with Personality Disorders, Intellectual Disability, or organic brain disorders are under stress. Antidepressants, steroids, stimulants, narcotic analgesics, and other substances can trigger obsessions and compulsions in patients with mental illness as well as in normal individuals. Furthermore, obsessions and compulsive behaviors may overlap with normal, culturally syntonic superstition, magical thinking, and "good luck" behaviors. For example, it is not normal for an adult to believe that "stepping on a crack" will actually cause his mother's back to fracture, but many sophisticated individuals avoid talking about future events to avoid "jinxing" themselves, or repeat affirmations in the hopes that saying their wishes will make them come true.

Please note that Obsessive-Compulsive Personality Disorder (DSM-5 301.4, ICD-10 F60.5) is a pervasive preoccupation with orderliness, perfection, and mental and interpersonal control. It is not a version of Obsessive-Compulsive Disorder (see *Mental Status Examination for Personality Disorders* in Chapter 8).

SECTION 15. STRESSFUL LIFE EVENTS:

Acute Stress Disorder (DSM-5 308.3, ICD-10 F43.0)

Posttraumatic Stress Disorder (DSM-5 309.81, ICD-10 F43.10)

In a traumatic event, a person is exposed to actual or threatened injury or sexual violation to self or others. Consider Acute Stress Disorder if the response has been present 3-30 days after the trauma and if the patient has at least nine of the following: recurrent, involuntary, and intrusive memories of the trauma; recurrent distressing dreams of the trauma; flashbacks of the trauma; distress and/or physiological reactions to reminders of the trauma; persistent inability to experience positive emotions (happiness, love, satisfaction); depersonalization (feeling detached from oneself) or derealization (feeling detached from one's environment); inability to remember an important aspect of the trauma; efforts to avoid feelings and thoughts about the trauma; efforts to avoid external reminders of the trauma; sleep problems; irritable behavior and angry outbursts; hypervigilance; poor concentration; or exaggerated startle response.

Consider Posttraumatic Stress Disorder if the response lasts more than one month and if the patient has all of these:

1. One or more of the following: recurrent, involuntary, and intrusive memories of the trauma; recurrent distressing dreams of the trauma; flashbacks of the trauma; distressing reminders of the trauma; or physiological reactions to reminders of the trauma.

2. One or more of the following: efforts to avoid feelings and thoughts about the trauma or efforts to avoid external reminders of the trauma.

3. Two or more of the following: an inability to remember an important aspect of the trauma; negative cognitions about oneself, others, or the world; unrealistic blame of oneself or others for the trauma; diminished interest or participation in important activities; feelings of detachment or estrangement from others; persistent negative emotions; or persistent inability to experience positive emotions.

4. Two or more of the following: irritable behavior and angry outbursts, reckless behavior, hypervigilance, exaggerated startle response, poor concentration, or sleep problems.

Both disorders must cause clinically significant distress or impairment in school, work, home or social function.

Adjustment Disorder with Depressed Mood (DSM-5 309.0, ICD-10 F43.21)

Adjustment Disorder with Anxiety (DSM-5 309.24, ICD-10 F43.22)

Adjustment Disorder with Mixed Anxiety and Depressed Mood (DSM-5 309.28, ICD-10 F43.23)

Adjustment Disorder with Disturbance of Conduct (DSM-5 309.3, F43.24)

Adjustment Disorder with Mixed Disturbance of Emotions and Conduct (DSM-5 309.4, ICD-10 F43.25)

Adjustment disorders are emotional or behavioral symptoms beginning within three months after a stressful life event that do not meet the criteria for another mental disorder. Adjustment Disorders are characterized by excessive distress and significant impairment in school, work, home, or social functioning that resolves within six months. They include Adjustment Disorder with Depressed Mood, Adjustment Disorder with Anxiety, Adjustment Disorder with Mixed Anxiety and Depressed Mood, Adjustment Disorder with Disturbance of Conduct, and Adjustment Disorder with Mixed Disturbance of Emotions and Conduct.

SECTION 16. DANGEROUS THOUGHTS: SUICIDALITY AND VIOLENCE

The consequences of suicide and violence are so serious that you must ask about them in every evaluation. If a patient thinks that their life is not worth living, you must ask if they have been having thoughts of ending their life, saying, for example, "Have you been thinking of suicide?" or "How often do you think of ending your life?" If your patient endorses suicidality, you must discover whether she has a plan and whether she has the means to carry out her plan. For example, if the patient plans to shoot herself, does she have access to a gun? Assign your patient a higher suicide risk if she has a plan, if she has the means to carry out the plan, and if her planned means of suicide is apt to be lethal. For example, hanging and jumping from a tall building are more likely to be lethal than vague threats of taking anxiolytic pills.

The strongest risk factor for suicide is a history of prior attempts (see Section 13). The presence of cognitive impairment, intoxication, access to weapons, emotional lability, or command hallucinations heightens the risk for suicide or violence. Mental disorders characterized by impulsivity, including unipolar Major Depressive Disorder, Bipolar Disorder, and Borderline, Narcissistic, Histrionic, Paranoid, and Antisocial Personality Disorders should arouse further concern. The presence of supportive friends or family members who will stay with the patient may reduce the potential for suicide. It is often useful to ask suicidal patients, "What is keeping you from killing yourself, now?" to find further avenues of support.

If the patient endorses thoughts of harming someone else, you must establish who that person is and determine the severity of the threat. You may ask, "Are you having violent thoughts about anyone?" or "Are you angry at anyone right now?" If the answer is positive, you should ask, "Are you thinking about harming this person?" If it seems that malicious thoughts or intentions are present, the interviewer should ask about the likelihood, imminence, and form of the planned violence. If you think the threat may be real, you might be required to notify and warn the person who is threatened. Make sure you know your legal and ethical responsibilities in such a situation.

SLEEP-WAKE DISORDERS

Insomnia Disorder (DSM-5 780.52, ICD-10 G47.00)

Hypersomnolence Disorder (DSM-5 780.54, ICD-10 G47.10)

Narcolepsy (sleep attacks) (DSM-5 347.0, ICD-10 G47.41)

Obstructive Sleep Apnea (DSM-5 327.23, ICD-10 G47.33)

Non-Rapid Eye Movement Sleep Arousal Disorder: Sleepwalking (DSM-5 307.46, ICD-10 F51.3)

Non-Rapid Eye Movement Sleep Arousal Disorder: Sleep Terrors (DSM-5 307.46, ICD-10 F51.4)

Nightmare Disorder (DSM-5 307.47, ICD-10 F51.5)

Restless Legs Syndrome (DSM-5 333.94, ICD-10 G25.81).

The main challenge in treating sleep disorders is to determine the physiological and/or environmental causes of the problem. There are many medical causes of sleep problems including heart failure, asthma, and chronic obstructive pulmonary disease. Note that disturbed sleep can also *cause* symptoms of dysphoria, anhedonia, fatigue, impulsivity, cognitive impairment, and poor judgment that can confuse diagnosis.

SUBSTANCE USE DISORDERS

Mild Alcohol Use Disorder (DSM-5, 305.00, ICD-10 F10.10)
Moderate or Severe Alcohol Use Disorder (DSM-5 303.90, ICD-10 F10.20)

Mild Opioid (Narcotic) Use Disorder (DSM-5 305.50, ICD-10 F11.10)
Moderate or Severe Opioid Use Disorder (DSM-5 304.00, ICD-10 F11.2)

Mild Cannabis Use Disorder (DSM-5 305.2, ICD-10 F12.10)
Moderate or Severe Cannabis Use Disorder (DSM-5 304.3, ICD-10 F12.20)

Mild Sedative, Hypnotic, or Anxiolytic Use Disorder (DSM-5 305.40, ICD-10 F13.10)
Moderate or Severe Sedative, Hypnotic, or Anxiolytic Use Disorder (DSM-5 304.10, ICD-10 F13.2)

Mild Cocaine Use Disorder (DSM-5 305.6, F14.10)
Moderate or Severe Cocaine Use Disorder (DSM-5 304.20, ICD-10 F14.20)

Mild Amphetamine-Type Stimulant Use Disorder (DSM-5 305.70, F15.10)
Moderate or Severe Amphetamine-Type Stimulant Use Disorder (DSM-5 304.4, ICD-10 F15.20)

Mild Hallucinogen Use Disorder (DSM-5 305.30, ICD-10 F16.10)
Moderate or Severe Hallucinogen Use Disorder (DSM-5 304.50, F16.20)

Mild Phencyclidine (PCP) Use Disorder (DSM-5 305.90, ICD-10 F16.10).
Moderate or Severe Phencyclidine Use Disorder (DSM-5 304.60, F16.20).

**Mild Tobacco Use Disorder (DSM-5 305.1, Z72.0),
Moderate or Severe Tobacco Use Disorder (DSM-5 305.1, ICD-10 F17.20)**

**Mild Inhalant (Solvent) Use Disorder (DSM-5 305.90, F18.10)
Moderate or Severe Inhalant (Solvent) Use Disorder (DSM-5 304.60, F18.20)**

In addition to being a significant clinical problem, Substance Use Disorders confound the diagnostic process by imitating the symptoms of many other mental illnesses. You should not diagnose other mental illnesses if substance use can explain a patient's symptoms. Instead, wait until the patient is clear of substance effects and reassess. If you misdiagnose a Substance Use Disorder, your patient will likely receive unnecessary treatment and be deprived of the treatment he needs. The primary substance diagnoses are Substance Use Disorder, Substance Intoxication, and Substance Withdrawal.

A Substance Use Disorder is defined as at least two the following within a 12-month period: the patient takes a substance in larger amounts for a longer period than intended; the patient tries or wants to reduce substance use; the patient spends considerable time obtaining, using, and recovering from the substance effects; the patient feels strong urges or cravings to use the substance; substance use causes impairment in school, work, home, or social function; use continues despite social problems attributable to the substance; school, work, home, or social activities are curtailed because of the substance; use continues despite physical danger attributable to the substance; use continues despite physical or psychological problems attributable to the substance; tolerance—increased amounts are needed and/or the effects of the substance decrease; and withdrawal—characteristic withdrawal symptoms and/or substances are taken to avoid withdrawal.

Consult *The Diagnostic and Statistical Manual of Mental Disorders* (DSM-5) or the *International Statistical Classification of Diseases and Related Health Problems 10th Revision* (ICD-10) to find the criteria needed to diagnose specific Substance Use Disorders, Intoxication, and Withdrawal.

PERSONALITY DISORDERS

Borderline Personality Disorder (DSM-5 301.83, ICD-10 F60.3)

Narcissistic Personality Disorder (DSM-5 301.81, ICD-10 F60.81)

Histrionic Personality Disorder (DSM-5 301.50, F60.4)

Avoidant Personality Disorder (DSM-5 301.82, ICD-10 F60.6)

Dependent Personality Disorder (DSM-5 301.6, ICD-10 F60.7)

Obsessive-Compulsive Personality Disorder (DSM-5 301.4. ICD-10 F60.5)

Schizoid Personality Disorder (DSM-5 301.20, ICD-10 F60.1)

Schizotypal Personality Disorder (DSM-5 301.22, ICD-10 F21)

Paranoid Personality Disorder (DSM-5 301.0, ICD-10 60.0)

Antisocial Personality Disorder (DSM-5 301.7, ICD-10 F60.2)

Patients with personality disorders account for a disproportionate share of mental health and other medical treatment resources in all countries. Personality disorders are enduring and inflexible patterns of emotions and perceptions of self and others that result in maladaptive behavior and impaired interpersonal relationships. These abnormalities originate in childhood and adolescence and continue throughout the lifetime and they are evident in a broad range of situations. The personality disorders include Borderline Personality Disorder, Narcissistic Personality Disorder, Histrionic Personality Disorder, Avoidant Personality Disorder, Dependent Personality Disorder, Obsessive-Compulsive Personality Disorder, Schizoid Personality Disorder, Schizotypal Personality Disorder, Paranoid Personality Disorder, and Antisocial Personality Disorder. Oppositional Defiant Disorder and Conduct Disorder in childhood are considered by many to be precursors to personality disorders in adulthood, and childhood Conduct Disorder is a prerequisite for the diagnosis of Antisocial Personality Disorder. Passive-Aggressive Personality, and Psychopathic Personality also describe clusters of maladaptive personality characteristics. For a full discussion of personality disorders, see the companion book in this series, *Mental Status Examination for Personality Disorders*.

CHAPTER 2
THE COGNITIVE EXAMINATION

In the modern treatment of mental, emotional, and behavioral conditions, it is not enough just to know what your clients think and feel. It is important to understand *how* they think and whether there are deficits in their abilities to perceive information, speak, remember, analyze information, and employ reason to make decisions. Unlike thoughts and feelings, your patients cannot simply tell you about their cognitive deficits. Instead, you must use tests and measures to determine this information. However, after successful cognitive testing, you will be able to tell your patients some of the reasons why they think and feel the way they do.

THE COGNITIVE EXAMINATION TEST BATTERY

Many clinicians are taught a loose collection of cognitive screening tests that can be performed in a few minutes during patients' evaluations. This book provides a comprehensive collection of new and traditional cognitive tests and explains what they mean and how to employ them in diagnosis and treatment planning. All of the patients described in this book were given the same Cognitive Examination. Key parts of this battery were published in *The American Journal of Psychiatry, Psychiatry Research, Biological Psychiatry, The International Journal of Neuroscience, Psychiatric Services, The Jefferson Journal of Psychiatry,* and *Mental Status Examination for Personality Disorders* (see Chapter 8). Follow along with the tests in Appendices III-VII as you read about each cognitive function.

In Appendix III, you will find the complete script for the Cognitive Interview. If you wish, you can simply read it to your patients and check off their responses after you complete your Diagnostic Examination. The Cognitive Interview covers all cognitive areas of *attention, language, memory, abstract thinking,* and *sequential thinking*. It is best to learn this script and stick to it as closely as possible so that every test presentation is the same.

In Appendix IV, you will find a Cognitive Questionnaire that your patients can complete by themselves. It covers the same cognitive areas of *attention, language, memory, abstract thinking,* and *sequential thinking* as the Cognitive Interview, although some subtests were omitted due to the limitations of the self-report format. You may hand out the Cognitive Questionnaire to your patients before their evaluation so that the results are waiting for you when you first see them. The interpretations in this book are based on Cognitive Questionnaires that patients completed in the waiting room without help—they were not sent out to be completed at home.

Appendix VI contains the Nonverbal Tests of Abstract and Sequential Thinking, which assess complex *abstract thought-processing* and *sequential thought-processing* skills independent of language. This brief battery is unique to this book. You can also use it for patients with poor communication skills, low native intelligence, low education level, aphasia, or language barriers.

Appendix VII contains the Luria Figure Drawing Test, a modification of the repetitive drawings A. R. Luria used to test for brain injury. The Luria Figure Drawing Test assesses *sequential thought-processing* (*executive function*) skills independent of language. You can also use it to evaluate patients with poor communication skills, low native intelligence, low education level, aphasia, or language barriers.

Original purchasers of this book are permitted to use and reproduce both forms of the Cognitive Examination without modification as long as proper credit is given.

Why Measure Cognition?

Cognitive deficits are important because they invariably cause functional problems in daily living. In mood disorders, depressive patients will often tolerate feelings of sadness but these patients quickly appear in our offices when cognitive impairment ruins their work performance. Similarly, parents frequently tolerate their children's hyperactive behavior but they seek professional help when cognitive deficits make their children's grades slip.

Major Neurocognitive Disorders, Mild Neurocognitive Disorders, and Delirium are important in all clinical practices. Assessing cognition is also important for the diagnosis of other mental disorders. For example, assessment of *attention* is necessary for the diagnosis of Bipolar Disorder, unipolar Major Depressive Disorder, Persistent Depressive Disorder, Generalized Anxiety Disorder, Attention-Deficit/Hyperactivity Disorder, Posttraumatic Stress Disorder, substance intoxication and withdrawal, Traumatic Brain Injury, Lewy Body Disease, and Vascular Disease. Changes in *language* are diagnostic features of Schizophrenia and other psychoses, Attention-Deficit/Hyperactivity Disorder, Autistic Disorder, and Frontotemporal Disease. Assessing *memory* is important for the diagnosis of Attention-Deficit/Hyperactivity Disorder, Posttraumatic Stress Disorder, Alzheimer's Disease, and Traumatic Brain

Injury. Measurement of *sequential thinking* is necessary for the diagnosis of Attention-Deficit/Hyperactivity Disorder, Obsessive-Compulsive Disorder, Frontotemporal Disease, and Parkinson's Disease.

Understanding patients' cognitive status is also essential in order to select the best treatment for them. Cognitively impaired patients may not be good candidates for pure cognitive therapy or medications that require a complex dosing schedule or special diet (such as MAO inhibitors). Rapid cognitive change can reveal emergency conditions like Delirium, brain trauma, cranial bleeding, or sudden cardiac decompensation while there is still time to correct them.

Standardized Test Batteries

You can obtain the most comprehensive assessment of cognitive function from lengthy, commercially available, standardized psychological evaluations such as the Wechsler, Luria, and Halstead-Reitan batteries. However, the time and effort they require renders them impractical for most clinical work. To obtain these tests it is best to refer patients to a testing specialist who does nothing but administer and evaluate one or more of these extensive batteries. Shorter batteries are commercially available, such as the Hartford-Shipley Test, the Peabody Picture-Word Vocabulary Test, and the Bender and Benton figure drawing tests. You could administer these in your office but they are usually impractical to use in Emergency Room, hospital, or busy clinic settings.

Monitoring Patients' Progress

Because all cognitive tests in this book generate a number from 0-8, they provide a quantitative measure of your patients' initial impairment and improvement during treatment. Improvements in cognitive function are usually more stable and less dependent upon immediate circumstances than patients' own reports of their emotions and thoughts. Patients *in extremis* may worry that they feel no better or that their treatment is not helping them but measurable improvements in cognitive function offer reassuring evidence that they are gaining ground in their fight for health. Better cognitive performance is easy for patients and their families to understand, whereas other symptoms of mental disorders may appear too variable or diffuse. Although manic patients might argue to retain their mania, or stoic depressives might play down their discomfort, all patients appreciate treatment that improves their cognition. After all, who wants to think and reason poorly?

Psychobiology of the Cognitive Examination

The present rationale for cognitive testing originated in the research of A. R. Luria, M.D. (see Chapter 8 and Appendix VII). Luria divided the work of the brain into hierarchical functions of *attention, language, memory,* and *abstract thinking,* to which we have added the category of *sequential thinking*, also known as *executive function*. Luria concluded that each of these functional domains represents an individual part of the brain with distinct types of neural activity. Moreover, each of these functions is dependent on the normal performance of the functions before it. For example, if the areas involved in *attention* are not intact, then patients may not be able to register *memory* or understand *language*. Because of this hierarchical relationship, when one of the functions is abnormal, then the testing results from all downstream functions may be affected.

We designed our Cognitive Examination to discover whether patients have significant, functional impairments in one or more of the five cognitive areas of *attention, language, memory, abstract thinking,* and *sequential thinking*. Each of the tests is expressed in a score from 0-8. For most of the subtests, you may consider scores of 7-8 to be Normal, scores of 6 to be Borderline, and scores of 0-5 to be Impaired.

This quantified Cognitive Examination measures mental function by comparing an individual with himself or herself, rather than with a standardized population mean. For example, if a patient does poorly on five tests of *memory* and well on all the other tests, then we can hypothesize that the brain areas supporting *memory* are deficient. However, if the patient does poorly on five tests distributed between *attention, language, memory, abstract thinking,* and *sequential thinking*, we can only conclude that the patient is not a good test taker.

Patients with mental illness often demonstrate pronounced cognitive deficits that you will detect by brief cognitive screening. However, because of the limitations of the clinical setting, you should follow up these screening tests with further testing and clinical observation whenever possible.

Attention

Attention is the ability to focus on a single stimulus, to maintain this focus over time, and to filter out distractions. *Attention* is necessary for us to maintain prolonged abstract or sequential analysis without intrusive, tangential thoughts. *Attention* also allows us to broaden our degree of focus to include as many as 5-9 simultaneous thoughts, or narrow it to just one thought at a time, while continuing to monitor surrounding events in the environment. *Attention* is associated with the prefrontal cortex, reticular activating system, thalamic nuclei, and other brainstem areas.

Tests of Attention

Level of Consciousness, Orientation, and Basic Verbal Comprehension are tests that quickly rule out severe attentional dysfunction. You can see severely disabled *attention* in psychosis, severe mood disorders, Panic Attacks, and after brain injury, stroke, metabolic abnormalities, poisoning, anoxia, and other serious brain insults. If severe impairment in these basic tests occurs suddenly, it may be necessary to begin emergency steps to diagnose and reverse the causes of Delirium. The Vigilance test measures the patient's ability to monitor their environment continuously. It is a quick way to acquire a finer measure of arousal than the other *attention* tests. See Appendices III-V.

Language and Aphasias

Language first requires *attention* to focus on language stimuli, and *memory* to remember and work with verbal information. In the nervous system, *language* is associated with the frontal cortex, temporal cortex, parietal cortex, and subcortical brain areas.

Basic Verbal Comprehension is necessary to complete most or all of the tests in our Cognitive Examination. Verbal comprehension is dependent on the posterior language area, also known as Wernicke's area.

Quality of Speech

Loudness is the interviewer's perception that patients are speaking louder than expected for a particular environment. Speech is very loud if it threatens to disturb others in that environment. *Mildly* rapid speech is just noticeable compared with the speech of other patients in the same environment, whereas *markedly* rapid speech may be so fast that it is unintelligible. Tangential speech is characterized by deviations from the point that interrupt the logical train of thought. Pressured speech is a torrent of words that interrupts the speech of others and is difficult to stop or "get a word in edgewise." Blocking is characterized by a sudden halt in the flow of speech. Blocking is associated with intrusive and tangential thoughts (and sometimes the presence of auditory hallucinations), although it can be produced in many conditions. You can find all these types of speech resulting from both organic pathology and mental illness, particularly Bipolar Disorder.

Scanning speech, where clients' conversation takes the form of rapid, staccato bursts, occurs in multiple sclerosis, although you will often observe mild scanning speech in individuals with Bipolar Disorder and Personality Disorders. Aprosodic speech with abnormal rhythm, stress, and intonation is often found in individuals with organic brain deficits, as well as in individuals who have not had the opportunity to hear cultural models, like the deaf. Dysarthric speech, including hoarseness, occurs after stroke or with injury to the nerves or muscles of the throat and larynx, as well as during local throat infections and inflammation.

Tests of Language

The Verbal Registration and Immediate Repetition test evaluates the language cortex surrounding the Sylvan fissure. A lesion or functional interruption of communication between receptive and expressive language areas, or the failure of either one, can also cause failure of the Verbal Registration and Immediate Repetition test. Many patients can perform the Verbal Registration and Immediate Repetition test even if more-complex *language* skills are impaired.

Full receptive and productive speech is more complex than repetition, because patients must register *and* translate the words they hear into personal meanings and experiences by passing them through an internal dictionary, possibly located in the inferior parietal lobe. Only when these words are given meaning can patients analyze them and produce a response. To reply, we translate our personal meanings and experiences through the internal dictionary into mental words and then into the motor patterns that identify the correct muscles necessary to speak the words.

Naming an object and its parts requires both recognition and discrimination of parts from the whole. The Object and Part Naming test often reveals covert *language* deficits in patients with otherwise intact *language* skills. It is quite surprising to discover patients who seem to be functioning normally but cannot recall the parts of common objects such as a watch, pen, or shoe. See Appendices III-V.

Aphasias and Language Syndromes

You can identify several classic patterns of brain deficits using the *language* tests in the Cognitive Examination.

In Global Aphasia, Basic Verbal Comprehension, Verbal Registration and Immediate Repetition, Object and Part Naming, reading, and writing are impaired. Global Aphasia often results from a stroke or brain injury. Speech Quality is poor, and the patient is often unable to speak spontaneously. There is often motor weakness and sensory loss on one side of the body.

In Broca's aphasia, Basic Verbal Comprehension and comprehension of the written word are intact but Verbal Registration and Immediate Repetition, plus Object and Part Naming are impaired. Quality of Speech in Broca's Aphasia, is halting, hoarse (dysarthric), and requires great effort on the part of the patient. Such patients mainly use nouns and verbs in an abbreviated style called telegraphic speech. Broca's aphasia arises in the anterior language cortex, in the perisylvian cortex and insula (Broca's area).

In Wernicke's Aphasia, Basic Verbal Comprehension, Verbal Registration and Immediate Repetition, Object and Part Naming, and writing are impaired. Nevertheless, Quality of Speech is good—speech is fluent, effortless, and well articulated. However, the speech is missing many substantive, meaningful words, lacks content, and may even be incomprehensible nonsense. Usually patients with Wernicke's syndrome are unaware of their problem. The syndrome is caused by a dysfunction in the posterior superior temporal gyrus of the language cortex (Wernicke's area).

Contrast Wernicke's speech with the rapid, tangential, high-content "Word Salad" of manic Bipolar Disorder, which initially sounds meaningful but is ultimately uninterpretable. Puns, made-up words, and interchanging words that sound similar (clang associations) are common in bipolar speech.

In Anomic Aphasia, only Object and Part Naming is impaired. Anomic aphasia produces speech that is usually fluent although marked by long, word-finding hesitations. Anomic Aphasia is not specific to any one area of the brain but it frequently results from injury to the second and third gyri of the temporal lobe. Inability to name (anomia) and comprehension errors can also involve subcortical brain locations.

In contrast, psychotic patients often show long pauses called "blocking" that represent distraction by voices, images or other hallucinations, often called "response to internal stimuli." Mild-to-severe word finding problems are present in dementias, especially in Parkinson's disease, but they are not specific to these disorders.

Memory

Memory can be divided into immediate or working memory, recent memory, and long-term memory. The process of *memory* first requires *attention*, which confers the ability to focus on and register stimuli so that patients can remember them. If verbal or written instructions, words, numbers, or other symbolic processes are needed for a *memory* task, then *language* abilities are also necessary.

The initial phase of instantaneous memory starts in the cellular memory of the sensory receptors of the eyes, ears, and other senses, and the brain areas immediately serving them. From the senses, we record a large volume of information, more than we can fit into available working memory. From all this information, we then select a limited number of stimuli to enter conscious, working memory. Working memory consists of a "scratch pad" that can hold just 5-9 channels of simultaneous information (about 3-4 bits of information—see Burgess and Spoor, Chapter 8). Intact working memory also requires the ability to keep information in or out of the working memory space. From working memory, information goes to other brain areas that perform specialized information processing. Generally, the information available in recent memory is available for a period of minutes to hours, unless it is rehearsed. Subsequent memory processes lay down longer-lived long-term memory traces that can last a lifetime. Much of *memory* consolidation occurs during sleep. Mental illnesses that interfere with sleep, such as unipolar Major Depressive Disorder and Bipolar Disorder, also interfere with the formation of long-term memory traces. In the nervous system, *memory* is associated with the functions of the hippocampus, dorsal medial thalamic nuclei, mammillary bodies, and language cortex.

Tests of Memory

The Digit Span test measures *attention*, basic stimulus registration, and the amount of information that can be contained in working memory on an eight point scale. Sometimes the task of spelling "world" backwards is substituted for Digit Span but many clinicians do not find this task as useful in clinical diagnosis. Naming Four Presidents measures distant or long-term memory heavily influenced by overall cultural awareness. Category Recall is a quantitative test of the ability to access and select information from long-term memory. Free Recall from a Story overloads working memory space and requires patients to be able to organize and consolidate information by context in order to keep enough of the story in their short-term working memory to analyze. See Appendices III-V.

Uncued Delayed Memory tests the patients' awareness of their surrounding environment and their ability to remember information spontaneously, without being forewarned that they will be tested on it. It measures patients' *memory* for the flow of events around them. Cued Delayed Memory tests learning—the ability to store and retrieve new information after being told to remember it. Patients are first checked to make sure they can register the target words (Red Ball, Blue Car, and the City of Chicago) in immediate memory and then told to remember the words later. Asking the patients to recall the targets at the end of the examination provides the delay. Although the choice of a few minutes delay, rather than hours or days, is purely practical, this interval is relevant for most human activities and communications in the everyday world.

If patients cannot recall the target information spontaneously, a series of questions can help ascertain whether the information was ever coded into *memory* at all. If patients fail to recall the words Ball, Car, or Chicago, they are first helped to remember through associations by saying, "One was red, one was blue, and one was a city." If patients still fail to remember Ball, Car, or Chicago, they are given a list of related words and asked to select the target words from among them. If patients still cannot remember the words, the clinician must suspect inattention or distractibility, because internal or external distractions can interfere with the encoding of registered information into longer-term memory stores. See Appendix III.

Memory Syndromes

Severely impaired short-term memory (Digit Span, Free Recall from a Story, Uncued and Cued Delayed Memory) results after prolonged thiamine (vitamin B_1) deficiency caused by chronic alcohol consumption, gastritis, frequent vomiting, and Crohn's disease damages the brain medial thalamus and mammillary bodies. Tests of long-term memory, like Four Presidents and Category Recall may be spared. When this memory deficit is accompanied by confusion, impaired eye movements, and motor incoordination, it is called Wernicke's Encephalopathy.

When the brain damage from thiamine deficiency and alcohol toxicity progresses and patients experience impaired short-term and distant memory, amnesia, false memories (confabulation), apathy, and reduced speech content, the condition is called Korsakoff's syndrome.

Abstract Thinking

Abstract thinking involves the comparison of several stimuli or bits of information together at the same time. *Abstract thinking* is also referred to as parallel or gestalt information processing. *Abstract thinking* operations are associated with the parietal lobe, particularly in the brain association areas located at the intersection of the parietal, temporal and occipital lobes (the so-called PTO association area).

Nonverbal *abstract thinking* is required for the observation and copying of figures in two-dimensional space as well as the observation and analysis of forms in three dimensions. For example, we use nonverbal *abstract thinking* to predict the volume and hidden sides of three-dimensional forms and for mental rotation of such forms in space. Verbal *abstract thinking* operations include the understanding of sets, the use of inductive reasoning, intellectual generalization, interpretation, and judgment. Simultaneous, gestalt perception and analysis also permit the appreciation of art and music.

It is necessary to have intact *attention* for successful *abstract thinking*, as well as intact *memory* in order to hold information in the mind for comparison. *Abstract thinking* ability improves as more bits of information can be held in *memory* storage at the same time. For example, in studying Vermeer's painting of the "Dutch Masters," it is necessary to simultaneously observe and interpret the light dancing off the elders' faces, the moisture on their skin, the texture of their clothes, the hardness of the table, the light and the dark shadows cast by the fire, the telling expressions on their faces, and the positions of their arms, legs and bodies all together, in order to appreciate the work. This is clearly a job for *abstract thinking*.

You will occasionally find patients who excel in *abstract thinking* but have very poor *sequential thinking* abilities. *Sequential thinking* is not necessarily required for *abstract thinking*, although many tasks require a mixture of both types. For example, to read and follow the sequential words of a book, it is necessary to have intact *sequential thinking*, whereas combining the information so gathered and comparing it together to understand the book requires *abstract thinking*.

Tests of Abstract Thinking

Simple Arithmetic operations require *abstract thinking* associated with the parietal lobe. If patients cannot demonstrate the capacity for Simple Arithmetic, then they will do poorly on more-complex arithmetic tasks, such as Serial Sevens and the Arithmetic Story Problem. See Appendices III-V.

The Proverb Interpretation test is a classic measure of higher cognitive function that is very useful in clinical evaluation. The Proverb Interpretation test has two parts. Comprehension of the original statement requires *language* and *sequential thinking*. The second part, which evaluates a patients' ability to generalize from a specific statement to its more global implications, involves *abstract thinking*. In "Don't cry over spilt milk," the patient must indicate that the spilt milk stands for some mistake or disappointment that happened in the past. For "Rome wasn't built in a day," the patient must show that the building of Rome stands for a monumental task that cannot be rushed. Patients with Schizophrenia, Intellectual Disability and many organic brain problems have difficulty making a generalization and produce literal or concrete interpretations. However, sometimes you will encounter patients with intact *abstract thinking* who lack the necessary *sequential thinking* ability to comprehend the proverb statement properly. Many patients with Bipolar Disorder fall into this category. They provide generalized answers that are irrelevant to the proverb or merely substitute another proverb or saying for the first. See Appendices III-V.

Set Analysis requires the ability to hold several bits of information in *memory* while simultaneously comparing the hierarchical relationship between them. For example, when asked about the difference between daisies and flowers, patients' correct response is to say that daisies are a type of flower. Because the recognition of inclusive and exclusive sets is an important part of analytical *abstract thinking*, the Set Analysis test provides valuable information about *abstract thinking* abilities not usually found in bedside cognitive testing.

Set Analysis consists of three questions arranged in order of simplicity, based on clinical experience. Sometimes the pattern of answers can be informative. For example, Set Analysis is preserved in some patients that seem low functioning because of poor verbal skills. Conversely, Set Analysis may unmask serious cognitive deficits in patients with good verbal skills who give the outward appearance of high cognitive functioning.

Visual spatial tasks require the comparison of many lines and surfaces together simultaneously to make sense of a figure. Many tests of figure drawing, typically called "constructions," are available for the evaluation of visual spatial relationships. However, many of the tests now in print add unnecessary, confounding *memory* components and time limitations.

The Greek Cross Figure Drawing provided in this battery is a simple, straightforward, and widely used visual spatial construction task. Reproducing the cross requires the simultaneous perception of many visual spatial elements in the drawing, the ability to hold this information together briefly in working memory, and the ability to translate this information into motor behavior to copy the figure on the page. The Greek Cross figure is composed of 12 lines of equal length—distortion of the figure results in changes of the lengths of the lines. A small circle added to the right of the cross tests the ability to discriminate parts from the whole of a drawing. Patients can complete the Greek Cross test with a minimum of verbal or written instruction. See Appendices III-V.

To score, measure each of the twelve lines in the patient's drawing with a ruler. Score one error for each line that is ¼ inch longer or ¼ inch shorter than the original. Also, score one error if the circle is drawn anywhere other than to the lower right of the copied Greek Cross, or if the circle is omitted. The total is eight minus the number of errors—the lowest score is zero.

The test of Judgment used in the Cognitive Examination has been a part of clinicians' mental status examinations for generations. In the current version, the physician asks the question, "Imagine you were watching a movie in a crowded theater and you discovered that the building had caught on fire. What would you do?" The correct answer has two parts: 1) to make sure the fire department has been called so the building does not burn up, and 2) to find a way for the audience in the theater to file out in an organized fashion without causing a panic that blocks the exits. Answering this question requires *abstract thinking* for the simultaneous assessment of these goals and their comparison with possible solutions. The traditionally correct answer is to call someone in authority to summon the fire department and help the audience file out of the theater. Nevertheless, with the ubiquity of cell telephones, it is now an equally a good plan for the patient to call 911 from the theater. Failing to call 911 and screaming "Fire!" are clearly serious errors with dire consequences for the entire audience. You will find that some patients justify their plan of immediate egress as the best way of saving their own skins but such disregard for the lives of the theater audience garners the lowest score for this solution. See Appendices III-V.

Another popular question traditionally used to test judgment is "What is the thing to do if you find an envelope on the street that is sealed, addressed and has a new stamp?" The traditional answer is "Put the letter in the mail immediately." Nowadays, you may give full credit for the responses, "Take the letter to the police station in case it was left by a terrorist" or "Just leave it alone because it might be dangerous."

If patients are too distracted to analyze either of these questions, you may ask them to explain what they think of a woman who runs into a store to buy something and leaves her baby out on the sidewalk. There are many correct answers to this test and there is no scale of quantification. Patients just have to give a plausible solution that would successfully protect the baby.

Lawrence Kohlberg's group provides a tool for more extensive judgment evaluation. *The Measurement of Moral Judgment* (see Chapter 8) outlines the use of test cases to evaluate nuances of the judgment process. For example, what should a man do if his dying wife needs a medicine right away but the only pharmacist is unavailable? Potential answers such as "break into the pharmacy," "go to the police," or "try harder to find the pharmacist," are scored in detail with commentary. You will find that simply discussing these stories with patients can be very helpful in finding out their capabilities for logic and judgment.

The Insight test avoids ethical and moral issues by using a simple question that virtually all patients can answer. Patients are simply told that telling the truth is good and asked to explain why. The test is designed to screen for lack of insight and to provide the examiner with some sense of the patients' view of themselves. The categories and relative weights given to the different answers reflect the patients' ability to generalize. Global or cultural values score higher than concerns about oneself or how others view us—whereas all of the above score higher than a values system based on punishment for disobeying the rules. The examiner is free to apply his or her own set of values to the problem and explore patients' answers further in the interview portion of the examination.

Parietal lobe dysfunction can also produce confusion of the Right versus Left sides, confusion of Parts versus the Whole of an object, and the inability to distinguish one finger from another, called Finger Agnosia. Clinicians call the pattern of these three deficits the Gerstmann syndrome.

Sequential Thinking

Sequential thinking, also called *executive function*, involves the ordering and execution of information and behaviors in a linear sequence, especially sequences with remembered elements, repeated elements, timing, or rhythms. The key attribute of *sequential thinking* is that the meaning of the current step in the series is dependent on recalling the meaning of the past step and anticipating the meaning of the next step. Linear operations are sometimes called serial information processing. The operations of *sequential thinking* are generally associated with the frontal lobe, particularly in the association areas of the inferior and dorsal lateral prefrontal areas, and the orbital frontal region.

Poor *sequential thinking* makes patients stray from the point in conversation and writing (tangentiality). Individuals with poor *sequential thinking* are also more likely to be overloaded by multiple stepwise tasks. Mathematic operations that require multiple steps and the use of variables are vulnerable to deficits in *sequential thinking* abilities. Difficulties in *sequential thinking* can make it difficult to start projects, to stay on task until project completion, to finish tasks, and to stop working when tasks are finished.

Logic operations suffer with *sequential thinking* deficits because logical thinking is a series of steps, each dependent on the last. Deductive reasoning and the sequential, ordered elements of reading and writing rely heavily on *sequential thinking*. Understanding the relationship between what has gone before and what is happening now or will happen in the future is an important part of *sequential thinking*. When clients act impulsively, they often demonstrate temporary unawareness of or lack of concern for the negative consequences of their actions in the future.

It is necessary to have intact *attention* for successful *sequential thinking*. Distractibility can interrupt the stream of sequential thought, causing the inability to stay on topic and task. It is necessary to possess intact *memory* for *sequential thinking* in order to remember the prior item in a sequence and to predict the next item. For example, in the command "bring the spoon and the fork" it is necessary to store the verb "bring" until the train of thought reaches "spoon" and "fork" in order to know what to do with them. However, it does not appear that *abstract thinking*, where many bits of information are compared at once, is essential for successful *sequential thinking*, where a thought only needs to be compared to those before and after it. Thus, you will find patients who appear to have intact *sequential thinking* and very poor *abstract thinking*.

Tests of Sequential Thinking

The Four-Step Sequential Command test is an extension of the Basic Verbal Comprehension test. Patients must be able to recall and arrange the four details of left ear, little finger, right hand, and smiling into the correct order. A common error is to omit the final action, sometimes called terminal drop. Be alert for patients who repeat, omit or transpose the steps and score these under Additional Sequential Information. See Appendices III-V.

Serial Sevens is a test that requires *attention* in order to persist in the operations, simple *abstract thinking* to complete the basic arithmetic operations, and *sequential thinking* to perform the sequential subtractions. You will find many patients who demonstrate the *abstract thinking* ability to perform arithmetic on the Simple Arithmetic task, but do not have the *sequential thinking* ability necessary to complete sequential Serial Sevens subtractions.

The Arithmetic Story Problem test requires *abstract thinking* to complete the basic arithmetic operations and *sequential thinking* to organize the information into the correct order to perform the arithmetic. You will find many patients that can perform the Simple Arithmetic equations but cannot perform the simplest sequential story problem, because they cannot put the operations in the correct sequential order.

The Luria Sequential Movement test is taken from the work of A. R. Luria (see Chapter 8), who demonstrated deficits in these sequential motor behaviors in patients with gross brain injuries. You can administer this test with a minimum of verbal instructions for patients with a language deficit or an inability to understand the clinician's native language. The hand positions in this test (forming a fist, making a flat palm, and forming the "OK" sign or ring with the first two fingers) are usually learned and encoded in childhood. If there is any doubt about the patient's motor ability to form the hand positions, demonstrate the hand positions by holding each of them up in the air after the test and allowing the patient plenty of time to form each of the positions, one at a time. Abnormal scores on this test are associated with deficits in the dorsal lateral prefrontal cortex of the brain. Compare the results of the Luria Sequential Movements in Appendices III-V with the Luria Figure Drawing Test of *sequential thinking* in Appendix VII.

Rhythm Reproduction requires patients to remember and repeat a sequence of long or short intervals. The sequence of six or nine movements cannot be comprehended as a gestalt. Instead, an awareness of the changes that come before and after each interval is required. We usually associate rhythms with music but maintaining the proper rhythms of speech, interactive communication, and repetitive body movements are essential to normal daily life. This is another test that requires a minimum of verbal instruction. See Appendices III-V.

Nonverbal Tests of Abstract and Sequential Thinking

This mini-battery of eight tests measures complex functions of abstract and sequential thought processing independent of language skills and may be used for patients with poor communication skills, low education level, aphasia, or language barriers, or as an adjunct to your usual Cognitive Examination. The *abstract thinking* tests measure the ability to compare several stimuli simultaneously to form a gestalt, while the *sequential thinking* tests measure the ability to use past information in a series to predict the next step in the series. This screening battery is short enough to use with impaired patients or when your time is limited.

Make a copy of the test in Appendix VI for each patient. Read the instructions on each page to the patient and point out how they are different. Then give the patient a blue ballpoint pen and collect the test when the patient is finished. If there are questions, just say, "Try to follow the instructions and use your best judgment. If you get stuck and cannot complete a question, just skip it and go on." There is no time limit.

Nonverbal Tests of Abstract Thinking

These tests measure the ability of patients to scan four figures simultaneously to find dissimilarities in shape or orientation. The test requires the ability to form inclusive and exclusive sets.

1. Triangles: The shape that does not belong is the circle, third in line. Every other shape is a triangle, albeit in different orientations.

2. Rectangles: The shape that does not belong is the triangle, the first in line. Every other shape is four-sided, albeit aligned in different orientations or with sides of different lengths.

3. Arrows: The shape that does not belong is the upward pointing arrow, second in line. Every other arrow is pointing horizontally.

4. Polygons: The shape that does not belong is the three-dimensional cube, last in line. Every other shape is two-dimensional.

Nonverbal Tests of Sequential Thinking

These tests measure the ability of patients to look at three steps of a sequence in order to determine the step that comes next. They require the ability to analyze a sequential trend, to learn from the past, and to use current information to predict the future.

1. Numeric Sequence: The shape that comes next is a square. The first shape (the circle) is composed of one line, the second shape (the cross) is composed of two equal lines, and the third shape (the triangle) is composed of three equal lines. A square composed of four equal lines comes next.

2. Sequential Rotation: The shape that comes next is a down pointing arrow. The arrows rotate 90 degrees in each sequential position. The first arrow points left (0 degrees), the second arrow points up (90 degrees), and the third arrow points right (180 degrees). The fourth shape should be an arrow pointing down, 270 degrees from the starting point.

3. Alternating Sequence: The shape that comes next is a large square. The first two shapes form a pattern: a small circle and a large circle. Because the third shape is a small square, the fourth shape must be a large square.

4. Arithmetic Sequence: The shape that comes next is a four-headed arrow pointing toward all compass points. The first arrow points in one direction (East); the second arrow points in two directions (East and West); and the third arrow points in three directions (East, West, and North). The fourth shape must have an arrow pointing in four directions (East, West, North, and South).

The Luria Figure Drawing Test of Sequential Thinking

The Luria Figure Drawing Test of *sequential thinking* (*executive function*) has been a regular part of neuropsych testing in my office for the last 20 years. This test of mental function is inspired by the drawing tests used by A. R. Luria, the father of neuropsychology, as reprinted in his books (see Chapter 8). This test specifically looks for sequential errors such as the *addition* of information to a sequence, the *omission* of information from a sequence, the *transposition* of elements within a sequence, and the *perseveration* of elements within a sequence. This brief test can be very helpful in evaluating *sequential thinking* in children, adults, cognitively impaired elders, and patients with language barriers.

Administering and Scoring the Luria Figure Drawing Test of Sequential Thinking

Make a copy of the Luria Figure Drawing Test in Appendix VII for each patient. Read the instructions to the patient while pointing out the target drawings and the area on the page where patients should make their copies. Then give the patient a blue ballpoint pen and collect the test when the patient is finished. If there are questions, just say, "Try to follow the instructions and use your best judgment. If you get stuck and cannot complete a question, just skip it and go on." There is no time limit.

Each correct subtest is worth one point for a total possible score of 8 points. The potential errors are listed under each subtest below. Do not subtract points for inconsistencies in size, tremulous lines, or slight variations in orientation.

1. mmmmmmmmmmmm. This question uses 12 identical letters to test for perseveration, addition, and omission. Patients fail the question if they repeat, add, or omit any letters, loops, or parts of letters from the series.

2. mnmnmnmnmnmn. This question alternates six pairs of two letters, adding the possibility of transposition errors. Patients fail the question if they transpose, repeat, add, or omit any letters, loops, or parts of letters from the series.

3. mmm mmn mnm nmn. This question alternates three letters in four groups, providing an additional level of sequential order and providing for more potential errors. Patients fail the question of they transpose, repeat, add, or omit any groups, letters, loops, or parts of letters from the series.

4. Arrowheads. These are simple, unconnected, straight-line analogs of the shapes in subsequent questions. Patients fail the question if they transpose, repeat, add, or omit arrowheads or lines from the series.

5. Square-Point-Square. This question provides a novel figure analog of Question 2, where eight square boxes and pointed spikes are alternated instead of familiar letters. Testees fail the question if squares or points are added or subtracted, repeated without alternation, if any lines forming squares or points are broken, or if any lines are added or omitted. A frequent error is to draw all or part of the preceding square or point again, instead of alternating between squares and points.

6. Double Vertical Loops. This question adds complexity by rotating the figures ninety degrees and requiring that the testee execute two loops per figure. Patients fail the question if they add or omit any double-looped figures, loops, or lines. A frequent error is the addition of a tiny loop or partial loop at the beginning or end of a line—any such tiny loop qualifies as a failure.

7. Half-Circle Loops. This question uses three groups of three simple, open curves oriented horizontally. Score a failure if any curves are added or omitted, or if curve orientation is transposed (if curves point up when they are supposed to point down), or if full or tiny loops or curves are added at the beginning or end of lines.

8. Double Horizontal Loops. This is an analog of the drawings in Question 6, with three groups of connected loops oriented horizontally. These groups of loops provide a strong stimulus for perseveration. Patients fail the question if the number of figures or loops within figures is wrong, if any loops are added or omitted, or if full or tiny loops or curves are added at the beginning or end of lines.

ADMINISTERING AND INTERPRETING THE COGNITIVE INTERVIEW AND QUESTIONNAIRE

The first step in performing the Cognitive Examination is to choose which form you wish to use for your patient. The one-on-one Cognitive Interview is personal and easy to use. If you need to save time in brief hospital or clinic appointments, give patients the Cognitive Questionnaire to fill out in the waiting area before they begin their appointment. I ask new patients to come for their appointment 20-30 minutes early for this reason.

The Cognitive Interview

Begin by making a copy of the Cognitive Interview in Appendix III for each patient. Record the patient's answers directly on the script, which also provides instructions for scoring. Calculate the scores for each question, and record them in the corresponding spaces marked, "Score:___/8." When you are done, transfer the scores for the Uncued and Cued Delayed Memory tests (Questions 23 and 24) to the *memory* section. Now you have a complete record of the patient's responses and you can proceed to analyze the results.

The Cognitive Questionnaire

Begin by making a copy of the Cognitive Questionnaire in Appendix IV and the Cognitive Questionnaire Score Sheet in Appendix V for each patient. Give the Questionnaire to patients to fill out in the waiting area before evaluation. If they ask questions, just say, "Try to follow the instructions and use your best judgment. If you get stuck and cannot complete a question, just skip it and go on." There is no time limit, but try to collect the papers promptly so that patients will not be tempted to go back over the form and change their answers. To prevent patients from changing their answers, make sure they complete the form with a pen, rather than an erasable pencil. I give blue pens to patients for completing the cognitive testing form—then any comments I make in my usual black ink are clearly discernible.

Now look at the completed Questionnaire. Notice that it does not contain scoring instructions or places to record final scores because this would be too confusing for patients filling out the form. The instructions for scoring and the places for recording the final scores are located on a second form, called the Cognitive Questionnaire Score Sheet, Appendix V. Follow the instructions to score the form. Now you are ready to analyze the results.

Interpreting Patterns of Response to the Cognitive Examination

Begin by comparing the scores between each of the sections of *attention, language, memory, abstract thinking,* and *sequential thinking.* If a patient performs significantly worse in one of the five categories compared with the other four, then this type of mental function and the brain areas underlying it are likely impaired. For example, if a patient does well in all the tests of *attention, language, memory,* and *abstract thinking* but fails most of the tests of *sequential thinking,* then *sequential thinking* is likely to be the problem and the brain areas underlying it are suspect.

Contrast the location of cognitive deficits in the brain with the results of physical and neurological examinations. This is also a time to request radiographic studies, scans, and other evaluations, if indicated.

If you feel you need additional information, consider administering *both* the Cognitive Interview and Questionnaire together, or adding the Nonverbal Tests of Abstract and Sequential Thinking (Appendix VI) and the Luria Figure Drawing Test (Appendix VII). You may wish to seek consultation from neuropsych testing specialists or request larger, more comprehensive testing batteries at this point.

Some patients will fail most of the tests in all five functions of *attention, language, memory, abstract thinking,* and *sequential thinking.* This pattern suggests problems upstream in attention or memory, or that the patient does poorly on cognitive tests, not that he has impairment in every area.

Look at how the cognitive tests overlap to understand patients' underlying functional deficits. For example, tests of Vigilance, Digit Span, Free Recall from a Story, Uncued and Cued Delayed Memory, Four-Step Command, Serial Sevens, the Arithmetic Story Problem, and Rhythm Reproduction all require holding information in working memory and are vulnerable to distractibility. If a patient seems distractible and fails these tests, he may be suffering from distractibility rather than some complex combination of *attention, memory,* and *sequential thinking* problems.

Failure on Serial Sevens or the Arithmetic Story Problem does not necessarily indicate problems in *sequential thinking* if your patient also failed Simple Arithmetic, because correct answers on Serial Sevens and the Arithmetic Story Problem require intact arithmetic skills.

Other comparisons are possible. For example, some patients will perform worse on the verbal compared with the nonverbal tests across the board, indicating an underlying *language* problem. Examine the tests in the *language* section to confirm this impression.

Please note that some of the test questions are easier than others, and in general, the *attention, language,* and *memory* tests are easier than the *abstract thinking* and *sequential thinking* tests. Within the *abstract thinking* domain, most patients find the Simple Arithmetic and Greek Cross tests to be easier than Proverbs and Set Analysis. Among *sequential thinking* tests, the Four-Step Sequential Command is usually easier than the Serial Sevens, Arithmetic Story Problem, Luria Movements, and Rhythm Reproduction tests. As an astute mental status examiner, it is important for you to be sure that patients who show poor performance on so-called tests of "higher functions" are not just normal patients who do poorly on any questions that are more difficult.

Tailoring the Cognitive Examination to Your Patient

You can tailor your cognitive testing battery to fit any of your patients. In addition to the tests in the Cognitive Interview and Questionnaire, you will find a novel Nonverbal Tests of Abstract and Sequential Thinking in Appendix VI, and the Luria Figure Drawing Test in Appendix VII.

Shortening the Examination

You will often have to evaluate patients with poor functional status or impaired consciousness due to Dementia, Delirium, Intoxication, stroke, or brain injury. Emergency room patients and new admissions are often excited or handicapped by impaired levels of consciousness. In emergency situations, your testing may be limited to the time it takes to wheel patients to the surgical theater. For the briefest examination, use Level of Consciousness, Orientation, Quality of Speech, and the Four-Step Sequential Command (which also measures verbal comprehension). If there is more time, add Simple Arithmetic, Digit Span, and Insight subtests, and plan to follow up your testing when and if you have the opportunity.

An Abbreviated Examination for Hospital and Clinic

You can abbreviate the Cognitive Examination by choosing one or two tests from each of the categories of *attention, language, memory, abstract thinking,* and *sequential thinking*. If your patient performs poorly on one of these, add more tests in that functional category for more information. For a brief examination, use Level of Consciousness, Orientation, Verbal Comprehension, Verbal Registration and Immediate Repetition, Quality of Speech, Digit Span, Four Presidents, Simple Arithmetic, Proverb Interpretation, Insight, a Four-Step Sequential Command, Serial Sevens, Luria Sequential Movements, and Cued Delayed Verbal Memory. You can perform these few tests in a brief time at the bedside or in the office.

For briefer examinations, use Level of Consciousness, Orientation, Verbal Registration and Immediate Repetition, Quality of Speech, Simple Arithmetic, and Cued Delayed Verbal Memory. These tests give little attention to abstract thought and ignore sequential processing altogether but they provide useful information, especially in patients who are acutely sick or injured.

Testing Patients with Poor Language Skills

Sometimes patients have poor communication skills due to language barriers, aphasia, or poor education. For these patients, consider using tests of Level of Consciousness, Verbal Comprehension, Quality of Speech, the Greek Cross, Luria Sequential Movements, and Rhythm Reproduction from the Cognitive Interview. If your patients have some grasp of the English language, try leading them through the Cognitive Questionnaire while giving a verbal explanation of the instructions. You may also try the Nonverbal Tests of Abstract and Sequential Thinking (Appendix VI) and the Luria Figure Drawing Test (Appendix VII), which require few instructions.

NEUROCOGNITIVE DISORDERS

Delirium Due to a Medical Condition (DSM-5 293.0, ICD-10 F05)

Delirium is a potentially fatal emergency that you must be able to recognize. Delirium is a rapid disturbance in *attention* and at least one other cognitive domain (*language, memory, abstract thinking, sequential thinking*) or perception that develops rapidly within the course of hours to days and tends to fluctuate during the course of a day. If a patient fails any of the first three tests of the Cognitive Examination—Level of Consciousness, Orientation, or Basic Verbal Comprehension—stop testing and look at the history, physical examination, or laboratory findings for evidence of nervous system dysfunction.

Delirium can result from cardiovascular disorders and stroke; bleeding, swelling, or tumor in the brain; toxicity from environmental poisons or liver failure; infection of the brain and spinal cord (meningitis); withdrawal of addictive substances; and many other conditions that can cause death or irreversible physical damage within seconds or minutes. Such patients need an immediate emergency medical workup with basic blood laboratories and radiographic imaging. The appearance of Delirium can also result from extreme intoxication, extreme fatigue, overwhelming traumatic events, and sudden awakening from a sound sleep. As a clinician, your job is to rule out potential causes of Delirium to the best of your ability and to seek help from other clinicians when you need it.

Mild Neurocognitive Disorder (DSM-5 331.83, ICD-10 G31.84)

Diagnose Mild Neurocognitive Disorder when there is a quantifiable decline in *attention, language, memory, abstract thinking, sequential thinking*, or social function that causes the patient to expend greater effort or use compensatory strategies to execute his or her daily activities. The cognitive deficits do not occur exclusively during a Delirium and they are not better explained by another mental disorder, such as Bipolar Disorder or Schizophrenia. Specify whether a behavioral disturbance accompanies the neurocognitive deficits.

Major Neurocognitive Disorder without Behavioral Disturbance (DSM-5 294.10, ICD-10 F02.80)

Major Neurocognitive Disorder with Behavioral Disturbance (DSM-5 294.11, ICD-10 F02.81)

Diagnose a Major Neurocognitive Disorder when there is a significant, quantifiable cognitive decline in *attention, language, memory, abstract thinking, sequential thinking*, or social function that interferes with the patient's ability to be independent in his or her everyday activities (e.g., paying bills or managing medications). The cognitive deficits do not occur exclusively during a Delirium and they are not better explained by another mental disorder, such as Bipolar Disorder or Schizophrenia. The following conditions may present with Neurocognitive Disorder:

Alzheimer's Disease (DSM-5 331.0, ICD-10 G30.9)

Diagnose Alzheimer's Disease when there is a gradual onset and a progressive impairment in *memory* and at least one other cognitive domain, without extended plateaus. There may be evidence of an Alzheimer's Disease genetic mutation from family history or genetic testing. The cognitive decline does not result from other neurodegenerative or cerebrovascular diseases, neurological, or mental disorders.

Traumatic Brain Injury (ICD-10 S06.2X9S)

Diagnose Traumatic Brain Injury (Sequelae of Diffuse Brain Injury with Loss of Consciousness) when there has been impact or movement of the head sufficient to displace the brain and either loss of consciousness, impaired *attention* (with disorientation and confusion), amnesia or impaired *memory,* or neurological signs (e.g., findings on neuroimaging, seizures, visual field deficits, loss of taste or smell, or one-sided weakness) that appear immediately after the trauma and persist after the acute post-injury period.

Frontotemporal Disease (DSM-5 331.19, ICD-10 G31.0)

Consider Frontotemporal Disease (Frontotemporal Lobe Degeneration) if there is a gradual onset and progression of either *language* impairment or behavioral symptoms (behavioral disinhibition; apathy or inertia; loss of sympathy or empathy; perseverative, stereotyped or compulsive/ritualistic behavior; or hyperorality and dietary changes) and prominent decline in *sequential thinking* (executive abilities) and/or social cognition. *Memory* and perceptual-motor function are relatively intact. The symptoms are not attributable to cerebrovascular disease, another neurodegenerative disease, the effects of a substance, or another mental disorder.

Prion Disease (DSM-5 046.79, ICD-10 A81.9)

Consider Prion Disease if there is gradual onset and rapid progression of motor symptoms, such as myoclonus or ataxia, or biomarker evidence of prions, combined with Mild or Major Neurocognitive Disorder.

Human Immunodeficiency Virus (HIV) Infection (DSM-5 042, ICD-10 B20),

Diagnose Human Immunodeficiency Virus (HIV) Infection if the presence of HIV virus has been documented. Mild or Major Neurocognitive Disorder should not be better explained by secondary brain diseases such as progressive multifocal leukoencephalopathy or cryptococcal meningitis.

Parkinson's Disease (DSM-5 332.0, ICD-10 G20)

Lewy Body Disease (DSM-5 331.82, ICD-10 G31.8)

Parkinson's Disease is typically diagnosed in the presence of pill-rolling tremor, slowness of movement, stiff and rigid muscles of the arms and legs, and impaired balance. Other symptoms include rapid shuffling walk with a bent-forward posture, dysarthria, mask-like facial expression, and depression. Cognitive impairment includes fluctuating *attention*, slowed processing speed, and deficits in *sequential thinking*.

When parkinsonism symptoms are present with fluctuating cognition, recurrent visual hallucinations, and possible rapid eye movement sleep disorder and neuroleptic sensitivity, consider Lewy Body Disease.

Huntington's Disease (DSM-5 333.4, ICD-10 G10)

Huntington's Disease may be determined by family history or genetic testing, or it may be diagnosed in the presence of random, jerky movements (chorea), posturing, speech and swallowing problems, sleep disturbance, compulsions, irritability, depression, and seizures. Cognitive impairment includes deficits in *language*, *memory*, *abstract thinking*, and *sequential thinking*.

VASCULAR DISEASE

Mild Neurocognitive Disorder (DSM-5 331.83, ICD-10 G31.84)

Major Vascular Neurocognitive Disorder without Behavioral Disturbance (DSM-5 290.40, ICD-10 F01.50)

Major Vascular Neurocognitive Disorder with Behavioral Disturbance (DSM-5 290.40, ICD-10 F01.51)

Consider Vascular Disease if cognitive deficits appear after cerebrovascular events (strokes) or if there is prominent decline in *attention* (including processing speed) and *sequential thinking* (frontal-executive function). There should be sufficient evidence of vascular disease in the history, physical examination, and neuroimaging to account for the measured cognitive deficits.

SUBSTANCE-RELATED NEUROCOGNITIVE DISORDERS

When neurocognitive impairments continue longer than the period of intoxication or withdrawal, consider Substance or Medication-Induced Mild or Major Neurocognitive Disorder. Deficits may or may not improve after a period of abstinence.

Intoxication with any substance can cause changes in *attention,* particularly in Level of Consciousness, resulting in confusion, stupor, or coma, at high doses. Attentional deficits can cause poor performance downstream in *language, memory, abstract thinking,* and *sequential thinking*. Substance intoxication can also directly impair *abstract thinking,* particularly the process of judgment, which can be determined by tests of judgment or by a history of poor judgment while intoxicated.

Intoxication with sedatives, including alcohol, benzodiazepines, barbiturates, opioids, and inhalants, typically impairs *attention*, causing errors on tests of Orientation, Basic Verbal Comprehension, and Vigilance. Sedatives also impair *language* Quality of Speech, causing slurred speech and dysarthria. *Memory* tests such as Digit Span, Free Recall from a Story, Uncued and Cued Delayed Memory, which depend on *attention* to register new information, are typically impaired. However, distant memory tests which do not require new information, like Four Presidents and Category Recall, may be spared. Chronic Alcohol Use Disorder is associated with impaired short-term memory in Wernicke's and Korsakoff's syndromes.

CHAPTER 3
THE MENTAL STATUS EXAMINATION IN THE EMERGENCY ROOM

In the fast pace of the Emergency Room, clinicians are challenged to marshal their total store of knowledge to assess, treat, and advocate for their patients. In the Emergency Room, clinicians see mental health patients as well as medical and surgical patients with mental health issues. Because of the emergent aspect of care, clinicians are often called upon to think and act quickly when their patients are in danger.

CASE 1
THE WOMAN WHO WAS STRUCK BY THE WRATH OF GOD

It was the middle of the afternoon at the Emergency Room of an East Coast medical center. A tired-looking Emergency Room nurse met me at the door escorting Mrs. H, an elderly Cuban woman. The nurse declined to enter my office but just pushed the patient through in a wheelchair accompanied by her paperwork. As he left, the nurse called over his shoulder, saying, "This one's crazy."

As soon as she entered my office, Mrs. H began screaming rapidly, "I'm in terrible pain! I've been struck by the wrath of God!" She stood up and paced the floor but she could not quiet herself. Mrs. H tried at one point to sit down but she immediately jumped up again as if struck.

"It has happened again," she roared. "I felt it coming for a week because my body did not feel right and so I knew I was going to be punished."

"Why do you think that God would want to hurt you, Mrs. H?" I enquired gently.

"Last week I got in an argument with my girlfriend and I've been angry ever since. I told her I had thoughts about cheating on my husband. I think she went and told the priest and now God is striking me down! It's a stupid question, anyway. How do I know why God does things? I was punished last night, that's all I know."

"Try to talk slower and tell me exactly what happened," I said, struggling to get a word in.

"I was in my kitchen last night when I saw the Holy Spirit. It looked like a ball of blue electricity. It came in through the window and flew around the kitchen. The light ran down my back and it felt like an electrical shock touching me. My back felt the burning of the fire. And when I looked on my body, I saw the burning mark of the Holy Spirit."

"Are you sure that you are not confused about what happened to you?" I asked.

Mrs. H was incensed. "You're just a doctor," she hissed. "What do you know about the Holy Spirit? Nothing! God has punished *me*, and I can see it and feel the pain of it!"

"Yes, but sometimes people can be confused about complicated things like God," I persisted weakly.

"You're clearly a big idiot," the elderly woman exclaimed, shaking her head in exasperation, "who has no experience with God. This is not the first time this has happened, you know. God punished me like this once before, two years ago. If you doubt my word, it is easy to prove I'm telling the truth. Just look at my back and you will see the mark of the Holy Spirit burned into my flesh!"

I did not believe her story of being marked by God but I was happy to look at her back if only to help build rapport with her. Although I tried to be gentle, she screamed in pain when I barely touched her shoulder. When I gently lifted up the back of her gown, I could not believe what I saw. Running across her back in a distinct straight line was an angry swollen red welt covered by blisters. I had never seen anything like it. All I could think was that she might have been struck by lightning. Or was I really witnessing an act of God?

Mrs. H appeared warm and her body temperature was elevated at 101 degrees Fahrenheit (normal=98.6 degrees).

In her Diagnostic Examination, Mrs. H demonstrated clear psychomotor agitation. She said she had not slept more than a few hours in the last seven days and she had not eaten for the last 10 hours. She said her heart had been pounding, she had been sweating excessively, and her hands were trembling continuously over the last week. Mrs. H agreed that she was irritable and angry but she denied emotions of sadness or elation. Mrs. H acknowledged paranoid thoughts and her thought content was fixed on her story about the Holy Spirit. She denied suicidal or violent thoughts or intentions.

On her Cognitive Examination tests of *attention*, Mrs. H failed a test of Orientation—she knew who she was but she gave the day and date when her episode had first occurred. When I asked her the time, she just shook her head, although there was a clock on the wall and she was wearing a watch. When I asked her *where* she was, she guessed she was in a church. When I asked her to hold up her left hand in a test of Basic Verbal Comprehension, she complied only half the time, even when I held up my hand as a model. On three occasions, she forgot about the Cognitive Examination altogether and she had to be reminded of what she was doing.

In tests of *language*, Mrs. H's Quality of Speech was poor—her speech was rapid and loud. Mrs. H could only repeat three of the six words read to her in English and Spanish in a test of Verbal Registration and Immediate Repetition. In the Object and Part Naming test, Mrs. H could name a watch, a pen, and a shoe with no problems, but she could not name their parts.

In *memory* tests, test, Mrs. H could only repeat two numbers out of seven on a test of Digit Span (working memory capacity). She failed Category Recall and she could not remember any words in tests of Uncued and Cued Delayed Memory. She declined any further testing.

CHALLENGE

Periodically we are faced with a paranoid patient who may actually be in danger. Clearly, Mrs. H had suffered some kind of severe and painful injury that she associated with her religious beliefs. I concluded that her reality testing was poor and that she was indeed psychotic. Because of her condition, however, it was necessary to elucidate what had really taken place to ensure there was no continuing danger to her health.

Your challenge is to diagnose Mrs. H's problem and to tie it in with her psychiatric picture. Here are some hints: Mrs. H's wounds were not self-induced as a result of religious mortification, personality disorder, or psychosis. She had not been scalded while cooking in her kitchen, nor was she the victim of lightning or home electrical problems.

SOLUTION

Mrs. H suffers from **Bipolar I Disorder, Most Recent Episode Manic with Psychotic Features** (DSM-5 296.44, ICD-10 F31.2) and **herpes zoster** (shingles, ICD-10 B02).

She met the following criteria for a **Manic Episode**:
A. The following have been present most of the day nearly every day:
1. Increased goal-directed activity or energy. Mrs. H had been agitated and staying up at night.
2. At least one of these:
   a. Elevated mood.
   b. Expansive mood.
   c. Irritable mood. Mrs. H was very angry in the examination, calling me "a big idiot." She said, "Last week I got in an argument with my girlfriend and I've been angry ever since."
These symptoms last at least one week or any duration if hospitalization is necessary. Mrs. H had been angry and agitated for a week and her condition was so serious that she was hospitalized.
B. At least three of the following symptoms (four if the mood is only irritable):
   1. Inflated self-esteem or grandiosity. It was grandiose for Mrs. H to think that she was so important that God would single her out for punishment by the Holy Spirit for having some impure thoughts. It was also grandiose and maladaptive to argue that she knew far more than her doctor did, whether true or not.
   2. A decreased need for sleep (needs <3 hours). Mrs. H had "not slept more than a few hours in the last seven days."
   3. Talking more than usual or interrupting others (pressured speech). Mrs. H was hyperverbal and left me "struggling to get a word in."
   4. Rapid or racing thoughts. When she came in my office, Mrs. H began "screaming rapidly" and her speech "was rapid and loud." I admonished her to "try to talk slower."
   5. Distractibility. "Mrs. H's Level of Consciousness was alert but distractible." "On three occasions, she forgot about the Cognitive Examination altogether."
   6. Increased goal-directed activity or psychomotor agitation. Mrs. H was agitated. Upon entering my office, "she stood up and paced the floor but she could not quiet herself." In her Diagnostic Examination, "Mrs. H demonstrated clear psychomotor agitation."
   7. Excessive involvement in activities that have a high potential for painful consequences (costly or risky impulsive actions).
Mrs. H was psychotic because she experienced hallucinations and delusions. Her report that she had seen the Holy Spirit as a ball of blue electricity that came in through her window and flew around the kitchen indicated hallucinations. Although her pain was real and probably felt like the wrath of God, she was focused on a delusional belief that the Holy Spirit had had burned her for having impure thoughts. Although we are all taught to respect others'

religious beliefs, Mrs. H's health was at stake and she needed her clinician to use objective reasoning to determine the diagnosis that would guide her successful treatment.

There are other nondiagnostic clues to the presence of Bipolar Disorder. Mrs. H said, "I felt it coming for a week because my body did not feel right." Patients often complain that they 'don't feel right in their body' before a bipolar episode, possibly because of increased adrenaline and endogenous stress hormones. Manic individuals frequently have decreased appetite and eventual weight loss—Mrs. H had not eaten in the last 10 hours.

Mrs. H's manic episode was exacerbated by a **herpes varicella zoster** infection, commonly called **shingles**. Shingles usually manifests as distinct bands of red, inflamed, and blistered skin on the back, distributed within a single sensory dermatome. The pain can be so intense that merely the pressure of clothing or bedclothes on the affected area is excruciating. The disorder is caused by the reactivation of dormant virus particles, causing inflammation and cell death in dorsal root ganglia of the spinal cord. Antivirals can be used to arrest the infection and prevent its spread. In severe cases, life-threatening encephalitis or vasculitis may occur.

Shingles originate from childhood chickenpox infections. After the initial infection, viral particles retreat to the spinal nerve ganglia where they remain dormant. The viral particles can then be reactivated by stress or unknown factors once or twice during the lifetime, or more frequently. Viral particles that settle in the cervical ganglia are the cause of cold sores of the mouth and lips.

Other Diagnostic Considerations

Some clinicians might consider the diagnosis of Schizophrenia upon seeing Mrs. H's hallucinations and delusions. However, delusions, hallucinations, and disorganized speech with derailment or incoherence are also characteristic of psychotic Bipolar Disorder, psychotic unipolar Major Depressive Disorder, and psychosis caused by other mental and medical conditions. According to DSM-5, Schizophrenia cannot be diagnosed in the presence of a Major Depressive Disorder or Bipolar Disorder.

Some clinicians might consider that Mrs. H was having a Panic Attack, based on her pounding heart, excessive sweating, and tremor. However, her dominant emotion was anger, not fear, and her symptoms were continuous and did not peak within minutes as required for Panic Disorder.

Mrs. H had Generalized Anxiety Disorder symptoms of restlessness, difficulty concentrating, and sleep disturbance, but she mentioned no uncontrollable worried thoughts about events or activities occurring most days for the last six months.

Mrs. H met some of the official criteria for Attention-Deficit/Hyperactivity Disorder, including problems sustaining attention, not listening to others, an inability to follow through on instructions on the Cognitive Examination, distractibility, forgetfulness, problems sitting in one place, restlessness, appearing to be "driven like a motor," talking excessively, and interrupting others' speech. However, she did not meet the necessary six criteria for either the Inattentive or the Hyperactive-impulsive Presentation. Attention-Deficit/Hyperactivity Disorder cannot be diagnosed when symptoms can be explained by a mood disorder such as Bipolar Disorder, which is diagnosed instead.

Bipolar Disorder explains all of Mrs. H's symptoms, including grandiosity, insomnia, abundant speech, pressured speech, flight of ideas, distractibility, agitation, anger, hyperreligiosity, and psychosis.

Cognitive Testing

Mrs. H's Cognitive Examination showed *attention* deficits resulting from the distractibility of Bipolar Disorder. Her mind was full of intrusive, repetitive, delusional thoughts that pushed other thoughts from her conscious working memory. Mrs. H's rapid speech reflected an overabundance of racing thoughts. She had to be reminded repeatedly to refocus on the testing. Her distractibility impaired other cognitive tests, particularly Digit Span, Category Recall, Uncued Memory, and Cued Delayed Memory, which are vulnerable to distraction because they require the patient to hold several items in conscious working memory at the same time. Distractibility is one of the diagnostic criteria for bipolar mania.

CLINICAL NOTES

When I was able to bring up Mrs. H's records, I found a long diagnostic history of Bipolar I Disorder that was usually well-controlled by medications. When Mrs. H experienced her painful shingles, she had stopped taking her medications, and her delusions began shortly afterward. After a short course of her usual antipsychotic and anticonvulsant mood stabilizing medicines in the hospital, Mrs. H's sensorium cleared and she was able to go home. The infectious disease resident started her on antivirals and followed Mrs. H as an outpatient.

CASE 2
MRS. BLACK IS TOO NERVOUS

I was called one afternoon to see a 39-year-old woman named Mrs. Black in the Emergency Room. When I arrived on the scene, the consult note simply read, "Rule out panic. Call the Psych." With this illuminating communication in mind, I went in to see the patient.

Mrs. Black was absent from her cubicle, having been taken to the bathroom. The nursing notes indicated that Mrs. Black had come in with an elevated pulse of 105 beats per minute (normal=60-100 bpm) and a high blood pressure of 165/97 millimeters of mercury (normal<120/80 mm Hg). There was an electrocardiogram (EKG) strip clipped to her chart that read "sinus tachycardia." A urine toxicology screen was negative for commonly abused drugs. The volume note on her nursing chart indicated that she got up from bed to void every half hour.

When Mrs. Black returned to her cubicle, I noticed that her face was flushed, her eyes were watery, she was perspiring, and her hands were shaking. She seemed excited and agitated and she had difficulty sitting still. She denied knowledge of any systemic health problems other than mild chronic insomnia.

Mrs. Black said that she had never smoked cigarettes or used any other form of tobacco. She said that drinking alcohol or using any addictive or illegal substances was against her religion. She denied the use of any prescription drugs. She said that she took an over-the-counter medication for her frequent headaches but she was unable to recall its name. When I asked her about drinking coffee, she looked at me sheepishly and said, "I only have two bad habits—chocolate and coffee. But I promise that I only drink two cups a day. And I drink it black. The rest of the time I just drink tea or cola."

In her Diagnostic Examination, Mrs. Black told me that she had come to the Emergency Room on the insistence of her daughter who felt that her mother was "just too nervous and hyper." Mrs. Black acknowledged that she looked hyperactive but she said, "That's the way I always look." When I asked her what she thought the problem was, she said, "Well, I'm sure I don't know." She denied any history of psychiatric disorders or hospitalizations and she indicated that she had not been irritable, or particularly happy or optimistic in the last week. She said that she was not suicidal or violent but she refused any further interview questions.

On her Cognitive Examination of *attention*, Mrs. Black was Oriented with good Basic Verbal Comprehension, but she failed a Vigilance task that required her to identify target numbers while distracted.

Mrs. Black's Quality of Speech was rapid and pressured but she did well on *language* tests of Verbal Registration and Immediate Repetition, and Object and Part Naming.

In her *memory* evaluation, Mrs. Black was only able to repeat back four of seven numbers in a Digit Span test. She did well on the Four Presidents and Category Recall tests but she was unable to recall any words after three minutes on a test of Cued Delayed Memory.

In tests of *abstract thinking*, Mrs. Black did well on the Simple Arithmetic and Greek Cross tests but she refused tests of Proverb Interpretation and Set Analysis.

In tests of *sequential thinking*, Mrs. Black did well on a Four-Step Sequential Command but she could only subtract 7 from 100 three times in the Serial Sevens test and she failed the Arithmetic Story Problem altogether. She refused tests of Luria Sequential Movements and Rhythm Reproduction.

I talked to Mrs. Black's daughter in the waiting area. The daughter told me that Mrs. Black took over-the-counter headache remedies two or three times daily. In addition to her two cups of coffee, which she obtained from the local convenience store, Mrs. Black also consumed three glasses of iced tea and three bottles of diet cola daily. She also consumed chocolate in the form of three dark chocolate bars each day.

CHALLENGE

All the clues necessary for diagnosis are available in the Mrs. Black's evaluation. See if you can choose a diagnosis that fits all of Mrs. Black's symptoms. Then propose a treatment for the diagnosis you have chosen.

SOLUTION

Mrs. Black suffers from **Caffeine Intoxication (DSM-5 305.90, ICD-10 F15.929)**:
A. **Recent consumption of caffeine, usually in excess of 250 mg (more than 2-3 cups of brewed coffee)**. Mrs. Black consumed coffee, strong iced tea, caffeinated cola, headache remedies containing caffeine, and dark chocolate bars containing caffeine and related alkaloid chemicals.

B. **Five (or more) of the following, developing during, or shortly after, caffeine use** (in general, these are signs of increased adrenaline and noradrenaline activity):
   1. **Restlessness**. "She seemed excited and agitated and she had difficulty sitting still."
   2. **Nervousness**. Her daughter felt that her mother was "just too nervous."
   3. **Excitement**. "In her examination, Mrs. Black "seemed excited."
   4. **Insomnia**. Mrs. Black acknowledged "mild chronic insomnia."
   5. **Flushed face**. "I noticed that her face was flushed."
   6. **Diuresis**—frequent urination. "Her nursing chart indicated that she got up from bed to void every half hour."
   7. **Gastrointestinal disturbance**.
   8. **Muscle twitching**.
   9. **Rambling flow of thought and speech**.
   10. **Tachycardia**—rapid heartbeat, or cardiac arrhythmia. Mrs. Black "had come in with an elevated pulse of 105 beats per minute." An electrocardiogram (EKG) read "sinus tachycardia."
   11. **Periods of inexhaustibility**.
   12. **Psychomotor agitation**. In her examination, "Mrs. Black acknowledged that she looked hyperactive."Her daughter characterized her as "hyper." I characterized Mrs. Black as "agitated."
C. **These symptoms cause clinically significant distress or impairment in school, work, home, or social function**. Mrs. Black's symptoms caused physical symptoms, upset her daughter, and precipitated a trip to the Emergency Room.

Other Diagnostic Considerations

There was no evidence that caffeine caused the recurrent failure to meet obligations, physical hazards, legal problems, social problems, interpersonal problems, or tolerance, that are required for a diagnosis of Substance Use Disorder. Although she experienced headaches and demonstrated problems *attention* problems on her Cognitive Examination, Mrs. Black did not exhibit other signs of Caffeine Withdrawal.

Other drugs can precipitate similar syndromes by intoxication or withdrawal but Mrs. Black denied drinking alcohol or using any addictive or illegal substances, she denied the use of any prescription drugs, and a urine toxicology screen was negative for commonly abused drugs. Other causes of increased adrenaline and serotonin, including undiagnosed hyperthyroidism, pheochromocytoma, and carcinoid tumor, could be ruled out with physical examination and blood tests.

Some clinicians might consider a diagnosis of Panic Attack because Mrs. Black exhibited symptoms of accelerated heart rate, sweating, and tremor, but these did not peak within minutes. Moreover, Panic Disorder cannot be diagnosed if Panic Attack symptoms are due to the direct physiological effects of a substance such as caffeine.

Generalized Anxiety Disorder is associated with restlessness and edginess, but the diagnosis requires that the patient have excessive anxiety and uncontrollable worries about activities or events occurring most days for at least six months.

Mania is associated with rapid, pressured speech; distractibility; and decreased sleep; but Mrs. Black showed no evidence of the elevated, expansive, or irritable mood required for the diagnosis of a Manic Episode.

Attention-Deficit/Hyperactivity Disorder is associated with distractibility, difficulty sitting still, and activated speech, but there was no evidence that these particular symptoms were causing impairment in school, work, home, or social settings, or that they had been present before seven years of age.

The diagnosis of Caffeine Intoxication explains all of the patient's symptoms.

Cognitive Testing

Mrs. Black's Cognitive Examination was consistent with distractibility due to increased adrenaline/noradrenaline activity. Her rapid, pressured speech showed an overabundance of racing thoughts. She made errors in Vigilance, Digit Span, Cued Delayed Memory, Serial Sevens, and the Arithmetic Story problem, which are vulnerable to distractibility because they require the patient to hold several items in working memory at the same time. Distractibility is also a well-known consequence of stimulant intoxication.

CLINICAL NOTES

One 7-oz cup of coffee usually contains 100-130 mg of caffeine. However, the two cups of coffee that Mrs. Black obtained from the local convenience store contained 32 ounces each, so she consumed the equivalent of nine regular cups of coffee containing 900-1100 mg of caffeine daily. During the rest of the day, she drank three glasses of iced tea (about 60 mg of caffeine) and three bottles of caffeinated diet cola (about 100 mg of caffeine). Most over-the-counter headache remedies contain caffeine. Mrs. Black took these pills 2-3 times each day for about 100-150 mg of caffeine daily. She also consumed chocolate in the form of three dark chocolate bars (about 90 mg caffeine) daily. I estimated that Mrs. Black consumed 1250-1500 mg of caffeine every day.

Caffeine, or 1, 3, 7-trimethylxanthine, is the most widely used stimulant in the world. Most adults find the stimulation of caffeine unpleasant at high doses and this limits caffeine's potential for abuse. The lethal dose of caffeine is between 5000-10,000 mg, although severe nervous system complications including seizures and arrhythmias can be seen after the ingestion of 1000 mg or more. Since toxicology screens usually do not include caffeine, it can easily be missed.

Theobromine is an alkaloid similar to caffeine. Three 1.5 oz dark chocolate bars contain about 300 mg of theobromine. Unknown amounts of theophylline, another stimulant alkaloid, were probably also present.

Caffeine, theobromine, and theophylline all compete for binding at the adenosine alpha-1 and alpha-2 receptors. Adenosine receptors are present in most cells and antagonizing them blocks the relaxing effects of adenosine. Caffeine increases the stimulating catecholamines epinephrine (adrenaline), norepinephrine (noradrenaline), and dopamine by blocking reuptake and decreasing catecholamine metabolism. Caffeine stimulates the heart, increases respiratory drive, and relaxes smooth muscle in both the circulatory and respiratory systems. It is also responsible for coffee's well-known diuretic effect.

Mrs. Black was cleared by the Cardiology staff and I taught her how to gradually taper off caffeine by reducing her intake by the equivalent of one-half cup of coffee (100 mg of caffeine) each day. By using this taper schedule, Mrs. Black could reach a more reasonable caffeine intake (250 mg) within about two weeks. An appointment was made for her in the outpatient psychiatric clinic to reinforce her recovery and address the reasons she had started ingesting so much caffeine.

CASE 3
WHERE IS ROBERTO?

In the gray of winter, I was called to the Emergency Room of a small local hospital to evaluate a young Hispanic man named Roberto. The nurse on the telephone simply said, "Come quick! He's been in a motorcycle accident!"

When I arrived at the Emergency Room, it was deserted. The medical doctors had the charts in a conference room where they were conducting morning rounds, the surgeons were in the surgery suite, and there was only one staff member to be seen, a harried male nurse. Before I could complete my introduction he said, "I'm from registry and I don't know any of these patients, so don't ask me." When I pressed him about Roberto's whereabouts, he waved me out into the hallway, where a hirsute, shirtless young man was wandering, fingering his skin, and laughing. A dirty splint was visible on his right leg. I could not coax him into a room so I was obliged to do my evaluation in the hall.

In his Diagnostic Examination, Roberto denied feeling sad, afraid, or angry and he denied thoughts of suicide or sensations of hearing voices. When I asked him why he was rubbing his skin, he merely fingered his arm and said, "Dirty."

On his Cognitive Examination of *attention*, Roberto's Level of Conscious fluctuated between alert and distracted. Roberto could only identify his name and his location on the Orientation test. When I called his attention to the time on a large wall clock, he commented that the clock looked like a face. His ability to hold up his hand on a test of Basic Verbal Comprehension was erratic and he failed a test of Vigilance where he was required to monitor a series of numbers to detect the numeral "5."

In *language* evaluation, Roberto's' Quality of Speech was poor—his flow of speech was halting, his words were slurred (dysarthric), and he showed strong perseveration, repeating words and phrases several times. On a test of Object and Part Naming, he could identify a watch, pen, and shoe but not their parts.

Roberto failed *memory* tests of Digit Span and Cued Delayed Memory. Although he could not remember any US presidents, he easily named several prominent members of the Mexican revolution, who he called "the streets" (because many Mexican streets are named for historical figures). He told me he had grown up in Guadalajara, and when I asked him how he liked the market in a small town nearby, he correctly told me that there was no market there. Thus, his long-term or distant memory was intact.

Roberto failed all the tests of *abstract thinking*. He was unable to perform a Simple Arithmetic test; his drawing of a Greek Cross showed only the left side of the figure; and he did not seem to be able to understand the instructions for Proverb Interpretation or Set Analysis.

Roberto also failed all the tests of *sequential thinking*. He could follow only three of the steps in a Four-Step Sequential Command and he failed Serial Sevens subtraction. In the Luria Figure Drawing Test (Appendix VII), Roberto's drawings, like his speech, were perseverative, with many repeated lines, loops, and figures. When I had exhausted Roberto, I repaired to a corner to try to make some sense out of the information I had collected.

CHALLENGE

This case illustrates the problems of trying to make an assessment with insufficient information. Using the information available, see if you can devise a tentative diagnosis for Roberto and decide what you would suggest for the next stage of his treatment. By the way, one solution would simply be to wait a day until more information was available from the chart or staff—do you want to wait?

SOLUTION

Roberto has **Delirium Due to Head Trauma** (DSM-5 293.0, ICD-10 F05), an emergency condition:
- **The patient has a rapid disturbance in *attention* that develops rapidly within the course of hours to days and tends to fluctuate during the course of a day.** Roberto failed *attention* tests of Orientation and Vigilance, as well as tests of Digit Span, Cued Delayed Memory, a Four-Step Sequential Command, and Serial Sevens subtraction that are dependent on sustained focus. It was noted that "Roberto's Level of Conscious fluctuated."
- **At least one other cognitive domain (*language, memory, abstract thinking, sequential thinking*) or perception is also affected.** (*Language*): Roberto failed a *language test* of Object and Part Naming. "His flow of speech was halting, his words were slurred (dysarthric), and he showed strong perseveration, repeating words and phrases several times." (*Memory*): "Roberto failed *memory* tests of Digit Span and Cued Delayed Memory." His ability to describe facts from distant, long-term memory confirms that his cognition used to be better. (*Perceptual disturbance*): Roberto "commented that the clock looked like a face."

There is evidence from the history, physical examination, or laboratory findings of a medical condition, substance intoxication or withdrawal, exposure to a toxin, or other medical cause of nervous system dysfunction. Because Roberto presented to the Emergency Room after a motorcycle accident, we can posit that trauma precipitated his cognitive changes.

Other Diagnostic Considerations

Without imaging and laboratory tests, we cannot be sure that Roberto's Delirium is not caused or complicated by other medical conditions such as cardiovascular dysfunction, stroke, or substance withdrawal. Conversely, acute brain trauma can mimic the symptoms of Major Neurocognitive Disorder, unipolar Major Depressive Disorder, Bipolar Disorder, psychosis, and anxiety disorders.

Cognitive Testing

Roberto failed most of the tests on his Cognitive Examination, although there was an indication that his baseline cognition was much better. Roberto's performance on the Greek Cross suggested brain damage to one hemisphere resulting in sensory neglect—patients with such damage draw figures that are missing elements on the left or right side. Similarly, perseverative speech and drawing and the misinterpretation of sensory information (such as seeing a clock as a face) are common findings in brain injury.

A. R. Luria, M.D., a founding father of neuropsych testing, conceived of cognitive function as a hierarchy of *attention* (prefrontal cortex and brainstem), *language* (left temporal lobe), *memory* (hippocampus, etc.), and spatial awareness (right temporal lobe). In this model, each functional component must be intact for the ones downstream to function normally. Thus, Roberto's impaired *attention* caused him to do poorly on downstream functions of *language* (Object and Part Naming), *memory* (Digit Span and Cued Delayed Memory), *abstract thinking* (Simple Arithmetic, Greek Cross), and *sequential thinking* (Four-Step Sequential Command and Serial Sevens).

CLINICAL NOTES

I was unable to locate or communicate with any other doctors in the Emergency Room, so I wheeled Roberto downstairs to the Imaging Department. When Roberto and I entered the Imaging Department, I found that his medical chart was already there. The resident doctor was quite happy to see us and told me that Roberto had been sent from the Emergency Room to the Imaging Department for an emergency brain scan to rule out traumatic brain damage. However, Roberto had simply wandered off before the scan could be completed. While the radiology staff had been trying to locate him, Roberto had walked back upstairs to the Emergency Room. After his scan, Roberto seemed sleepy and he was transferred immediately to the surgical suite for treatment of intracranial bleeding from a subdural hematoma.

Closed head injuries produce brain damage as a result of abrupt movement of the head with impact of the brain upon the inside of the skull. Trauma is most likely to occur in the prefrontal and parietal areas where the brain is tightly contained within skull curvature. Closed head injury is common—hospital records suggest that over five hundred thousand new cases occur per year. Risk factors include alcohol and drug abuse, age, and male gender.

Ultimately, localization of injury requires a computerized tomography (CT) scan or magnetic resonance imaging (MRI) study of the brain, which should be done as soon as possible. Some doctors believe a blood test called serum S-100B is useful in detecting intracranial damage in patients who have a normal MRI.

Cognitive abilities begin to return rapidly after closed head injury. Attention and memory impairment from mild or moderate injuries often resolve during the first week or two after injury. Even with severe injuries, the greater part of total recovery is usually completed within six months after brain trauma. I saw Roberto a week later, just before he was discharged from the hospital. At that time, he was fluent in English and Spanish, conversed logically, and performed normally on my Cognitive Examination.

CASE 4
MR. SMITH HAS VOODOO WORMS!

The beliefs of different cultures influence patients' understanding of the meaning of disease and clinicians' ability to heal. We are trained to combat problems with knowledge and facts, whereas patients' cultural understanding can transcend the logic of our own clinical culture. When the facts are unknown or the patient cannot accept our explanations, then the approach to the problem may become more important than the solution. This somewhat terrifying case involves the approach to a confounding medical problem and the need to make a psychological interpretation that the patient can accept.

This case took place in the Emergency Room of an East Coast hospital that serves a broad range of cultures including Native American, Caribbean, and Cuban. Around 3:00 A.M., I was called to see a 32-year-old man of Caribbean birth named Mr. Smith. Mr. Smith's accompanying papers vaguely listed "urinary problems" as his chief complaint.

When I came into the cubicle where he was sitting, Mr. Smith looked up and said, "Doctor, I've been cursed." When I looked confused, he explained further.

"There's a Santeria woman on my block and this man I know paid her to curse me. She has got a St. John the Conqueror root and she cursed me with it. Yesterday this curse made me fall down and today this woman has filled my body with red worms," he said.

"Yes. And how do you know this?" I said, trying not to sound critical.

"I know it because I *see* the worms!" he said, as if I was a dunce. "They come out in my piss. I know that's not right. When I saw them swimming out, I came right to the hospital."

I agreed with Mr. Smith that his condition certainly did not seem to be right and handed him a cup to provide a urine sample. Then I excused myself to look up more information about the patient. I could find no previous medical or psychiatric records and there was no indication that he had ever come into our Emergency Room before. His complete blood count, electrolytes, creatinine, and blood urea nitrogen were all normal.

Suddenly I heard a shout from his cubicle and I ran in to see Mr. Smith looking hysterical. He held his urine cup at arm's length as if it contained the plague. I could see that it was partially full of a clear fluid.

"Look!" he screamed, "I just peed out a worm!"

I peered over Mr. Smith's shoulder to stare down into the cup. To my horror, I saw a thin, bright red object the size of a short piece of spaghetti that was swishing around in the sample cup. It certainly looked to me like a thin, red worm swimming around in the fluid.

In his Diagnostic Examination, Mr. Smith said that his appetite, sleep, and activity were normal. He denied physical symptoms of restlessness, edginess, muscle tension, pounding or racing heart, shortness of breath, choking, chest pain, stomachache, nausea, excessive sweating, chills, hot flushes, trembling, shaking, tingling, fatigue, dizziness, lightheadedness, a sense of detachment, poor concentration, or his mind going blank. Mr. Smith denied experiencing recent elation, sadness, hopelessness, anxiety, irritability, or anger. He denied thoughts of suicide and violence and he said that he had no fears of losing control, dying, or going crazy. He denied delusions or hallucinations in any sensory modality. Mr. Smith's Cognitive Examination was normal for all tests of *attention, language, memory, abstract thinking,* and *sequential thinking.*

CHALLENGE

It would take lots of luck for you to figure out the nature of Mr. Smith's medical problem, although you are welcome to try. Your job is to develop a psychological approach to the patient that will help him cope with his frightening magical experience and still allow him to accept help from mainstream medicine.

SOLUTION

Mr. Smith suffers from **hematuria** (ICD-10 R31), probably resulting from physical trauma from his recent fall.

When I looked at the thin, red worm under a microscope, I clearly saw a line of red blood cells in a gelatin-like matrix that held them in a worm-like shape. Mr. Smith, it seemed, had blood in his urine (hematuria) and the resultant blood cells had conformed to the dimensions of the urethra until they were dislodged.

Other Diagnostic Considerations

"Culture-bound" refers to syndromes where cultural understanding intersects with medical pathology. Dissociation and violence characterize such syndromes as amok, ataque de nervios, boufee delirante, and zar. Spells, root work, mal puesto, and voodoo include hexing and charms that may have magical, spiritual, and religious overtones. African slaves brought Santeria, the Cuban equivalent of Haitian voodoo, to the Americas, where it was influenced by Catholicism. Mr. Smith's belief in Santeria, which may seem strange to most clinicians, was normal within his culture and did not represent any illness that needed treatment.

Mr. Smith was anxious but he did not have an anxiety disorder. For example, he denied symptoms of Panic Disorder, including pounding or racing heart, excessive sweating, trembling, shaking, chills, hot flushes, shortness of breath, choking, chest pain, nausea, stomachache, dizziness, lightheadedness, tingling, a sense of detachment, or fears of losing control, dying, or going crazy.

He also denied symptoms of Generalized Anxiety Disorder, including sleep problems, restlessness, edginess, muscle tension, fatigue, poor concentration, his mind going blank, or irritability. There was no evidence of at least six months of uncontrollable worried thoughts about activities such as work or school performance.

Although Mr. Smith's initial presentation suggested hallucinations and paranoid delusions, his examination showed no evidence of psychosis.

CLINICAL NOTES

Hematuria with blood cells in the urine is usually due to damage to the bladder, ureters, or urethra, which can often be seen after a bad fall or a motor vehicle accident. Microscopic blood in the urine (microhematuria) can be detected by laboratory analysis of the urine. The most common causes of microhematuria in individuals younger than 40 years of age are kidney stones and urinary tract infections. Strenuous exercise can result in urinary bleeding—over 20% of marathon runners exhibit hematuria. Other causes of acute hematuria include the use of aspirin, antibiotics, blood thinners, and phenytoin (Dilantin), as well as diabetes, hypertension and cancer.

For me, hematuria was a satisfying explanation of my patient's problem, but I began to think that it would be of little help for Mr. Smith. Without knowledge of the nature of blood cells and the urinary system, my cross-cultural explanation could very well sound like mumbo-jumbo.

There is no single correct solution for reassuring Mr. Smith and making the clinician's viewpoint meaningful in the context of his culture. After a bit of thought, I decided to start from the truth. I did not believe in the power of voodoo to cause physical trauma but I did believe that modern health care could provide a healing force for both mind and body. With this mindset, I went back to Mr. Smith.

First, I tried to give Mr. Smith a brief but clear explanation of his pathology. I explained that he had blood in his urine, probably from his recent fall, and his blood cells had stuck together. I told him that I had looked at the object very carefully in the microscope and I was positive that it was just a bunch of blood and not a worm or any other creature. I offered to let him see the object in our microscope, but he declined.

"But what about the Santeria?" he shot back. "I know that she's cursing me and you can't do anything about that."

I told Mr. Smith that I believed that modern health care *could* fight against magic. I told him that I did not exactly know how this occurred and that it might not be completely effective against curses. However, I told him that I was positive that I had seen modern health care work against magic before and I asked him if he had ever seen or heard of this.

After a moment, Mr. Smith scratched his head and admitted that, in fact, he had seen two circumstances where medicine seemed to make curses better. He agreed with me that health care could help against Santeria although it might not be able to eliminate all of the curse's power. That was good enough for me.

As Mr. Smith prepared to leave, I made an appointment for him in the genitourinary clinic the next day. Before he walked out, I encouraged him to return if he had any further problems and expressed my expectation that he would soon be feeling better.

CASE 5
JANE AND THE NIGHT VISITORS

One cold winter morning at 4:00 A.M., a friend named Tom and his girlfriend Jane came to the rural Emergency Room where I was working. Jane dispensed with pleasantries and spoke out first.

"Tom and I had a horrible experience last night and I just have to tell someone about it," she announced.

"Is this really an emergency?" I began, tiredly. "Perhaps you would feel better discussing your experience later, in the daytime."

"That's OK," Jane brushed aside my objections. "Tom said you would want to hear this story because you are his friend."

Last night we were studying at my house. I live in a little house on the outskirts of town, out in the middle of nowhere. Sometimes it gets a little scary when I'm there on my own because, you know, anything could happen. Anyway, about 1:00 A.M., we heard sounds outside the front door. It seemed like the shuffling of army boots or maybe security dogs. When Tom and I tried to look under the door, we saw shadows moving and I heard some sounds that could have been voices.

"At first we did not think much of it, but the sounds kept on and on for almost half an hour and we became more and more scared," Jane bowled on with her story. Tom wanted to open the door, but I wanted to get a better idea of who they were, first. So I kept pressing my ear to the door until I could make out what they were saying."

"What were they saying, Jane?" I asked.

"I have remarkable hearing," Jane continued, "and when I put my ear to the door, I could hear my name and Tom's name and something that sounded like 'killer' or 'kill her.' I know I heard the word 'kill' several times.

"When I told that to Tom, we both got really scared. Tom wanted to go out and confront them, but at that point I was too afraid. We decided that we would shout at them through the door and tell them to go away. I shouted as loud as I could, 'You'd better go away because I have a gun!' After that, the sounds went away. Tom couldn't see anything when he looked under the door. Even though I told him not to, Tom finally opened the door and the men had gone, although I thought I could see some scratches on the ground outside the door."

I turned my attention toward my friend. "So what do *you* think of all this, Tom?"

"Well, Jane is right," Tom replied. "It sounds like we were both loaded but we were sober and there were definitely sounds. I didn't see why Jane was so worried until she told me about the Navy. Then I was really scared."

"What was it about the Navy?" I queried.

"Well, Jane was in the Navy years before she started graduate school. She had many jobs carrying papers back and forth between high-ranking officers. Later on, she found out that some of these papers contained top security information. She's sure that the Navy officers had her carry the secret papers because they thought she wouldn't look suspicious, but she said there was a real danger that agents from other countries might kidnap her and torture her to tell them what was in the papers if they ever found her."

"That does sound scary," was all I could think to say.

Jane assured me that she and Tom had no need of a formal Diagnostic Examination or Cognitive Examination. She said, "I've never had any problems with my mind. And I'm sure Tom hasn't. The problem is the people who were threatening us!"

Nevertheless, I realized that at least Tom must have considered the possibility of mental illness or they would not have been seeing a psychiatrist at four o'clock in the morning.

CHALLENGE

Jane told quite a story. It was clear to me that both she and her boyfriend believed in the reality of their experience. The possibility that miscreants from her prior career might be involved was even more disturbing to them.

See if you can come up with an explanation of their experience that makes good psychological sense. Then decide what treatment, if any, you would render.

SOLUTION

Jane suffers from **Delusional Disorder** (DSM-5 297.1, ICD-10 F22.0) and Tom has **Induced Delusional Disorder (Other Specified Schizophrenia Spectrum and Other Psychotic Disorder, Delusional Symptoms in the Partner of an Individual with Delusional Disorder)** (DSM-5 298.8, ICD-10 F24).

Jane met the criteria for **Delusional Disorder:**

A. **Delusions have been present for at least one month.** Jane believed that she was in danger from enemy agents who wanted to kidnap and torture her for top-secret information she had handled "years before she started graduate school."
B. **Schizophrenia Criterion A has never been met.** Jane showed no evidence of hallucinations, disorganized speech, grossly disorganized or catatonic behavior, and I knew of no such history.
C. **Apart from the impact of the delusion, functioning is not impaired and behavior is not odd or bizarre.** Jane was doing well in graduate school and in her relationship with Tom. She did not appear odd or bizarre.

Tom had **Induced Delusional Disorder**:

An established delusion in one individual is induced in another who shares close emotional ties. (*Established delusion*): After exposure to Jane's beliefs, Tom also became convinced that Jane was in danger from enemy agents and that there was a threatening presence at the door. (*Close emotional ties*): Tom and Jane were boyfriend and girlfriend.

Note that the second individual may not meet full criteria for delusional disorder, and his or her delusion may disappear when the individuals separate.

Other Diagnostic Considerations

There are many other causes of delusions and hallucinations. Persecutory delusions and paranoid hallucinations are commonly seen in Schizophrenia, Bipolar Disorder, psychotic unipolar Major Depressive Disorder, Substance-Use Disorders, brain diseases, and central nervous system toxicity. Some delusions in Obsessive-Compulsive Disorder are persecutory in nature—although the patient usually knows that his thoughts are unreasonable, he still acts as if they are real. I have also seen persecutory delusions in patients suffering from Borderline, Paranoid, Histrionic, Schizoid, and Schizotypal Personality Disorders, as well as in individuals with Intellectual Disability, especially during times of stress (see *Mental Status Examination for Personality Disorders*, Chapter 8). I had no evidence that Tom suffered from any of these disorders, but I did not know about Jane.

CLINICAL NOTES

Also called *Folie á Deux,* Induced Psychotic Disorder has been called "a mental illness shared by two people," and "a single psychotic event shared by another." In Induced Psychotic Disorder, one person develops a new delusion in the context of a close relationship with another person who already has the delusion established. *Folie á Deux* is one of many disorders that figure prominently in textbooks and reference volumes but appear to be rare in clinical practice.

At the time of their evaluation, neither Tom nor Jane was experiencing any hallucinations or immediate feelings of danger. I counseled my friend Tom not to worry about fears that materialize in secluded, scary environments. Jane had harbored this persecutory belief for a long time, and I suggested that she consult a professional in the community to handle her "stress." Two months after this episode, Jane had her first psychotic break. While in the hospital, she was given a diagnosis of Schizoaffective Disorder, Bipolar Type (DSM-5 295.70, ICD-10 F25.0). The incident at her door was probably a prodromal warning sign anticipating her break. Six months later, after schizophrenic medications had failed to control her symptoms, she had a severe, disruptive Manic Episode and her diagnosis was changed to Bipolar I Disorder, Most Recent Episode Manic (DSM-5 296.4, ICD-10 F31.12). She cleared with anticonvulsant medications.

Clinicians often hesitate to make a diagnosis in an effort to give their patients the benefit of the doubt. I have frequently heard, "Well, it *could* be true, I guess," in reference to delusional stories. However, giving your patient the benefit of the doubt will not help her get better. In this case, common sense is helpful. The notion that "enemy agents" are after a young graduate student sounds more like a movie plot than real life. The concept is overly dramatic and its interpersonal tone is narcissistic and grandiose, making Jane seem like a very special person, indeed. It seems unlikely that high-ranking officials in the Navy would put secure documents in the hands of a woman who would pose a security risk. Moreover, I have worked with many individuals who had high security clearances and dealt with secure documents but none has expressed the fear that they would be kidnapped and tortured by agents from other countries.

Months later, I talked to Tom alone about the incident. I explained to him how vague sensory impressions can be mistaken for meaningful events under the right circumstances. He said that, although he had originally believed in the reality of his experience, over time he had come to doubt his judgment. He now no longer believed that he had heard miscreants threatening murder outside his ex-girlfriend's door. However, he told me that he was still convinced of the truth of Jane's story about carrying top-secret Navy information and he believed it possible that Jane might someday be in danger.

CASE 6
SAM AND DAVE MAKE A PACT

Purposeful deaths of two or more people together, usually called suicide pacts or double suicides, are not mental health disorders. Nevertheless, suicide pacts cause concern and make headlines when they do occur. It is often difficult to reconstruct the underlying story after the event, so good clinical detective work is necessary wherever a suicide pact is suspected. This is a story of such a case where the participants were identified and treated before any mortality resulted.

Sam and Dave presented to the Emergency Room at 4:00 A.M. with suicidal ideation. The emergency nurse suspected substance use and urine was collected for a toxicology screen. Then both men were directed to my office. I looked at them over my desk and inquired, "So, why are we here together this morning?"

Sam replied for both of them. "You see, doctor, Dave and I are partners—he's all I've got—and we made a suicide pact a month ago. We were both living on my disability, we didn't have jobs, and my place was a dump. We were hopeless and really depressed. So, we decided we would make an antidepression plan. We put all our eggs in one basket and decided that we'd do everything we could to make our life bearable for a month. Then, if we still felt bad at the end of the month, we would both kill ourselves. Life is just too short to be unhappy, right? Well, tomorrow is our last day. But we are both really depressed and we were worried that we would jump the gun and do it too soon. We spent all our money and we don't have any friends or family, so we came in here."

I was curious to hear Dave's story. "How about you, Dave? Is that about the way you see things?"

"Uh. Yeah," was Dave's soft reply. "It's like Sam says." I asked Sam to leave so that I could speak to him alone in the hall. Dave initially objected, pulling closer to Sam, but Sam just stood up and walked out of the room and I followed.

Sam and I sat down in the hall to talk quietly. In his Diagnostic Examination, I found that Sam was a gaunt 60-year-old man who had worked in the distant past in retail stores and now subsisted on disability income. Sam's face was florid and he wore brightly colored, flamboyant clothes. Sam's pupils were dilated and he appeared agitated. Sam said he did not sleep much and did not eat much. He endorsed problems with pounding heart, excessive perspiration, nausea, poor attention, impulsivity, and hyperactivity. Sam said he felt like he was "on top of the world!" and he endorsed emotions of anxiety and irritability. His mood was expansive and his manner was very sociable. He denied the presence of hallucinations in any modality but he said that he might have had experienced something like them before.

On his Cognitive Examination of *attention*, Sam was distractible and he failed a Vigilance test where he had to hold up a finger whenever the numeral "5" was read to him.

In *language* tests, Sam's Quality of Speech was poor—his speech was loud and rapid and it was difficult to inject a word into his monologue. Sam was hoarse (dysarthric) and he slurred his words. His other *language* tests were normal.

In tests of *memory*, Sam failed Digit Span, Uncued Delayed Memory, and Cued Delayed Memory for six words after one minute.

In tests of *abstract thinking*, Sam could do Simple Arithmetic but his Proverb Interpretations were irrelevant. For example, in response to, "There's no use crying over spilt milk," Sam said, "Life is too short to be crying. The hell with the bastards!" In response to "Rome wasn't built in a day," Sam said, "The hell with the Romans! They're just a bunch of generals who want to push people around." Sam was similarly deficient in Set Analysis.

In tests of *sequential thinking*, Sam accurately followed a Four-Step Sequential Command and he did well on Serial Sevens subtraction. However, after failing the Arithmetic Story Problem he refused further testing.

When I walked back into my office, 18-year-old Dave was sitting silently and his thin body was hunched down in his chair. A baseball cap was pulled down over his eyes and he seemed lost in the folds of a gray sweatshirt that was much too big for him. He wore no socks and the large holes in his tennis shoes revealed his toes beneath.

"Are you depressed, Dave?" I asked.

"I guess I am if Sam said so. Do you have anything to eat?" he added. "I'm really hungry. Sam says that soon we'll go to Mexico. He says Mexico is warm all the time and food is really cheap." Dave declined further participation in his Diagnostic Examination.

On his Cognitive Examination of *attention*, Dave's Orientation and Basic Verbal Comprehension were good but he could not understand the instructions for the Vigilance test. In the *language* section, Dave's production of speech was minimal and his voice was just a whisper. He did adequately on the Verbal Registration and Immediate Repetition test but he became confused on a task of Object and Part Naming.

In *memory* testing, Dave could remember only three of seven digits on the Digit Span test. He could not name Four Presidents nor could he understand the instructions on the Category Recall and Free Recall from a Story tests. After one minute, Dave could not even remember that I had given him any words to recall on the test of Cued Delayed Memory. Subsequently, Dave said he was too fatigued to continue testing.

At that moment, a technician arrived with two charts and the drug screens, which showed alcohol and cocaine in Sam's urine, apparently the consequences of his "antidepression plan."

CHALLENGE

Your challenge in this case is to envision a scenario that fits all the available information and makes sense. See if you can develop a diagnostic solution for each party that explains all you have heard. You will find that neurophysiological, psychological, and social factors all play a role.

SOLUTION: SAM

Sam is experiencing **Alcohol Intoxication** (DSM-5 303.00, ICD-10 F10.929) and **Cocaine Intoxication** (DSM-5 292.89, ICD-10 F14.929).

Sam met the following diagnostic criteria for **Alcohol Intoxication**:
A. **Recent use of alcohol**. Sam's blood test showed that he had recently consumed alcohol.
B. **Clinically significant maladaptive behavioral or psychological changes (such as inappropriate sexual or aggressive behavior, mood lability, or impaired judgment, that developed during, or shortly after, alcohol ingestion**. (*Mood lability*): After drinking, Sam said that he was "really depressed." Then he said he felt "on top of the world." (*Impaired judgment*): Sam said he was worried that he "would jump the gun" and kill himself.
C. **One or more of the following signs developed during or shortly after alcohol use**:
   1. **Slurred speech**. Sam "slurred his words" on his Cognitive Examination.
   2. **Incoordination**.
   3. **Unsteady gait**.
   4. **Nystagmus** (repetitive vertical or horizontal movements of the eyes.)
   5. **Impairment in attention or memory**. Sam earned abnormal scores on *attention* measures of Level of Consciousness and Vigilance and on *memory* tests of Digit Span, Uncued Delayed Memory, and Cued Delayed Memory.
   6. **Stupor or coma**.

Sam also exhibited the following symptoms of **Cocaine Intoxication**:
A. **Recent use of cocaine**. Sam's blood test showed that he had recently used cocaine.
B. **Clinically significant maladaptive behavioral or psychological changes (such as euphoria or affective blunting; changes in sociability; hypervigilance; interpersonal sensitivity; anxiety, tension or anger; stereotyped behaviors; impaired judgment; or impaired school, work, home, or social function) that developed during, or shortly after, use of cocaine**. (*Euphoria*): Sam said he felt like he was "on top of the world!" (*Anxiety, tension, or anger*): Sam endorsed emotions of anxiety and anger. (*Impaired judgment*): Sam said he was worried that he "would jump the gun" and kill himself. (*Impaired function*): Sam could not have attended school, gone to work, or handled family or social responsibilities in his intoxicated mental state.
C. **At least two of the following developed during or shortly after alcohol use**:
   1. **Tachycardia or bradycardia** (too rapid or too slow heartbeat.)
   2. **Pupillary dilation**. "Sam's pupils were dilated."
   3. **Elevated or lowered blood pressure**. Sam's face was "florid" but Vital Signs were not taken.
   4. **Perspiration or chills**. Sam endorsed problems with "excessive perspiration."
   5. **Nausea or vomiting**. Sam complained of "nausea."
   6. **Evidence of weight loss**. Sam was "gaunt."
   7. **Psychomotor agitation or retardation**. Sam appeared "agitated."
   8. **Muscular weakness, respiratory depression, chest pain, or cardiac arrhythmias**.

9. **Confusion, seizures, dyskinesias (abnormal movements), dystonias (abnormal muscle contractions), or coma**.

Other Diagnostic Considerations

There was no evidence that Sam's alcohol or cocaine use caused the recurrent failure to meet obligations, physical danger, legal difficulties, tolerance, or withdrawal required for a diagnosis of Substance Use Disorder.

Sam exhibited symptoms of a bipolar Manic Episode, such as irritability, expansive mood, and elevated mood, plus insomnia, pressured speech, rapid speech, distractibility, and impulsive use of stimulants with alcohol. However, Bipolar Disorder could not be diagnosed while he was intoxicated. In fact, his past clinic notes characterized him as "overly dramatic" but there was no mention of Bipolar Disorder. His disability income was not based on psychiatric problems but rather from a back injury that he had sustained in an accident on a loading dock.

Some clinicians might have considered the diagnosis of Major Depressive Disorder because of Sam's suicidality and possible anhedonia. Diagnoses of Panic Disorder or Generalized Anxiety Disorder reference Sam's physical symptoms of activation. Attention-Deficit/Hyperactivity Disorder might be suggested because of Sam's distractibility, impulsivity, and agitation. However, all these symptoms can be caused by substance use. When a patient is intoxicated, further diagnosis should be deferred until the patient is again at baseline.

Cognitive Testing

Sam's *language* skills were intact, but he failed the Vigilance test of *attention*, the Uncued and Cued Delayed tests of *memory*, the Proverb Interpretation and Set Analysis tests of *abstract thinking*, and the Arithmetic Story Problem test of *sequential thinking*. There was no focal pattern to these deficits—they probably just reflected Sam's poor test-taking ability while intoxicated.

SOLUTION: DAVE

Dave has mild **Intellectual Disability** (DSM-5 319, ICD-10 F70):

A. **Intellectual deficits in *memory* and learning, *abstract thinking*, reasoning and planning, confirmed by both clinical assessment and standardized intelligence testing.** In his daily life, Dave seems to have shown poor insight and planning. In his Cognitive Examination, Dave made errors in tests of *attention, language,* and *memory*. When Dave's chart finally arrived, it contained standardized psychological tests performed at age 15 that revealed significant cognitive deficits.

B. **Failure to meet developmental and sociocultural standards for personal independence and social responsibility in one or more activities of daily life, such as communication, social participation, and independent living across school, work, home, and social environments.** (*Independence*): Dave seems to have been dependent on Sam for direction. (*Responsibility*): Being drawn into a suicide pact is not very responsible. (*Communication*): Dave's "production of speech was minimal and his voice was just a whisper." "Sam usually talks for me," Dave said. (*Social participation*): It seemed that Dave spent all his time with Sam and had no other social or interpersonal life. (*Independent living/work*): We have no work history for Dave but he was not working at the time of his evaluation. (*Independent living/home*): Dave lived with Sam but we do not know what responsibilities he shared.

C. **The deficits begin in childhood.** Dave's life appears to have been stable for a while, and he is now 18 years-of-age. His records contained psychological testing performed at age 15.

Other Diagnostic Considerations

Intellectual Disability can mimic many other psychiatric conditions, especially when individuals are fatigued or under stress. However, Dave's symptoms could all be explained by his impaired cognition and socioeconomic condition.

Cognitive Testing

Dave made errors in tests of *attention, language,* and *memory*. Dave's cognitive testing showed more deficits than I would have expected, even from a young boy interviewed at 4:00 A.M. He was exhausted at the time of his evaluation and he should be retested when he is at baseline.

CLINICAL NOTES

I decided to send Sam to a locked unit for the night, to be evaluated again in the morning. When I read the ward doctor's morning chart note, his evaluation mentioned anxiety and shakiness but no symptoms of mania or depression. Sam denied suicidal ideation and said he had decided to live. His liver enzymes were elevated and physical examination showed edema, mild jaundice, and loss of some peripheral light touch sensation, consistent with alcohol use. Sam was sent from his ward to a program to be detoxified from alcohol.

When I interviewed Dave further, he revealed that he had been 16 years of age, homeless, and living on the street when he was first picked up by Sam. Sam brought Dave to his house, fed and cared for him, and generally assumed the joint roles of a father figure and a boyfriend.

I soon realized that Dave had no idea what a suicide pact was or that Sam had planned a mutual suicide. He considered himself lucky, because after he joined up with Sam, he had more to eat and he was warm inside Sam's house. When asked about the alcohol and cocaine, Dave was at a loss. "I just eat and drink what Sam gives me," he said.

I chose to let Dave sleep the remaining few hours of the night in the Emergency Room. In the morning, I walked him over to the Social Services Department and explained his situation to a case manager.

In the end, the suicide pact had existed only in Sam's mind. I shudder to think what would have happened if he had actually carried out his plans. Now, whenever I hear about a suicide pact, I am especially watchful for pairs with one strong, active member and another very passive one.

CASE 7
ROGER GOES THROUGH THE ROOF

I arrived to work at a large Eastern medical center for my late night shift. As I walked through the door, I noticed that the emergency psych nurse was wearing a grim expression. When I approached, she just shook her head and led me by the arm into the Emergency Room. I soon noticed a muffled screaming and a sound like the sky was falling. This commotion seemed to move around until I heard it coming in my direction. In the corner of the room, the ceiling began to quiver and bounce, accompanied by unintelligible epithets from above. This disturbance continued across the ceiling and exited at the opposite corner of the room. It felt like a moose was in the attic.

The nurse explained, "A 21-year-old black man named Roger came in tonight with an elevated heart rate of 115 beats per minute (normal=60-100 bpm), a high blood pressure of 155/85 millimeters of mercury (normal<120/80 mm Hg), and muscle rigidity. He looked intoxicated—his speech was hoarse and slurred and he was weaving around like he was drunk. Also, his eyes looked weird, shifting back and forth real fast.

"This man was really tall and skinny," she continued. "He looked like a basketball player. And he was fast. Roger seemed agitated, so we put him in an observation room and managed to give him an intramuscular injection of the benzodiazepine lorazepam (Ativan), but it was ineffective. Ten minutes later, Roger became belligerent and potentially assaultive, so we gave him another intramuscular injection of benzodiazepine together with an intramuscular injection of the atypical antipsychotic risperidone (Risperdal) but that didn't quiet him down, either. After that, Roger became so agitated that he broke away from us and started running through the Emergency Room. We called Security but when Roger saw them coming, he jumped straight up into the air until his head and shoulders went through the suspended ceiling. He pulled himself up into the space between the suspended ceiling and the top of the room, and he has been crawling around up there ever since, screaming his head off. There was blood on the tiles where he cut himself on the sharp ceiling wires but that didn't seem to bother him. When we get him down it'll be your turn. What do you think we should do?"

Roger was not available to do a Diagnostic Examination or Cognitive Examination.

CHALLENGE

Put yourself into the unenviable position of the Emergency Room clinician. Try to determine Roger's diagnosis, noting which previous treatments did not work, and then devise a treatment strategy that will quiet the patient.

SOLUTION

Roger is experiencing **Phencyclidine (PCP) Intoxication** (DSM-5 292.89, ICD-10 F16.929):
A. **Recent use of phencyclidine**. Roger's urine toxicology screen came back positive for phencyclidine.
B. **Clinically significant maladaptive behavioral changes (such as belligerence, assaultiveness, impulsiveness, unpredictability, psychomotor agitation, impaired judgment, or impaired social or occupational functioning) that developed during or shortly after phencyclidine use**. (*Belligerence/assaultiveness*): The nurse noted that Roger "became belligerent and potentially assaultive" after his first benzodiazepine injection. (*Impulsiveness/unpredictability*): Roger's choice to jump into the ceiling shows both impulsiveness and unpredictability. (*Psychomotor agitation*): Initially, "Roger seemed agitated," and then he "became so agitated that he broke away from us and started running through the Emergency Room." (*Impaired functioning*): Roger could not have attended school, gone to work, or handled family or social responsibilities in his intoxicated mental state.
C. **Within an hour, two or more of the following signs**:
   1. **Vertical or horizontal nystagmus** (repeated rhythmic eye movements). The nurse noted that Roger's "eyes looked weird, shifting back and forth real fast."
   2. **Hypertension or tachycardia** (high blood pressure or rapid heartbeat). (*Hypertension*): Roger's blood pressure was high at 155/85 mm Hg. (*Tachycardia*): His heart rate was elevated at 115 bpm.
   3. **Numbness or diminished responsiveness to pain**. "He cut himself on the sharp ceiling wires but that didn't seem to bother him."
   4. **Ataxia** (poor coordination). "He was weaving around like he was drunk."
   5. **Dysarthria** (hoarse, slurred, or uncoordinated speech). "His speech was hoarse and slurred."
   6. **Muscle rigidity**. The nurse commented that Roger showed "muscle rigidity."
   7. **Seizures or coma**.
   8. **Hyperacusis** (sensitivity to loud sounds).

Other Diagnostic Considerations

Roger's symptoms match the symptoms of Phencyclidine Intoxication. There was no evidence that Roger's use of phencyclidine had made him unable to meet life obligations or caused the physical danger, legal problems, social problems, interpersonal problems, tolerance, or withdrawal that are required for a diagnosis of Substance Use Disorder. Assessment of other mental conditions must be deferred until acute intoxication has passed.

Use of the popularized mnemonic device RED DANES (**R**age, **E**rythema, **D**ilated pupils, **D**elusions, **A**mnesia, **N**ystagmus, **E**xcitation, and **S**kin dryness) will result in diagnostic errors, because it only describes three of the 9 criteria necessary for the diagnosis of phencyclidine intoxication.

CLINICAL NOTES

Suspect phencyclidine intoxication when patients look intoxicated but are alert, activated, agitated, and violent. Some Emergency Rooms will receive more phencyclidine-intoxicated patients than others, depending on their geographic location.

Roger's treatment proceeded from his diagnosis. The initial phase involved patient management and basic psychotherapeutic principles. When security staff pulled Roger from the ceiling, I had him brought to a holding area that was separated from the general Emergency Room and where light and sound were attenuated (because phencyclidine makes patients sensitive to loud noises). A security guard was posted across the room from Roger so that he did not feel threatened. These measures were taken to reduce Roger's danger to others and to reduce his sensory input and provide an environment of safety, calmness, and control.

In a few minutes, an experienced psych technician entered the room and offered Roger some orange juice and gentle conversation. Then, after Roger had calmed down, I entered the room in the presence of the nurse and security guard. I spoke in a calm voice to Roger and I offered him a choice of an oral or intramuscular dose of the antipsychotic haloperidol (Haldol). Roger agreed to take oral haloperidol and soon this, plus the calming effects of the environment, helped Roger relax. Roger was then led into a dim, quiet observation room where he slept until morning.

The behavioral interventions of separation, containment, decreased sensory input, and gentle social contact were a successful strategy to minimize Roger's agitation so that staff could help him. Frequently, proffering a "peace offering" of juice, gum, or a cigarette helps reduce resistance to working with the staff. Conversely, abrupt handling; exposure to the bright, loud, hectic Emergency Room environment; and aggressive use of intramuscular agents can feed into patients' paranoia. Fortunately, this Emergency Room had well-trained nurses, technicians, and security personnel as well as access to a quiet room to help Roger cool off. Although many clinicians have been trained to use a show of strength to control patients' behavior, Roger's size and physical strength, plus the stimulant effects of phencyclidine, would have made a direct confrontation potentially dangerous for both Roger and the staff.

The pharmacological properties of phencyclidine explain why Roger's initial medications were ineffective. In receptor-binding studies, phencyclidine binds to the glutamate NMDA—MK-801 receptor. However, benzodiazepines reduce phencyclidine symptoms poorly because their sites of action are on the GABA receptors—they do not bind to NMDA (phencyclidine) receptors. Similarly, atypical antipsychotics clozapine (Clozaril), olanzapine (Zyprexa), quetiapine (Seroquel), risperidone (Risperdal), and ziprasidone (Geodon) cannot reverse phencyclidine effects because they do not bind to NMDA (phencyclidine) receptors, either. Fortunately, haloperidol is active at the glutamate NMDA receptor and it can directly turn off phencyclidine action, reducing the symptoms of phencyclidine intoxication. Other medications that bind to the phencyclidine NMDA-MK801 receptors include the atypical antipsychotic aripiprazole (Abilify), the antidepressant venlafaxine (Effexor), and the narcotic analgesic pentazocine (Talwin).

Roger awoke the next morning with little recall of his night's escapades and no apparent symptoms. He was sent home with an admonition to stay away from phencyclidine and other street drugs for the sake of his health and that of others. I later heard that he was a power to be dealt with on the city's basketball courts.

CASE 8
LITTLE JUDI SCREAMS IN TERROR

Jay and Marti came to the Emergency Room with their 8-year-old daughter Judi. They had been married for twelve years and Judi was their first and only child. Both parents appeared fatigued and there were dark circles under their eyes. They left Judi in the waiting room with her grandmother while they discussed their problem with me.

"Doctor, Judi has this awful problem and we don't know what to do," Jay began. "It started a few months ago and we haven't been able to get a good night's rest ever since."

"We always put Judi to bed at 9:00 P.M.," said Marti. "She is really good about her bedtime and she always goes right to sleep in a few minutes. Usually I just sit quietly in her room or stand outside the bedroom door until she falls asleep."

"Marti and I usually go to bed at 11:00 P.M.," Jay continued. "But if it's going to be a bad night, we're suddenly awakened around 12:00 A.M. with this blood-curdling scream from Judi's room. We run into her room expecting the worst but there is nothing in her room except her sitting up in bed screaming."

"Jay's right," Marti confirmed. "We run into Judi's room and she's sitting up in bed looking so frightened. Not just a little frightened but she's shaking with fear. When I hold her, she's panting, her poor little heart is pounding, and her body is wet with fear. Even when she's fully awake, I can't calm her down, no matter what. At first, we thought she was just having nightmares but this is too much for nightmares. There's never been a nightmare that could strike fear into the heart of a child like this."

"At first I thought there was a prowler or someone trying to get in the house," continued Jay. "I put in an alarm system, which we needed anyway, but we never caught anybody. Then I wondered if Judi could be seeing scary things in her room. The most frustrating thing is that Judi has amnesia. She can't tell us what happened—she doesn't even remember waking up screaming, and she claims that everything is OK. Marti and I talked about this just being a bad dream, but she won't tell us what she was dreaming about. She swears that she hasn't been dreaming at all."

Judi's Diagnostic Examination revealed a normal 8-year-old girl with appropriate affect, clear and measured speech, and the ability to answer my questions with ease. There had been no other signs of emotional or behavioral problems other than her nighttime episodes, which she said she did not remember. She and her parents denied any problems with attention, hyperactivity, sadness, anhedonia, elevated mood, or irritability. Overall, Judi's attitude about the affair was light and unconcerned. When I administered an age-appropriate Cognitive Examination, she performed well on tests of *attention, language, memory, abstract thinking,* and *sequential thinking*.

CHALLENGE

What's wrong with Judi? What will you tell the parents about her condition and what treatment will you recommend? Make up your mind and then go on to the Solution to see what happened.

SOLUTION

Judi is experiencing **Sleep Terrors (Non-Rapid Eye Movement Sleep Arousal Disorder, Sleep Terror Type, DSM-5 307.46, ICD-10 F51.4):**

A. **Repeated episodes of incomplete wakening from sleep; usually occurring during the first third of the sleep period.** (*Waking*): Judi's father said, "If it's going to be a bad night, we're suddenly awakened around 12:00 A.M." If Judi usually gets up at 7:00 A.M., 12:00 A.M. is about one third of the way through Judi's sleep cycle.

Abrupt arousal usually beginning with a panicky scream, with intense fear and signs of autonomic arousal, such as tachycardia (rapid heartbeat), rapid breathing, pupillary dilation, and sweating during each episode. The patient is usually unresponsive to attempts to comfort him or her. (*Panicky scream*): The parents were "awakened with this blood-curdling scream from Judi's room." (*Intense fear*): Judi's mother found her daughter "sitting up in bed looking so frightened." (*Autonomic arousal*): Judi's heart was "pounding," she was "panting," and her body was "wet with fear." (*Unresponsive*): Judi's mother could not "calm her down, no matter what."

B. **Little or no dreaming is recalled.** "She swears that she hasn't been dreaming at all."
C. **There is amnesia for the episode**. Jay said, "Judy has amnesia."
D. **The episodes cause clinically significant distress or impairment in school, work, home, social, or other important areas of functioning**. Judi's symptoms were disrupting her home and family situation. Her parent's

were frightened, they did not know what to do, and they had not been able to get a good night's rest for "a few months."

Other Diagnostic Considerations

Sleep Terrors originate in deep, non-dreaming, Stage IV sleep. Children are often confused and disoriented for up to ten minutes, probably reflecting the time it takes to wake from deep sleep. Electroencephalogram (EEG) recordings show increased delta waves before an episode and an alpha pattern during the attack. There is a significant release of adrenaline during the episode that causes rapid heartbeat, panting, tremor, and perspiration, mimicking fear. Purposeless movements of the hands and face (automatisms) may be seen. In DSM-5, Sleep Terrors share a diagnosis with Sleepwalking as Non-Rapid Eye Movement Sleep Arousal Disorders.

Sleep Terrors should be distinguished from Nightmares (DSM-5 307.47, ICD-10 F51.5), which occur during rapid eye movement (REM) sleep stages in the second half of the night. In Nightmares, children usually awake rapidly, become alert and oriented quickly, and show little physical arousal. Unlike Sleep Terrors, children with Nightmares have dreams that they can usually recall immediately after waking.

Sleep-related seizures can also cause confusion and disorientation on waking and they may be associated with both automatisms and dramatic body movements. Unlike Sleep Terrors, seizures are most common in the first two hours of sleep and the last two hours before waking. Seizures are suspect in children with an established history of epilepsy. Otherwise, unless a professional witnesses the episode, it may be necessary to refer children for a sleep electroencephalogram for seizure diagnosis.

CLINICAL NOTES

Sleep Terrors have a prevalence of about 3% in children 4-12 years of age. Males are more frequently affected than females. The illness rarely continues through adolescence. Children with Sleep Terrors usually have a normal Diagnostic Examination and Cognitive Examination. Because Sleep Terrors usually go away on their own, the usual treatment is to reassure the parents. As you have seen, this childhood disorder can have marked emotional effects on parents.

I explained the benign nature of Sleep Terrors to Jay and Marti. Jay had immediate insight into the condition when he remembered that one of his sisters walked in her sleep for a brief period in her early childhood. Marti was still not comfortable about her daughter's health. However, I pointed out to Marti that the episodes did not appear to have any negative effects on her daughter and I invited her to confirm this by continuing to notice her daughter's good state of physical and mental health.

CASE 9
DR. FRANK STUDIES ASIAN MEDICINE

Twenty-seven-year-old Frank Z, Ph.D., walked into my cubicle in the Emergency Room, exclaiming, "Doctor, I can't take this any more!"

"Six days ago I was feeling on top of the world," began Frank breathlessly, "but over the last five days, my heart has been racing and pounding in my chest and I am perspiring all the time, even in a cold room. My hands are shaking uncontrollably and I can't get my breath. My chest hurts from my heart pounding. I'm so sick to my stomach, I can't eat, and I feel so dizzy that I think I'm going to faint. My body feels really weak and I haven't been able to sleep for three days.

"Do you think I'm going to die, Doctor?" Frank whined plaintively. "I've started asking everybody I know what could be wrong. I've called up my regular doctor a hundred times and finally he told me to go to the Emergency Room and ask to see a psychiatrist. No one wants to talk to me anymore—that hurts my feelings. And I'm really anxious! This whole situation pisses me off no end!"

"Does anything make your condition better or worse?" I asked, when Frank stopped for air.

"Nothing makes me feel any better," Frank hurried on, "but some things make me feel even worse. Like if I drink just a little coffee or even cola, my heart starts racing harder and I get more agitated. Even eating chocolate makes me feel worse.

"I work as a medical research scientist but I have not been able to go to the university to do my work. I am taking courses in Oriental Medicine at a local Asian college, but I can't go to school like this!"

Throughout his evaluation, I noticed Frank blinking his eyes compulsively. He looked around the room as if he expected something dangerous and he could only stay seated for a few seconds before rising and pacing the floor.

Frank's pulse was elevated between 100-120 beats per minute (normal=60-100 bpm) and his blood pressure was elevated at 140/95 millimeters of mercury (normal<120/80 mm Hg).

On his Cognitive Examination, Frank's *attention* was intact.

His Quality of Speech was loud, rapid, and pressured but he did well on all *language* tests.

In the *memory* section, Frank made errors on the Digit Span test. He could remember the most recent Four Presidents but he failed tests of Free Recall from a Story and Uncued and Cued Delayed Memory.

In *abstract thinking* tests, Frank failed a test of Judgment.

In *sequential thinking* assessment, Frank omitted the last step in a Four-Step Sequential Command and he failed a test of Serial Sevens subtraction.

Frank denied taking any medications other than aspirin. He said that he had stopped all drinking and smoking a year ago after becoming interested in Asian Medicine. Frank denied abusing drugs. He was taking multivitamins, ginseng extract, and a chelated mineral supplement "to improve my health."

CHALLENGE

Frank's symptoms overlap the spectrum of anxiety disorders and mood disorders. Use your best diagnostic logic to find the best diagnosis and eliminate the wrong ones, then decide how you would treat Frank.

SOLUTION

Frank suffers from ***Panax ginseng*** **Intoxication** (DSM-5 292.89, ICD-10 F15.929).

Frank met the following criteria for **Stimulant Intoxication**:
A. **Recent use of a stimulant**. (Frank said he was taking ginseng extract.)
B. **Clinically significant maladaptive behavioral or psychological changes (such as euphoria or affective blunting; changes in sociability; hypervigilance (an enhanced sense of danger in the immediate environment); interpersonal sensitivity; anxiety, tension (arousal or uneasiness that motivates action or anger); stereotyped behaviors such as tics or dyskinesias; impaired judgment; or impaired school, work, home, or social function that developed during, or shortly after, use of amphetamine or a related substance**. (*Sociability*): Frank indicated that his interpersonal contacts became more frequent and more intense, saying, "I've started asking everybody I know what could be wrong," and "I've called up my regular doctor a hundred times." (*Hypervigilance*): Frank "looked around the room as if he expected something dangerous." (*Interpersonal sensitivity*): Frank complained of hurt feelings, saying, "They don't want to talk to me any more—that hurts my

feelings." (*Anxiety*): Frank said, "I'm really anxious!" (*Tension*): Frank was so distraught that he began to seek help from friends and professionals. (*Anger*): Frank said, "This whole situation pisses me off no end." (*Stereotyped behavior*): I noticed Frank blinking his eyes compulsively. (*Impaired judgment*): Frank "failed a test of Judgment" on his Cognitive Examination. More importantly, Frank worked as a medical research scientist and was studying Asian medicine, yet he could not figure out that he needed to reduce or stop his dose of ginseng. (*Impaired function*): Frank could not go to work or attend school in his intoxicated mental state.

C. **Two (or more) of the following, developing during, or shortly after, use of amphetamine or a related substance**:
1. **Tachycardia or bradycardia** (heartbeat that is too rapid or too slow). "Frank's pulse was elevated between 100-120 beats per minute (normal=60-100 bpm)."
2. **Pupillary dilation**.
3. **Elevated or lowered blood pressure**. Frank's "blood pressure was elevated at 140/95 millimeters of mercury (normal<120/80 mm Hg)."
4. **Perspiration or chills**. Frank said, "I am perspiring all the time, even in a cold room."
5. **Nausea or vomiting**. Frank told me, "I'm so sick to my stomach, I can't eat."
6. **Evidence of weight loss**.
7. **Psychomotor agitation or retardation**. Frank "could only stay seated for a few seconds before rising and pacing." His hands were "shaking."
8. **Muscular weakness, respiratory depression, chest pain, or cardiac arrhythmias**. (*Muscular weakness*): "My body feels really weak." (*Respiratory depression*): "I can't get my breath." (*Chest pain*): "My chest hurts from my heart pounding."
9. **Confusion, seizures, dyskinesias (abnormal movements), dystonias (abnormal muscle contractions), or coma**.

Other Diagnostic Considerations

There was no evidence that Frank's ginseng use caused the recurrent unmet obligations, physical danger, legal difficulties, tolerance, withdrawal, or other problems during a 12-month period that are required for a diagnosis of Substance Use Disorder.

Frank's experience resembled a Manic Episode, with brief euphoria, irritability, insomnia, talkativeness, pressured speech, distractibility, and an increase in goal-directed activity. However, Frank did not exhibit a week-long episode of euphoria, expansiveness, or irritability and his symptoms were better explained by his substance use.

Frank exhibited many of the symptoms of a Panic Attack, including heart palpitations, rapid heart rate, sweating, tremor, shortness of breath, chest pain, nausea, dizziness, and fear of dying. However, these arousal symptoms were present continuously over the prior five days—they did not reach a peak within minutes as in a Panic Attack. Moreover, Panic Disorder cannot be diagnosed if the symptoms are due to the use of a substance.

There was no need to consider the diagnosis of Anxiety Disorder Due to *Panax ginseng* Intoxication, because anxiety is included in the criteria for stimulant intoxication.

If there is any doubt about other diagnoses, Frank should be reevaluated when he has reached baseline.

Cognitive Testing

Frank's Cognitive Examination was notable for distractibility. His rapid and pressured speech is evidence of racing thoughts, which tend to overload conscious working memory. The Digit Span test, Free Recall from a Story, Uncued Delayed Memory, Cued Delayed Memory, Four-Step Sequential Command, and Serial Sevens are all vulnerable to distractibility because they rely on keeping several stimuli in conscious working memory at once. Stimulant intoxication is associated with distractibility.

CLINICAL NOTES

Frank's problem was initially misdiagnosed. Frank later told me that he had seen another clinician a few hours before he came to see me in the Emergency Room. This doctor gave Frank the diagnosis of Bipolar I Disorder, Most Recent Episode Manic, and had attempted to hospitalize him under that diagnosis. However, Frank did not accept that diagnosis and sought a second opinion from me.

Panax ginseng and other types of ginseng have strong stimulant effects that are additive with the effects of caffeine and other stimulants. Ginseng seldom causes problems at regular doses like 100 mg daily, but nutritional advisors and the popular press often recommend the use of larger doses. Common side effects are adrenaline-like in nature, including insomnia, tachycardia, and palpitations. However, high-dose ginseng has been known to trigger Manic Episodes in individuals with underlying Bipolar Disorder.

The advertised benefits of *Panax ginseng* are many, including improved stress tolerance, better cognitive function, enhanced athletic abilities, and better sexual performance. Taken together with other stimulants, ginseng can cause life-threatening heart arrhythmias. *Panax ginseng* inhibits liver enzymes (CYPD-2D6) and it can elevate serum levels of antidepressants and antipsychotics. *Panax ginseng* can reduce platelet aggregation and cause excess bleeding in patients taking "blood-thinners" such as warfarin (Coumadin). Because ginseng is not a prescription medication, there was no legal requirement that Frank be informed of any of the dangers of taking it.

I gave Frank a mild sedative and sent him home to rest and sleep. He was advised to stop taking ginseng and to refrain from consuming caffeine, tea, cola, or chocolate for the next three weeks. Frank was referred to his primary care physician for a cardiac checkup and EKG at the doctor's discretion. Within one week, Frank's condition was mostly a memory.

Currently there is no system in place to ensure that the individuals who buy health supplements are given enough information to make an informed choice about their use. It is left to clinicians to sort out the consequences of unexpected effects and drug interactions.

CASE 10
JOHNNIE WANTS TO KILL HIS FRIENDS

I was called to see 13-year-old Johnnie Columbine in the pediatric Emergency Room of a large hospital. His mother began the interview.

"This morning, Johnnie took a knife from our kitchen drawer and told me that he was hearing voices telling him to go to school and kill all his classmates. He also threatened to kill himself. When I tried to intervene, Johnnie cut me so deep that I had to go to the doctor." She showed me a bandage on her left arm.

Johnnie's father continued. "Before last week, Johnnie was just an angry boy. Sometimes he would clear up for a couple of months, then he was back to being sullen all the time. We couldn't get him interested in school or any other activities. Usually I could get him out of his funk with a joke, but after an hour he would be as sullen as ever.

"At home, Johnnie argued constantly with me, his mother, and his sister. He was always hard to get along with because he would never admit when he was wrong and he would never stop talking. You see, Johnnie overate when stressed, and he became quite overweight, but he couldn't stand to be teased about it. Unfortunately, his feelings were easily hurt—then he would pick fights at school and get in trouble."

"We never used to have any problem getting Johnnie to bed," Johnnie's mother noted, "but it was always hard to get him up in the morning. He usually slept most of the day on weekends, too. Despite all this sleep, Johnnie seemed to be tired all the time—he spent most of his time on the couch and seemed almost paralyzed. We thought that tiredness might be why Johnnie had problems concentrating in classes. He would simply get distracted and zone out for 10-20 minutes at a time. Johnnie was always a procrastinator and handed in assignments late, but sometimes he worked around the clock on a project that interested him. We couldn't calm him down. One day he was caught shoplifting candy from a neighborhood store and that was the last straw.

"We were sick of his bad behavior," said Johnnie's mother. "So a month ago, I took him to see another therapist. This one said Johnnie was depressed—that had never occurred to us before because we never saw him being sad. The therapist called a psychiatrist she worked with to get him medications, but we thought that this specialist was outrageously expensive. We called our family physician and he was nice enough to phone in a prescription for an antidepressant without charging us anything. Unfortunately, it made Johnnie worse and we discontinued it after about a week. That was two weeks ago.

"This last week was the worst ever. Johnnie flew into rages, had tantrums, and broke things. He was sent home from school three days in a row for arguing with his teachers in the classroom and fighting with other kids out on the playground. At home, he stayed up all night watching television. He started getting physical and hitting his sister. When we confronted him about it, he threatened to kill himself if we didn't let him do whatever he wanted. Then he cut me and that's what brought us here."

Johnnie came to me with a screen for prescription drugs and abused substances in the blood, which was negative.

In his Diagnostic Examination, Johnnie denied problems with exercise, appetite, and weight. He did not seem tired and he ran around my cubicle while we talked. When I asked him about his sleep, he laughed and said that he purposely kept himself up at night to have more fun watching his favorite shows. Johnnie denied any physical symptoms and he laughingly told me that he didn't need a doctor because he knew what was best for him. Johnnie's mood was animated, optimistic, and sometimes inappropriate, and he endorsed feelings of irritability and anger.

On his Cognitive Examination of *attention*, Johnnie was alert and oriented but he failed a Vigilance test requiring him to raise a finger whenever the numeral "5" was read.

Johnnie did well on all tests of *language*, but his Quality of Speech was very rapid and he interrupted the clinician frequently.

In tests of *memory*, Johnnie could only remember four of the seven numbers in the Digit Span test of working memory. He easily remembered the last Four Presidents but this is not a sensitive test of distant memory in schoolchildren who should be able to remember recent presidents. Johnnie failed tests of Uncued and Cued Delayed Memory.

In *abstract thinking* tasks, Johnnie failed Proverb Interpretation because his replies consisted of other proverbs and sayings. For example, for "Don't cry over spilt milk," he said, "Don't worry, be happy." For "Rome wasn't built in a day," Johnnie said, "While the cat's away the mice will play," and laughed. Johnnie could not understand the instructions for Set Analysis but he explained at length why it was a good thing to tell the truth on a test of Insight.

In tests of *sequential thinking*, Johnnie could only subtract 7 from 100 three times in a test of Serial Sevens. He failed the Arithmetic Story Problem, despite demonstrating arithmetic ability on a test of Simple Arithmetic. He refused further testing.

CHALLENGE

Suicides and violence by children are serious concerns in our society. See if you can figure out what is happening with Johnnie.

SOLUTION

Johnnie's final diagnosis was **Bipolar I Disorder, Most Recent Episode Manic, Severe** (DSM-5 296.43, ICD-10 F31.13).

Unfortunately for Johnnie, his diagnosis took a roundabout route. Before receiving the antidepressant, Johnnie met the following criteria for a unipolar or bipolar **Major Depressive Episode**:

At least five of the following symptoms nearly every day for at least two weeks:
1. **A sad, depressed mood (can be irritable in children and adolescents).** Johnnie's parents described his irritable, angry mood. It is also evident in his past history of sullenness; arguing with his father, mother, and sister; and picking fights with the children at school.
2. **A loss of interest or pleasure in most activities (anhedonia).** Johnnie's father noted that, "We couldn't get him interested in school or any other activities."
3. **A significant change in appetite or weight (e.g., a change of more than 5% of body weight per month).** The father noted that, "Johnnie overate" and "he became quite overweight."
4. **Insomnia or hypersomnia.** (*Hypersomnia*): Johnnie's mother noted that "it was always hard to get him up in the morning. He usually slept most of the day on weekends."
5. **Psychomotor depression or agitation.** (*Retardation*): Johnnie's mother said, "He spent most of his time on the couch and seemed almost paralyzed."
6. **Fatigue or low energy.** We were told that "despite all this sleep, Johnnie seemed to be tired all the time."
7. **Thoughts of guilt or worthlessness.**
8. **Difficulty concentrating or making decisions.** "Johnnie had problems concentrating in classes. He would simply get distracted and zone out for 10-20 minutes at a time."
9. **Recurrent thoughts of death, suicide, or a suicidal attempt or plan.** There was no evidence of these before Johnnie received the antidepressant.

The symptoms must cause a significant impairment in school, work, home, or social life; and they must include either depressed mood or anhedonia.

At this time, Johnnie also met the criteria for **Atypical Features**, which many associate with *bipolar* depression:
A. **Mood reactivity** (mood brightens in response to actual or potential positive events). Johnnie's father said, "Usually I could get him out of his funk with a joke but after an hour he would be as sullen as ever."
B. **Two (or more) of the following features**:
   1. **Significant weight gain or increase in appetite**. "Johnnie overate when stressed and he became quite overweight."
   2. **Hypersomnia**. "It was always hard to get him up in the morning. He usually slept most of the day on weekends, too."
   3. **Leaden paralysis** (heavy leaden feelings in the arms or legs). Johnnie's mother noted that he "seemed to be tired all the time—he spent most of his time on the couch and seemed almost paralyzed."
   4. **A long-standing pattern of interpersonal rejection sensitivity that results in school, work, family, or social impairment**. "His feelings were easily hurt—then he would pick fights at school and get in trouble."

Although he was mostly immobilized with fatigue and leaden paralysis, Johnnie already showed several diagnostic symptoms of a **Manic Episode** before receiving any antidepressant medication:

A. The following have been present most of the day nearly every day:
Increased goal-directed activity or energy. Mostly, Johnny was tired and immobilized but when he became interested in a project, "We couldn't calm him down."

Plus at least one of these:
  a. **Elevated mood.**
  b. **Expansive mood.**
  c. **Irritable mood.** Johnnie had a long history of irritable and angry moods. His father said that Johnnie was "an angry boy" who "argued constantly with me, his mother, and his sister."
These symptoms last at least one week or any duration if hospitalization is necessary. Although Johnny would sometimes "clear up for a couple of months," Johnny's symptoms had been present most days for a long time.
B. **At least three of the following symptoms (four if the mood is only irritable):**
  1. **Inflated self-esteem or grandiosity.** We knew Johnnie suffered from grandiosity because "he would never admit when he was wrong."
  2. **A decreased need for sleep (needs <3 hours).**
  3. **Talking more than usual or interrupting others (pressured speech).** His father said that Johnnie "would never stop talking."
  4. **Rapid or racing thoughts.**
  5. **Distractibility.** "Johnnie had problems concentrating in classes" because "he would simply get distracted."
  6. **Increased goal-directed activity or psychomotor agitation.** (*Goal-directed activity*): Although Johnnie did not like schoolwork and procrastinated, "sometimes he worked around the clock on a project that interested him." (*Psychomotor agitation*): At these times his parents "couldn't calm him down."
  7. **Excessive involvement in activities that have a high potential for painful consequences (costly or risky impulsive actions).** "One day he was caught shoplifting candy from a neighborhood store." Shoplifting candy is an example of an activity that has a high potential for painful consequences.

After being given exposed to an SSRI antidepressant for a week, Johnnie's mania worsened and he developed command auditory hallucinations telling him to "go to school and kill all his classmates." He exhibited these additional symptoms of a **Manic Episode**:

A. **The following are present most of the day nearly every day:**
Increased goal-directed activity or energy. Johnny was hyperactive and sleepless at home and he "did not seem tired and ran around my cubicle while we talked."
Plus at least one of these:
  a. **Elevated mood.** Johnnie now laughed frequently and inappropriately throughout his examination, despite the seriousness of his circumstances.
  b. **Expansive mood.** "Johnnie's mood was animated [and] optimistic."
  c. **Irritable mood.** Now, Johnnie "endorsed feelings of irritability and anger." Johnnie's anger became so severe that "he flew into rages, had tantrums, and broke things" and "he started getting physical and hitting his sister." Also, he "was sent home from school three days in a row for arguing with his teachers in the classroom and fighting with other kids out on the playground."
These symptoms last at least one week or any duration if hospitalization is necessary. The antidepressant made Johnnie's symptoms so severe that he had to be hospitalized.
B. **At least three of the following symptoms (four if the mood is only irritable):**
  1. **Inflated self-esteem or grandiosity.** In addition to his previous grandiosity, Johnnie's parents said that now "he threatened to kill himself if we didn't let him do whatever he wanted." He told me that "he didn't need a doctor because he knew what was best for him."
  2. **A decreased need for sleep (needs <3 hours).** Now Johnnie "stayed up all night watching television."
  3. **Talking more than usual or interrupting others (pressured speech).** Now, Johnnie "interrupted the clinician frequently."
  4. **Rapid or racing thoughts.** Now, Johnnie's "speech was very rapid."
  5. **Distractibility.** Now, Johnnie's distractibility was so severe that he failed tests of Vigilance, Digit Span, Uncued and Cued Delayed Memory, Serial Sevens and the Arithmetic Story Problem on his Cognitive Examination.
  6. **Increased goal-directed activity or psychomotor agitation.** (*Goal-directed activity*): Now, Johnnie "purposely kept himself up at night to have more fun." (*Psychomotor agitation*): Despite staying up all night, Johnnie "did not seem tired and ran around my cubicle while we talked."

7. Excessive involvement in activities that have a high potential for painful consequences (costly or risky impulsive actions). After receiving an antidepressant, Johnnie became violent. He "took a knife from our kitchen drawer," "threatened to kill himself," and cut his mother "so deep that I had to go to the doctor."

Other Diagnostic Considerations

Despite the presence of numerous manic symptoms, Johnny's inactivity lead him to receive the diagnosis of Major Depressive Disorder. Bipolar depression is pharmacologically, physiologically, and neuroanatomically different from unipolar Major Depression, and the antidepressant that Johnnie was given for presumed unipolar Major Depressive Disorder made Johnnie's preexisting manic symptoms so severe that Johnnie, his family, and his friends were endangered.

Some clinicians would have initially considered a diagnosis of Attention-Deficit/Hyperactivity Disorder. However, Johnnie's symptoms of difficulty sustaining attention, distractibility, difficulty keeping his seat, and intruding on others' conversations were caused by his underlying Bipolar Disorder. Attention-Deficit/Hyperactivity Disorder cannot explain the anger, anhedonia, violence, fatigue, weight change, sleep change, hypersomnia, suicidality, hallucinations, or thoughts of killing his classmates that are symptomatic of Bipolar Disorder. According to DSM-5, Attention-Deficit/Hyperactivity Disorder cannot be diagnosed if the patient's symptoms can be explained by Bipolar Disorder.

Whenever clinicians are faced with new psychosis or sudden mental and emotional changes, Substance-related Disorders should always be considered. For example, methamphetamine can cause distractibility, facilitate rage and disinhibition, and even trigger a psychotic break. However, a drug screen performed in the Emergency Room demonstrated no abused or prescribed substances in Johnnie's blood.

Cognitive Testing

After exposure to the antidepressant, Johnnie's speech was very rapid and he interrupted the clinician frequently, indicating racing thoughts. Racing thoughts are diagnostic symptoms of bipolar mania.

Johnnie also failed tests of Vigilance, Digit Span, Uncued and Cued Delayed Memory, a Four-Step Sequential Command, and Serial Sevens. These tests all require the patient to hold multiple items in conscious working memory and are therefore vulnerable to distractibility. Distractibility is another diagnostic symptom of bipolar mania.

I have frequently seen patients suffering from Bipolar Disorder interpret proverbs with other proverbs and sayings.

CLINICAL NOTES

After the episode of psychotic violence, assault, and suicidality, it finally became clear that Johnnie had a diagnosis of Bipolar I Disorder. This diagnosis explains all of Johnnie's symptoms and the worsening of his condition after receiving the antidepressant.

We are finding that Bipolar Disorder is common in children. Some estimates suggest that at least one million children suffer from the disorder and the number could be much higher. The majority of children suffering from Bipolar Disorder present with depressed rather than manic symptoms and so, like Johnnie, they are vulnerable to misdiagnosis and inappropriate treatment.

In Bipolar Disorder, antidepressants can cause several undesirable effects: 1) they can be partially or completely ineffective, 2) they can worsen depression, 3) they can trigger or worsen mania, and 4) they can trigger psychotic episodes, suicide, and violence. There is also evidence that antidepressants and consequent Manic Episodes can irreversibly worsen the lifetime course of Bipolar Disorder, particularly in children. Johnnie's psychotic experience probably could have been avoided if he had originally been given a mood-stabilizing medication such as lithium salts, carbamazepine (Tegretol), or other anticonvulsant instead of an antidepressant—these are first-line treatments for Bipolar Disorder.

I placed Johnnie in the hospital and started an appropriate mood stabilizer for his symptoms of mania, bipolar depression, and psychosis. Within a few days, Johnnie was much improved, although he still found it hard to sleep. After a week, Johnnie was released to the care of an outpatient doctor.

CASE 11
ZEBRA BOY

One morning, a social worker brought a seven-year-old Asian boy named Toma to the Emergency Room to evaluate potential child abuse.

First, the social worker saw me alone in my cubicle to discuss Toma's case. She had been called to see Toma at school, where his teacher informed her that he was a good student with exemplary classroom behavior. His social interactions with his schoolmates were normal. Toma's parents, who jointly operated a business, had never attended parent teacher conferences and the teacher did not know them. The teacher had no further information about the parents, family, or home environment.

After recess that morning, Toma had returned to the classroom hot and sweating from his exercise and experienced difficulty when he tried to take off his pullover sweater. One of his classmates tried to help him and succeeded in pulling both the sweater and the boy's shirt over his head, leaving his torso bare. At that moment, the children and teacher noticed the presence of multiple bruises in the form of dark Zebra-like stripes across Toma's back. When asked about these marks, the boy told his teacher that his parents were responsible, but in the resultant turmoil, he refused to discuss the issue further. Suspecting child abuse, the principal called Social Services and a social worker came and picked up Toma from school. My examination was to be followed by an X-ray for broken limbs and a detailed examination by a pediatrician to check for physical and sexual abuse.

After the boy was brought into my office, the social worker lifted his shirt to show me nine dark red bruises on his back, radiating laterally from the spine. These zebra stripes showed inflammatory redness, swelling, and warmth, and they blanched under pressure of my thumb.

I examined the rest of Toma's body and I could find no further bruises, burns, or scars. His weight, height, growth and development appeared normal for his age. I lightly palpated his ribs, limbs, and fingers without finding any withdrawal response that might have suggested strains, sprains, or breaks. His neurological examination, which might have revealed nervous system injury, was normal.

The child understandably appeared avoidant and afraid. He denied that anyone was trying to hurt him but declined to answer the questions in his Diagnostic Examination. He was more cooperative on his Cognitive Examination, demonstrating normal *attention, language, memory,* and *abstract thinking.* He declined to do further cognitive testing and I did not try to induce him to do so at that time.

CHALLENGE

What has happened to this boy? Does this presentation suggest child abuse or some other condition? What will you recommend to the social worker?

SOLUTION

This is a classic presentation of "**coining**." Coining is a traditional folk remedy in Asian countries including China, Vietnam, Indonesia, Korea, Java, Laos, and Cambodia where it is variously called *goh kyol, cao gio, gua sha, kos khyol,* or *kerikan.*

Other Diagnostic Considerations

Child abuse is so unconscionable that clinicians may err on the side of suspicion whenever they find physical signs that may indicate abuse. Faced with a reticent child bearing dark red bruises, officials were right to seek additional information. However, in Toma's case, his injuries resulted from misguided attempts to help him, not hurt him.

CLINICAL NOTES

Coining involves repeated rubbing or scratching the skin of the forehead, back, or chest with a smooth-edged coin, ceramic soup spoon, or metal cap with a rounded edge. Oils, Tiger Balm, herbal preparations, skin lotion, or water may also be applied to the skin. This rubbing or scraping creates linear, painful-looking bruises ranging from pink to red to dark blue-black. These marks have led teachers, social service workers, mental health clinicians, and medical doctors to think that children bearing these marks have been beaten.

Coining bears some similarity to other folk practices involving pinching and cupping the skin. Cupping refers to using a set of heated cups to apply suction to the skin. The intent of the coiner is certainly to benefit the child, not to abuse him, and so coining should not be labeled child abuse. Reported incidents where children were removed from their parents represent a significant misunderstanding of the purpose of the practice.

Coining is described in the popular press as a "safe, highly reputable technique" that "serves to prevent any need for further medical intervention by a medical professional." Another popular media source reports that coining is "commonly used to treat fever, asthma, bronchitis, urinary symptoms, gynecological problems, and food poisoning," "precluding any need for medical treatment."

Despite its cultural relevance, folk medicine is not appropriate for the treatment of potentially serious infections; pulmonary, urinary, gynecological, or gastrointestinal illness; or potentially fatal poisoning, and such comments are irresponsible and dangerous. The literature contains many case histories of children who have died from reliance on folk medicine to treat serious health problems. Furthermore, coining, pinching, and cupping have been known to produce physical injury and lasting scars.

I explained the coining procedure to the social service worker and advised her to follow through with a full pediatric examination to make sure that no serious underlying medical problem was present. I told her that I found no evidence of intent to abuse the child. I suggested that she meet and debrief the parents as planned and check back with the child within one or two weeks to make sure the lesions had healed.

CHAPTER 4
THE MENTAL STATUS EXAMINATION IN THE HOSPITAL

Hospital-based clinicians may be called upon to diagnose and treat their own inpatients, detect undiagnosed medical problems, and request consultation and advice from clinicians in other departments. They may provide consultation to inpatients on medical wards and act as a liaison between departments.

CASE 12
KEEP KENNETH OFF OUR UNIT!

When I was called to evaluate Kenneth G at a moderate-sized city hospital, I was surprised to find him in the Cardiac Intensive Care Unit. "I wanted you to catch him while he is here," the resident told me. "We only keep Kenneth in the CICU until we have ruled out a myocardial infarction, so he will probably go home tomorrow."

"Did you call a psychiatry consult because you think he has an emotional or mental disease?"

"Oh no!" the resident assured me. "He's not a psych case—he is a nice guy. Really, you'll like him."

I changed the direction of my questioning. "So how did he come to be in the Cardiac Intensive Care Unit?"

"Kenneth's always in the CICU," the resident told me. "He's been here 10 times this year and we don't know what to do about him. He always comes in with the outward signs of a myocardial infarction, and he has cardiac risk factors, so we have to put him in the Cardiac Intensive Care Unit. Even though we always rule out a myocardial infarction, we don't feel that we can just reassure him and send him home. Who knows whether the next time really will be a life-threatening heart attack?"

"Why did you call the psychiatrist?"

"We called the psych because we've already had a consult from everyone else and you are the last one on our list. We want you to find a way to keep him off our unit. Don't feel bad—I'm sure it feels just as uncomfortable for you to be on a cardiac ward as it does for us to have a psych here among us."

With this resounding vote of confidence, I went to see the patient.

Kenneth was a 60-year-old man with hypertension who had suffered a small myocardial infarct two years before. He lead an active life, smoked eight cigars per day and consumed three drinks of Scotch whisky daily. His father and mother had both died of heart disease and his older sister had died after a stroke. Kenneth described the events leading to his hospitalization as follows: "Everything happened at once. I was in my living room and I noticed my heart was beating too loud and strong, like it was going to explode out of my chest. I began to stumble around like I was drunk. Then my breathing got real fast and I started to get numb in my face and hands. I began to sweat and shake like a leaf. Finally, I started to get a terrible pain right over my heart and I couldn't get my breath. At that point, I felt out of control and I pushed the emergency button built into my home security system. When the ambulance came, they took me to the hospital. I kept having the symptoms for a while after I got to the hospital, but by the time I came up to this heart care place, I was feeling better."

"Has it happened like this before, Kenneth?"

"That's how it always happens, Doctor. It's been like this for two years. I can't get it out of my mind." Kenneth looked grim.

In his Diagnostic Examination, I found that Kenneth looked his age. He was wearing a hospital gown and he sat calmly in his hospital bed throughout our interview. He mentioned that he usually woke several times during the night with worries on his mind. Kenneth was euthymic and there was no evidence of thought disorder or other psychotic processes. However, he was very frightened about his health, and he told me that he had been thinking of killing himself this year if the doctors could not find out what was wrong with his heart.

"I never used to feel this way, but lately it's been getting worse. Each time I come into the hospital, the doctors tell me I had another heart attack, but the next day they say I didn't have one and I should go home. When I ask the doctors what is wrong with me, they all say they don't know. That seems suspicious to me. I know the way I feel is not natural. Since I can't get any doctor to tell me I'm OK, I think I must have some disease that's so bad that they will not tell me about it. I figure I'm about to die but they won't tell me for fear I'll kill myself."

On his Cognitive Examination, Kenneth did well on all tests of *attention, language, memory, abstract thinking,* and *sequential thinking.*

CHALLENGE

The cardiologists felt compelled to readmit Kenneth repeatedly to repeat a workup that never showed any pathology. Based on the limited information in his examination, what is wrong with Kenneth and how can you help him?

SOLUTION

Kenneth has **Panic Disorder** (DSM-5 300.01, ICD-10 F41.0):

Four of the following symptoms peak within minutes: Kenneth said, "everything happened at once"):

1. **Pounding or racing heart.** Kenneth said, "I noticed my heart was beating too loud and strong, like it was going to explode out of my chest."
2. **Excessive sweating.** In describing his problem, Kenneth said, "I began to sweat."
3. **Trembling or shaking.** Kenneth said that he began to "shake like a leaf."
4. **Shortness of breath.** Kenneth said that "I couldn't get my breath."
5. **Choking.**
6. **Chest pain.** Kenneth told us that "I started to get a terrible pain right over my heart."
7. **Nausea or stomachache.**
8. **Dizziness, lightheadedness, or unsteadiness.** Kenneth said, "I began to stumble around like I was drunk."
9. **Chills or hot flushes.**
10. **Numbness or tingling in the fingers or face (paresthesias).**
11. **Feeling detached from self (depersonalization) or environment (derealization).**
12. **Fear of losing control.** Kenneth noted that "I felt out of control."
13. **Fear of dying.** Although Kenneth told us that "I figure I'm about to die," he does not mention this fear as a part of his panic episode. Nevertheless, he pushed the emergency button in his living room to summon an ambulance.

These attacks must be followed by one month of worry about additional Panic Attacks and/or maladaptive attempts to avoid having additional Panic Attacks. Kenneth said, "I can't get it out of my mind." He "was very frightened about his health," to the point of considering suicide.

Other Diagnostic Considerations

The Cardiac Intensive Care Unit noted that Kenneth's symptoms overlapped the symptoms of myocardial infarction but they had repeatedly ruled out medical causes for his attacks. These extensive workups help us eliminate other physical causes for panic symptoms, including hyperthyroidism, Cushing's disease, pheochromocytoma, and other medical conditions that increase adrenaline and noradrenaline.

Some clinicians consider that Kenneth may have another anxiety disorder. However, Kenneth does not exhibit the poor concentration, mind going blank, fatigue, muscle tension, restless sleep, restlessness, edginess, or feelings of being keyed-up that are required for a diagnosis of Generalized Anxiety Disorder.

Kenneth has recurrent thoughts about his attacks and negative cognitions that he will die, but he does not mention any other symptoms of Posttraumatic Stress Disorder such as recurrent dreams, flashbacks, distressing reminders, efforts to avoid thoughts, feelings, or reminders, amnesia, self-blame, persistent negative emotions, diminished participation in important activities, feelings of estrangement from others, or inability to experience positive emotions, irritable behavior, angry outbursts, hypervigilance, exaggerated startle response, or sleep problems.

He does not fear that panic symptoms will embarrass him in front of others as in Social Anxiety Disorder, nor does he describe the obsessions or compulsions of Obsessive-Compulsive Disorder.

Some of Kenneth's symptoms overlap the diagnosis of Alcohol Withdrawal, including sweating, rapid pulse, hand tremor, psychomotor agitation, and anxiety. Withdrawal is precipitated by a rapid cessation or reduction in *heavy* alcohol use—therefore, it is useful to know how much alcohol Kenneth was consuming daily. The average drink contains 1.5 oz of distilled liquor, meaning that his three drinks of Scotch whisky contained a total of about 4.5 oz of whisky. Eighty-six proof liquor contains 43% ethyl alcohol—thus, Kenneth was consuming about 2 oz of ethyl alcohol per day. Two ounces of alcohol was probably not enough to precipitate full-blown withdrawal. Moreover, withdrawal only accounts for some of Kenneth's symptoms, whereas Panic Disorder accounts for all of them.

CLINICAL NOTES

Panic Disorder occurs in about 0.5% of the world's population. Although the onset may occur at any age, most cases begin between adolescence and 30 years. Women are twice as likely as men to develop panic disorder.

Panic Disorder can be genetically inherited—if one of a pair of identical twins has Panic Disorder, the other has a 50% likelihood of having Panic Disorder, also. Stimulants, including caffeine and nicotine, can also trigger Panic Attacks and these substances should be avoided by individuals with Panic Disorder. Although many individuals take alcohol and sedatives to block the onset of panic symptoms, alcohol and sedative withdrawal stimulates adrenaline activity and may also worsen panic symptoms.

Hyperventilation reduces the concentration of carbon dioxide in the bloodstream, causing the blood to become too alkaline and the fluid surrounding the brain and spinal cord to become too acidic. This process causes increased release of epinephrine and norepinephrine, producing numbness of the face and fingers, sweating, tremor, and triggering Panic Attacks. Conversely, slow breathing can hasten the recovery from a panic episode. Other treatments for Panic Disorder include medications, stress reduction exercises, and Cognitive Behavioral Therapy.

Unfortunately, Kenneth did have risk factors for heart disease and I could not prove to the cardiologists that he would not someday present with a heart attack. Kenneth refused Behavioral Therapy but he accepted alprazolam (Xanax) 1 mg daily. After starting the alprazolam, Kenneth did not show up in the Emergency Room for the rest of the year. The cardiologists were impressed by this medical breakthrough and told me that I would be welcome in their Cardiac Intensive Care Unit anytime. In December, Kenneth voiced his appreciation by sending me a quart of Scotch whisky and a box of cigars.

CASE 13
DR. RALPH HAS THE WORST TRIP OF HIS LIFE

Miss Hamilton was a 75-year-old woman who was hospitalized with a diagnosis of **Major Depressive Disorder, Single Episode, Severe** (DSM-5 296.23, ICD-10 F32.23). She had stayed for months on the locked inpatient psychiatric ward at a Veteran's Administration Medical Center without any improvement. Repeated work-ups by the Internal Medicine residents showed no internal problems. There were outstanding charts from an outlying hospital but they appeared to have been lost.

Miss Hamilton was quite overweight. She usually spent her days sleeping on a wooden bench in the dayroom, clad in her slippers and a thin, white hospital gown. One day the nursing aids forgot to take her out to the dayroom and she slept all day in her bed.

When I saw her on the hospital ward for a Diagnostic Examination, Miss Hamilton was sitting motionless, as if she were paralyzed—it seemed to take her an inordinate effort just to straighten up and talk with me. In her faint voice, she told me that she had lived her life all alone in a small, isolated farmhouse in the country. She said that she had no family or friends. In recent years, she had lost her land and savings for mortgages and taxes and she had fallen deeply into debt.

Miss Hamilton seldom looked happy. When I tried telling her a joke to brighten her mood, she initially smiled and laughed. However, after a few moments, she said, "Anyway, it doesn't matter. I'm going to die here soon." She refused to answer any further questions on the Diagnostic Examination.

Miss Hamilton had difficulty keeping her mind on her Cognitive Examination. She seemed slowed and confused, and her attention wandered. Miss Hamilton's Quality of Speech was poor—she appeared nearly mute, and when she did speak, it was in an almost inaudible whisper. Her response to all my other testing efforts was to ignore me.

After failing many antidepressants, I wondered if a trial of a monoamine oxidase inhibitor (MAOI) would help. There were few dietary risks because the hospital nutritionist preplanned all her meals and there were few compliance risks because her medicine was organized and given by nursing staff. If she developed hypotension, we would know because the nursing staff took her blood pressure every day. I wrote a prescription for phenelzine (Nardil) because, at that time, it was the MAOI with which I had the most experience.

Miss Hamilton's subsequent progress was quite satisfactory. She brightened in the first week and began talking volubly. She began spending her free time in the day room, listening to her small radio so intently that staff had to come get her for dinner. One morning, the staff found her awake in bed after listening to her radio throughout the night. By the end of three weeks, Miss Hamilton demonstrated a clearly upbeat outlook. She spoke up in her therapy group and we saw a new, irritable side to her character that we had never seen before. She followed male staff and attempted to pinch them on several occasions.

After another week of this, we received a call from Miss Hamilton's son, who was living in Iowa, and I learned more about her history. Initially Miss Hamilton had a large family and many friends who she eventually alienated by her bad temper and holier-than-thou attitudes. Her son remembered the police being called on many occasions during her wild parties. Known as a workaholic, she had made and lost several fortunes before burning out in her fifties.

Her son was relieved that his mother had "finally settled down," and based on her stability, he agreed that the hospital would discharge her into his care. My colleague, Dr. Ralph, jumped at the opportunity to fly with her to the Midwest to ensure her safe arrival (and to have some fun away from the ward at the government's expense).

I was pleased with this result. I had seen a lonely, elderly woman through her bout of severe depression. My choice of phenelzine had apparently been the solution to her suffering that my fellow physicians had overlooked. This poor woman had been given a new lease on life and she was now going to live out her years in peace and happiness with her son and his family.

Therefore, I was sorely surprised to hear, on Dr. Ralph's return, that Miss Hamilton's trip had gone horribly wrong.

CHALLENGE

Do you agree with Miss Hamilton's diagnosis and treatment? See if you can guess the nature of the unexpected event that happened to Miss Hamilton on her flight home. It is a common enough occurrence in mental health treatment. It was not caused by any cardiovascular problems, such as a stroke or embolism that might be encountered at high altitudes. She did not have any unexpected reaction to the food on the plane and she did not relapse back into her depression.

SOLUTION

The day that Dr. Ralph left, we were finally able to download Miss Hamilton's belated medical records. In the past she had repeatedly been treated for **Bipolar I Disorder, Most Recent Episode Depressed, Severe** (DSM-5 296.53, ICD-10 F31.4), a diagnosis we had overlooked.

Dr. Ralph discovered this misdiagnosis soon after his plane took off. As soon as the plane reached flying altitude, Miss Hamilton flew into a full-blown bipolar Manic Episode, laughing loudly, talking rapidly, calling names, groping, and making inappropriate comments to male passengers. It was very difficult to keep her in her seat and she grabbed handfuls of little liquor bottles from the passing cart for which my colleague had to pay. The situation only worsened after she consumed the alcohol.

In our hospital, Miss Hamilton initially met the criteria for a **Major Depressive Episode** which we assumed was evidence of unipolar **Major Depressive Disorder**:
At least five of the following symptoms nearly every day for at least two weeks:
1. **A sad, depressed mood.** We learn that "Miss Hamilton seldom looked happy."
2. **A loss of interest or pleasure in most activities (anhedonia).** Before her MAOI antidepressant, Miss Hamilton did not appear to enjoy anything in her hospital environment, saying, "It doesn't matter. I'm going to die here soon."
3. **A significant change in appetite or weight (e.g., a change of more than 5% of body weight per month).** In my evaluation, I noticed that Miss Hamilton "was quite overweight."
4. **Insomnia or hypersomnia.** (*Hypersomnia*): Before receiving her MAOI antidepressant, "Miss Hamilton "usually spent her days sleeping on a wooden bench in the dayroom, clad in her slippers and a thin, white hospital gown. One day the nursing aids forgot to take her out to the dayroom and she slept all day in her bed." (*Insomnia*): After beginning her antidepressant, "the staff found her awake in bed after listening to her radio throughout the night.
5. **Psychomotor depression or agitation.** (*Retardation*): Miss Hamilton "usually spent her days sleeping on a wooden bench" or "sitting motionless."
6. **Fatigue or low energy.** "It seemed to take her an inordinate effort just to straighten up and talk with me." "One day the nursing aids forgot to take her out to the dayroom and she slept all day in her bed."
7. **Thoughts of guilt or worthlessness.** (*Worthlessness*): Miss Hamilton complained that "she had no family or friends," "she had lost her land and savings for mortgages and taxes," and "she had fallen deeply into debt."
8. **Difficulty concentrating or making decisions.** Miss Hamilton "seemed slowed and confused, and her attention wandered."
9. **Recurrent thoughts of death, suicide, or a suicidal attempt or plan.** (*Death*): Miss Hamilton said, "It doesn't matter. I'm going to die here soon."

Miss Hamilton's depression was characterized by **Atypical Features**, which many clinicians associate with *bipolar* depression:
A. **Mood reactivity** (mood brightens in response to actual or potential positive events). When I told Miss Hamilton a joke, "she initially smiled and laughed," but returned rapidly to her depression.
B. **Two (or more) of the following features**:
   1. **Significant weight gain or increase in appetite**. In my evaluation, I noticed that Miss Hamilton "was quite overweight."
   2. **Hypersomnia**. "Miss Hamilton "usually spent her days sleeping on a wooden bench in the dayroom, clad in her slippers and a thin, white hospital gown. One day the nursing aids forgot to take her out to the dayroom and she slept all day in her bed."
   3. **Leaden paralysis** (heavy leaden feelings. "Miss Hamilton was sitting motionless, as if she was paralyzed—it seemed to take her an inordinate effort just to straighten up and talk with me."
   4. **A long-standing pattern of interpersonal rejection sensitivity, not limited to episodes of mood disturbance that results in school, work, family, or social impairment**.

Miss Hamilton also met the following additional criteria for a **Manic Episode** which were enhanced by her antidepressant:

A. The following have been present most of the day nearly every day:
Increased goal-directed activity or energy. Miss Hamilton exhibited no increased energy until she received her MAOI antidepressant. Then she became active on the ward during the day and stayed up at night.
Plus at least one of these:
    a. Elevated mood. After receiving her antidepressant, Miss Hamilton began "laughing loudly" on the airplane.
    b. Expansive mood. While still in the hospital, after receiving her antidepressant, Miss Hamilton's mood "brightened' and she "demonstrated a clearly upbeat outlook."
    c. Irritable mood. On the ward, after beginning her antidepressant, "we saw a new, irritable side to her character that we had never seen before." Miss Hamilton's son indicated that she had a prior lifetime history of anger episodes that had alienated her family and friends.
These symptoms last at least one week or any duration if hospitalization is necessary. Miss Hamilton's condition was so severe that she required hospitalization, even before receiving her antidepressant.
B. At least three of the following symptoms (four if the mood is only irritable):
    1. Inflated self-esteem or grandiosity. (*Inflated self-esteem*): Her son told us of Miss Hamilton's history of a "holier-than-thou attitude," which is equivalent to inflated self-esteem. (*Grandiosity*): It is grandiose to imagine that you can pinch hospital staff on the hospital ward or steal liquor bottles, call names, grope, and make "inappropriate comments" to fellow passengers on the airplane without being held responsible for your behavior.
    2. A decreased need for sleep (needs <3 hours). After starting her antidepressant, "the "staff found her awake in bed after listening to her radio throughout the night."
    3. Talking more than usual or interrupting others (pressured speech). After starting her antidepressant, Miss Hamilton "began talking volubly."
    4. Rapid or racing thoughts. On the plane, Miss Hamilton began talking rapidly.
    5. Distractibility. On the ward, even before receiving her antidepressant, "Miss Hamilton had difficulty keeping her mind on her Cognitive Examination" and "her attention wandered."
    6. Increased goal-directed activity or psychomotor agitation. Miss Hamilton's son said that, in the past, she had been "known as a workaholic." (*Sexually*):
    7. Excessive involvement in activities that have a high potential for painful consequences (costly or risky impulsive actions). In the hospital, after her antidepressant, Miss Hamilton "followed male staff and attempted to pinch them on several occasions." On the plane, Miss Hamilton threw tantrums, stole liquor, groped, and "made inappropriate comments to male passengers." In the past, her son "remembered the police being called on many occasions during her wild parties."

Other Diagnostic Considerations

We should have been suspicious of our diagnosis of unipolar Major Depressive Disorder after Miss Hamilton did not respond to the usual antidepressants despite adequate and lengthy trials. Bipolar I Disorder, Most Recent Episode Depressed, is very frequently misdiagnosed as unipolar Major Depressive Disorder. Studies have shown that bipolar depression seldom relapses after treatment with antidepressants: instead, antidepressants can have no effect, cause increased depression, trigger mania, or create psychosis when given to patients with Bipolar Disorder.

Antidepressant medications increase the brain availability and response to serotonin, norepinephrine, and dopamine—disorders like Bipolar Disorder that are not caused by an insufficiency of these neurotransmitters generally do not respond to antidepressants at usual therapeutic doses. Other common causes of depression that do not necessarily respond to antidepressants at usual doses include Personality Disorders and Substance Use Disorders.

Personality Disorders, especially Borderline Personality Disorder, present with chronic depression. However, Miss Hamilton did not exhibit other symptoms of Borderline Personality Disorder, such as chronic feelings of emptiness, fear of abandonment, chronic and intense anger, idealization and devaluation of other people, unstable identity, frequent suicidality or self-mutilation, or brief episodes of paranoia or dissociation.

Miss Hamilton's slowed cognition and behavior could have resulted from Cerebrovascular Disease with depressed mood and irritability. However, there were no signs of strokes in her history or physical examination. Although there was evidence of attention problems, these were a result of the distractibility of Bipolar Disorder. Miss Hamilton showed no evidence of impaired *sequential thinking,* poor planning, or disorganization that would indicate frontal-executive dysfunction.

Substance Use Disorder was unlikely, considering that Miss Hamilton had been on a locked inpatient psychiatric ward for four months.

Cognitive Testing

Miss Hamilton was distractible ("her attention wandered," "she had difficulty keeping her mind on her Cognitive Examination") and she seemed slowed and confused. Distractibility is a diagnostic symptom of manic Bipolar Disorder.

CLINICAL NOTES

Just one Manic Episode is enough to confirm a lifetime diagnosis of Bipolar I Disorder. However, we did not search hard enough for evidence of mania and we overlooked many clues to Miss Hamilton's correct diagnosis. For example, she had not responded to the usually effective treatments for unipolar Major Depressive Disorder. Miss Hamilton exhibited Atypical depressive symptoms that are often associated with *bipolar* depression. Her son's call revealed that she had a history of manic symptoms in the past. If we had waited for her medical records, we would have found that Miss Hamilton had carried a past diagnosis of Bipolar Disorder with Depressed Episodes that would have precluded the use of antidepressants.

After Miss Hamilton became unmanageable on the plane, Dr. Ralph, the flight attendants, and several passengers urged the pilot to turn back. However, this was impossible. When the plane finally landed, Dr. Ralph faced many critical remarks from the other passengers. Then he was left with the task of explaining to Miss Hamilton's family why the hospital had decided that this wild woman was well enough to come home. Eventually, the son calmed down and agreed to take Miss Hamilton to the local Veteran's Administration Hospital. The last thing that Dr. Ralph saw was the son's family forcing Miss Hamilton into their car and driving away.

It is an ongoing challenge for clinicians to discriminate between unipolar Major Depressive Disorder and Bipolar Disorder, Most Recent Episode Depressed (bipolar depression). In Miss Hamilton's case, severe depressive symptoms, overlooking available information, delayed receipt of past records, and the staff's assumption that she had treatment-resistant unipolar Major Depressive Disorder contributed to her misdiagnosis and mistreatment.

CASE 14
MRS. TEMPE SUCKS HER SPOON

One night, I received a message from a community physician asking me to visit his patient, Mrs. Tempe, a middle-aged woman who had just arrived on the medical ward of a small Northern California hospital. I was unable to reach the admitting physician by telephone. When I arrived on the ward, the medical chart gave "changing medications" as the reason for her hospitalization—otherwise it was bereft of a diagnosis or other notes and there were no prior records available. The staff looked concerned and rushed me into her hospital room.

When I came to her bedside, I noted that Mrs. Tempe had the handle of a plastic spoon hanging out of her mouth. She appeared to be sucking on it like a lollypop. Her affect appeared somewhat lighthearted for her current situation, and her demeanor seemed distant and unconcerned.

"Why are you here in the hospital today, Mrs. Tempe?" I asked hopefully.

"Well, I don't really know," Mrs. Tempe replied. "I can't remember what the doctor called my condition. I know that I've been taking a medicine called valproate (Depakote) for several years but it hasn't been working very well lately. This is the slow season for my accounting business and my doctor invited me to come here so that he could start some new medication. I wish I could remember what it was. My husband and my family had agreed that they could do without me for a weekend, so I came here while they went off on a camping trip.

"Also, I haven't really been feeling like myself for the past few weeks. I think something is about to happen but I don't know what it is," she told me. "Sometimes my mind seems to stop and time passes and I can't remember what I was doing before. My husband Bob told me that my hands had been shaking but they don't seem to be doing that now." Mrs. Tempe looked at her hands, which were not shaking.

"It's the oddest thing," Mrs. Tempe continued, flatly. "In the last few weeks, I've been hearing voices outside my window at night. I don't remember that ever happening before. The voices sound like they're coming from two men and one woman, or two women and one man. Sometimes their whispering keeps me up 'till late at night. I heard them just a moment ago."

I looked outside Mrs. Tempe's window and found no one. "Do you think that these people are up to no good, or do you think they might wish you some harm?" I asked.

"I don't have the slightest idea why they are there. I can't remember what they said, if I ever knew. I don't think they mean to harm me—I think they are just outside my window, whispering."

In her Diagnostic Examination, Mrs. Tempe endorsed normal activity and sleep but she complained of disturbing, intensely colored dreams during the past two weeks. "Sometimes I feel like there's a golden halo around my head, like you see in religious paintings," she confided. Other than these details, Mrs. Tempe denied physical symptoms, concentration problems, suicidal thoughts, or thought disorder.

On her Cognitive Examination, Mrs. Tempe performed well on tests of *attention, language, memory, abstract thinking,* and *sequential thinking.* Twice during the evaluation, Mrs. Tempe stared vacantly into space while her fingers picked at her clothing, bedclothes, and a saint's medallion that she wore on a silver chain around her neck. At that time, I noted that she was perspiring, although the room was cool. When I turned to leave the room I saw that she had put the saint's medallion in her mouth.

CHALLENGE

We are used to having a wealth of information available on the patients we see. In addition to our patient interview, we may refer to medical records, consult with other physicians, or speak directly with family members. There is usually plenty of information to complete a task like a brief hospital consultation. However, in this case, our available data were severely limited. Using the facts you have heard, see if you can anticipate the patient's actual diagnosis.

SOLUTION

Mrs. Tempe suffers from **temporal lobe epilepsy** (ICD-10 G40.2) and **Psychotic Disorder Due to Temporal Lobe Epilepsy, with Hallucinations** (DSM-5 293.82, ICD-10 F06.0).

When Mrs. Tempe "stared vacantly into space while her fingers picked at her clothing and bedclothes," she was having a **temporal lobe seizure**. A temporal lobe seizure usually lasts 30 seconds to two minutes. During that time, the patient may sit quietly, staring into space, with small movements of the mouth and face and picking movements of the fingers. Increased heart rate and perspiration may be noted. Most patients are partially conscious during the seizure, followed by brief dizziness, confusion, and amnesia after the seizure has passed. When her medical charts arrived in the morning, they confirmed that Mrs. Tempe had **temporal lobe epilepsy**.

Even where there was no apparent seizure, Mrs. Tempe demonstrated a flat and "inappropriate affect," time distortion, "hearing voices," feeling "a golden halo" around her head, and "a tendency to put items in the mouth." Patients may experience feelings of déjà vu, or they may see their own body (autoscopy). An electroencephalogram (EEG) might have revealed abnormal, interictal spikes during these periods.

Temporal lobe epilepsy can mimic many mental disorders. The patient may experience flat affect with auditory, visual, tactile, or gustatory illusions and hallucinations reminiscent of Schizophrenia. There is often euphoria, anger, inappropriate affect, hyperreligiosity, obsessive writing and drawing (hypergraphia), and hypersexuality that suggest Bipolar Disorder. There may be emotions of fear or panic suggesting Panic Disorder. Depersonalization and derealization symptoms similar to those of Posttraumatic Stress Disorder may occur. There can be overperfectionism with a tendency to overvalue details, rules, and order that overlap the symptoms of Obsessive-Compulsive Personality Disorder. Like other seizure patients, individuals with temporal lobe epilepsy often experience symptoms of Major Depressive Disorder.

Mrs. Tempe's experiences hearing voices outside her window were consistent with **Psychotic Disorder Due to Another Medical Condition**:

A. **Prominent hallucinations or delusions**. Mrs. Tempe said, "I've been hearing voices outside my window at night," and "sometimes I feel like there's a golden halo around my head."
B. **There is evidence from the history, physical examination, or laboratory findings that the psychosis is the direct physiological consequence of a general medical condition**. Mrs. Tempe's presentation was consistent with temporal lobe seizures (see above), and this diagnosis was confirmed by her medical charts.
C. **The disturbance is not better accounted for by another mental disorder**.
D. **The disturbance does not occur exclusively during the course of a Delirium**.

In coding disorders due to another medical conditions, the clinician should record the name of the specific condition, "Temporal Lobe Epilepsy," rather than the words "Another medical Condition."

Other Diagnostic Considerations

It is natural to consider Frontotemporal Disease (Frontotemporal Lobe Degeneration) in a patient with temporal lobe pathology. Mrs. Tempe exhibited some stereotyped picking movements and hyperorality, but she showed no cognitive problems in *language* or *sequential thinking* on her Cognitive Examination, and her behavioral inhibition and interpersonal behavior were intact. She showed no loss of apathy, inertia, sympathy, or empathy needed for the diagnosis of Frontotemporal Disease.

Mrs. Tempe's flat affect, hallucinations, and odd behaviors suggested Schizophrenia, but there was no evidence that her symptoms had been present continuously for at least six months.

Her symptoms of euphoria, anger, inappropriate affect, grandiose illusions, obsessive writing and drawing (hypergraphia) suggest Bipolar Disorder, but Mrs. Tempe showed no evidence of a week-long period of increased activity, euphoria, expansiveness, or irritability; or increased speech, pressured speech, racing thoughts, or impulsive actions with potentially painful consequences that would be necessary for that diagnosis.

Mrs. Tempe did not exhibit either the sadness or anhedonia needed to diagnosis unipolar Major Depressive Disorder.

CLINICAL NOTES

Temporal lobe epilepsy occurs in about 0.3% of the general population. The onset is usually between childhood to adolescence. Causes include genetic inheritance, early brain injury, infections, trauma, brain tumors, and brain or blood vessel malformations.

I wrote a note explaining how the symptoms of temporal lobe epilepsy could mimic those of many mental disorders. I noted that these symptoms usually waned when medical treatment was optimized and discussed this with the night staff, who were greatly relieved. Over the next week, her neurologist gradually changed her anticonvulsant, after which Mrs. Tempe was discharged. The last thing I heard, she was living at home without symptoms and doing well in her accounting business.

CASE 15
"RULE OUT PSYCH"

It was 6:00 A.M. when I arrived at the small Health Maintenance Organization hospital. When I checked my mailbox, I found out a consult that read, "See Mr. Jones on Medical Ward C sometime today. Rule out psych." Arriving on the ward, I found that Mr. Jones had come in at 3:00 A.M. the previous night because of dizziness and a fall. He was admitted from the Emergency Room by a cardiology resident. The chart was missing from the nursing station, so I went to Mr. Jones' room to perform a mental status examination.

When I entered the room, I saw a graying, middle-aged man with a chalky complexion, lying motionless upon his bed. The covers were tucked in around him and were smooth as if they had not been disturbed all night. I called out Mr. Jones' name but he did not wake up. I spoke quite loudly and shook him gently by the arm but there was no response.

Mr. Jones' current pulse was rapid at 110 beats per minute (normal=60-100 bpm) but his blood pressure was normal at 110/75 millimeters of mercury. His skin was pale and clammy and his conjunctiva and nail beds were gray. When I pinched a knuckle on his hand, Mr. Jones reflexively pulled his arm away but he still did not wake up.

I found that his pupils were fixed and equal bilaterally. There was no facial asymmetry. A gag reflex was present and equal on both sides of the throat. A quick check of the deep tendon reflexes in his knees and forearms found them brisk and equal on both sides of the body.

As I turned to leave the room, I found the door blocked by a tired, pudgy young resident holding Mr. Jones' medical chart. He was wearing a loose-fitting white coat and he had an expensive cardiologist stethoscope slung around his neck. His name badge said "Dr. Kaufman."

"You're the psych?" he said. "I'm glad I called you. Mr. Jones's pretty sluggish this morning."

"Comatose would be a better word," I replied. "Does that concern you?"

"Well, it's really strange," Dr. Kaufman said. "He was looking pretty good last night when he came to the Emergency Room. He was sitting up, joking, and talking to everyone. I checked him before I went to sleep an hour ago and he was talking a little weird, so I sent you the consult. But maybe that's normal for an older man who spent the night in the Emergency Room. So, I sent you a consult just to be complete. But when I saw him last night, he was sitting up in bed and moving. Not like this. What do you think?"

"I do not think this is normal, even for an older man," I bristled, because the patient and I were of similar age. "Why is he in the hospital?"

"He came in last night with dizziness after a fall, but his examination, laboratory tests, computerized tomography (CT), and magnetic resonance imaging (MRI) scans were normal. However, we had a bed open so I thought it would be good to observe him overnight," Dr. Kaufman replied. "His physical exam was normal, but his blood pressure was 150/114, so I started him on some new antihypertensive medications and brought his blood pressure back to normal. I bet this old guy hasn't had a normal blood pressure in *years*. I thought he would wake up healthier than before and jump out of bed, ready to go home. It doesn't make sense."

The young doctor's optimism seemed dubious in the face of a patient who could not be aroused.

CHALLENGE

Your challenge is to examine the available information, determine what happened to Mr. Jones, and suggest the next step in his treatment.

SOLUTION

Mr. Jones is experiencing **Delirium Due to Hypotension and Hypoxia** (low blood pressure and insufficient oxygen; DSM-5 293.0, ICD-10 F05), **cerebral anoxia** (ICD-10 G93.1), and **iatrogenic hypotension** (ICD-10 I95.2), resulting from rapid lowering of blood pressure with medications.

Mr. Jones showed the following symptoms of **Delirium**:

The patient has a rapid disturbance in *attention* that develops rapidly within the course of hours to days and tends to fluctuate during the course of a day. (*Attention*): Mr. Jones was not aware of his environment at all. He could not focus, sustain, or shift attention. (*Rapid and fluctuating*): Between 5:00-6:00 A.M., Mr. Jones' level of consciousness had changed drastically. According to Dr. Kaufman, Mr. Jones "was looking pretty good last night when he came to the Emergency Room" at 3 A.M., "sitting up, joking, and talking to everyone." When the resident "checked him before" going to sleep at 5:00 A.M., "he was talking."

At least one other cognitive domain (*language, memory, abstract thinking, sequential thinking*) or perception is also affected. Mr. Jones' was in a coma—all his cognitive abilities were affected.

There is evidence from the history, physical examination, or laboratory findings of a medical condition, substance intoxication or withdrawal, exposure to a toxin, or other medical cause of nervous system dysfunction. Between 3:00-6:00 A.M., Mr. Jones' blood pressure had been rapidly lowered with antihypertensive medications. Without enough blood pressure to oxygenate his brain, Mr. Jones lost consciousness.

Other Diagnostic Considerations

In addition to hypoxia, Delirium can result from brain injury, tumor, cardiovascular disorders, stroke, bleeding, infection (meningitis), metabolic imbalance, liver failure, or other medical illnesses affecting the brain. Extreme intoxication, withdrawal, or overdose can cause or mimic Delirium. Dr. Kaufman's examination, laboratory tests, and scans would have revealed the presence of many of these alternate diagnoses.

The symptoms of mild-to-moderate Delirium can also resemble Cerebrovascular Disease (stroke), Catatonia, or other psychotic symptoms but Mr. Jones had experienced complete loss of consciousness.

CLINICAL NOTES

A healthy heart can supply the brain with plenty of oxygen at a normal blood pressure below 120/80 millimeters of mercury. However, Mr. Jones' arteries were so constricted that his heart needed to maintain a high blood pressure of around 150/114 in order to transport enough oxygenated blood from his lungs to his brain. When the resident doctor lowered Mr. Jones blood pressure too rapidly, Mr. Jones' heart could not supply enough aerated blood to his brain and he lost consciousness.

Pound for pound, the brain uses as much energy as the heart. It needs a constant supply of oxygen. The first signs that the brain is receiving insufficient oxygen are confusion, cognitive impairment, and lethargy. These may have been the symptoms that the resident observed in Mr. Jones before going to bed at 5:00 A.M. Mild-to-moderate oxygen depletion causes brain dysfunction but not permanent brain injury. More severe oxygen depletion kills brain cells in the hippocampus, cerebellum, and neocortex of the brain. If oxygen is completely cut off for 10 minutes or more, consciousness may not return.

After discussing this situation with Dr. Kaufman, he gave Mr. Jones supplemental oxygen and intravenous glucose and allowed him to returned to his usual higher blood pressure. Shortly afterward, Mr. Jones regained consciousness and left the hospital. He was seen as an outpatient by Dr. Kaufman who corrected his blood pressure more prudently than before.

CASE 16
MULTICOLORED DANCING GOLF BALLS

I was asked to consult on Andi, a 55-year-old woman staying in the medical ward of a large hospital. I examined her chart, but it was not very helpful. It said that Andi was a surveyor who presented with myoclonic jerks of the upper limbs and vague complaints about her eyes. Screening laboratories were normal. There was a toxicological screen from the Emergency Room that was negative for alcohol or any other substances of abuse. A test for heavy metals was negative. There was no history of significant illness or prior hospitalization.

I interviewed Andi in bed. She jumped slightly when I came in her hospital room, as if she was startled.

"Tell me about the circumstances that brought you here, Andi."

"Well, doctor, I returned this week from a long trip to Zaire, Africa. My company had sent me to look at possible mining sites in several unpopulated areas. After I came back, I had some funny experiences, so I came to the hospital."

"Tell me about those experiences," I invited.

"Right after I returned from Africa, I went out golfing with my friends," Andi replied. "When I started out, I had some trouble seeing the ball, but I blamed my glasses and I kept playing. When I looked for my ball on the fourth hole, I was very surprised to see that it was yellow. Not just a yellow tinge, mind you, but bright yellow like a school bus. You see, it hadn't been yellow before, so that was strange. Then, when I bent down to pick it up, it broke out in purple polka dots. I mean it was as yellow as before, but now it was covered with bright purple polka dots.

"Then, all around me, the grass was suddenly filled with golf balls of all colors. There were lime green ones, electric pink ones, bright red ones, and so forth. They were dancing around like they were having a gay old time. And I was very amused. I just stood there laughing at these golf balls hopping around. I thought it was very funny.

"Of course my friends gathered around to see why I was laughing. I acted like a complete innocent and I told them all about what I was seeing. I sort of hoped that they might see it too. When they became concerned, it dawned on me that I was not having a normal experience. Then I got scared and I went home.

"At home that night I had a big row with my husband, which is unusual for me. The next day I started seeing the golf balls again. My husband said I needed to go to the hospital and here I am!" Andi concluded brightly.

During her Diagnostic Examination, I noticed that Andi's face was rather expressionless and I observed several jerking movements of her arms that she could not explain. Andi complained about insomnia and a sleep study revealed shortened sleep duration, disorganized electroencephalogram (EEG) tracings, and virtual absence of random eye movement (REM) sleep. Andi complained of physical symptoms of headaches and body weakness. Andi also said she felt sad, anxious, and recently irritable. Overall, she had become disinterested in her life.

On her Cognitive Examination, Andi showed normal *attention, memory,* and *abstract thinking*.

Andi performed normally in cognitive tests of *language,* but her Quality of Speech was poor—her speech was hoarse and sometimes difficult to understand.

In tests of *sequential thinking*, Andi forgot the last step in a Four-Step Sequential Command, failed Serial Sevens subtraction, and could not repeat the sequences of Luria Sequential Movements or Rhythm Reproduction.

The next day, when I revisited Andi at her bedside, she did not recognize me until I mentioned my name.

CHALLENGE

There is a broad differential diagnosis for this patient. The psychiatry consultation was predicated on her reported visual hallucinations, but these particular hallucinations did not resemble anything I had seen in Schizophrenia, unipolar Major Depressive Disorder, or Bipolar Disorder. In the absence of any prior mental illness, the abruptness of these symptoms suggested an organic origin. There was no evidence of stroke, head injury, or the ingestion of hallucinogens. What is wrong with Andi?

SOLUTION

Andi has **Prion Disease due to Creutzfeldt-Jakob disease** (DSM-5 046.79, ICD-10 A81.9) with **Major Neurocognitive Disorder** (DSM-5 294.10 ICD-10 F02.80) and **Psychotic Disorder Due to Creutzfeldt-Jakob disease, with Hallucinations** (DSM-5 293.82, ICD-10 F06.0).

Andi met the following criteria for **Prion Disease**:

A gradual onset and rapid progression of motor symptoms, such as myoclonus or ataxia, or biomarker evidence of prions. (*Rapid progression*): Andi's symptoms developed within the course of a week, a very rapid progression for most neurocognitive disorders. (*Motor symptoms*): Andi demonstrated dysarthric speech, an exaggerated startle response, and jerking movements of her arm. (*Biomarker evidence*): Laboratory evidence eventually confirmed the presence of Creutzfeldt-Jakob Disease.

Major Neurocognitive Disorder:

A significant quantifiable decline in *attention, language, memory, abstract thinking, sequential thinking*, or social function. Initially, Andi showed only dysarthric speech and impaired *sequential thinking*. Within a day, she could not recognize her physician.

These deficits interfere with the patient's ability to be independent in everyday activities. Andi could not living normally if she was hallucinating and could not recognize the individuals in her life.

Andi also met the following criteria for **Psychotic Disorder Due to a Another Medical Condition**:
A. **Prominent hallucinations or delusions.** Andi was seeing multicolored dancing golf balls.
B. **There is evidence from the history, physical examination, or laboratory findings that the disturbance is the direct physiological consequence of a general medical condition.** Andi had Creutzfeldt-Jakob disease.
C. **The disturbance is not better accounted for by another mental disorder.**
D. **The disturbance does not occur exclusively during the course of a Delirium.** Andi did not have a Delirium.

When coding Psychotic Disorders Due to a Another Medical Condition, always list the specific name of the condition: Psychotic Disorder Due to Creutzfeldt-Jakob disease.

Other Diagnostic Considerations

Andi's brief, two-day symptom duration did not allow the diagnosis of other conditions that produce hallucinations and delusions, such as Schizophrenia and Schizophreniform Disorder (which require the presence of symptoms for one month), psychotic unipolar Major Depressive Disorder (which requires two weeks of symptoms), and Manic Episode (which requires one week of symptoms). Brief Psychotic Disorder can be diagnosed in the presence of hallucinations and delusions present for just one day, but like most mental health diagnoses, it cannot be made if the disturbance is due to a another medical condition like Creutzfeldt-Jakob disease.

Cognitive Testing

Patients with Creutzfeldt-Jakob disease typically have problems with speech fluency, facial recognition, and Digit-Symbol Substitution, a test of *sequential thinking*. Vocabulary, Digit Span, and *abstract thinking* are usually intact. On her Cognitive Examination, Andi had poor Quality of Speech and she did poorly in tests of Four-Step Sequential Command, Serial Sevens subtraction, Luria Sequential Movements, and Rhythm Reproduction, demonstrating a deficiency in *sequential thinking*. She did not recognize me when I returned to visit her.

CLINICAL NOTES

Creutzfeldt-Jakob disease, also known as spastic pseudosclerosis, is a prion disease. Prion diseases are also called transmissible spongiform encephalopathies and include Gerstmann–Sträussler–Scheinker syndrome, fatal familial insomnia, and kuru. Mad cow disease (bovine spongiform encephalopathy) is a prion disease of cattle. Dr. Hans Creutzfeldt and Dr. Alfons Jakob first described prion diseases in humans in the 1920s. The infectious particle in prion diseases is a single protein that is able to replicate itself without additional DNA or RNA.

Patients with early stages of Creutzfeldt-Jakob disease lack strong facial expressions and appear to have flattened affect. Their speech is hoarse and dysarthric. They complain of insomnia and studies show brain wave disorganization on the electroencephalogram and an absence of random eye movement sleep. Creutzfeldt-Jakob disease patients frequently complain of headaches, muscle weakness, anhedonia, dysphoria, and anxiety. They may exhibit social withdrawal.

Myoclonic jerks are an early sign of nervous system deterioration. Up to half of patients develop auditory or visual hallucinations, paranoid delusions, and formal thought disorder. Late stages may bring Major Neurocognitive Disorder, body rigidity, and mutism.

Creutzfeldt-Jakob disease can be acquired in a variety of ways. Prions attack the tissue of the nervous system first and most aggressively, and ingestion of food contaminated with infected brain and spinal cord tissue can transmit infectious Creutzfeldt-Jakob disease. However, Creutzfeldt-Jakob disease eventually infects every tissue in the body and any tissue containing the prions can transmit Creutzfeldt-Jakob disease through ingestion or by intravenous routes. Creutzfeldt-Jakob disease can also be transmitted iatrogenically from infected corneal transplants, growth hormone injections, brain membrane grafts, and infected needles. Boiling or radiation sterilization procedures do not inactivate infectious prions.

Creutzfeldt-Jakob disease and other prion diseases can be inherited from parents carrying the diseases. There is also a spontaneous form of Creutzfeldt-Jakob disease (called sporadic Creutzfeldt-Jakob disease) that is probably caused by a random change in protein folding comparable to an isolated genetic mutation. This form has an incidence of one case per million persons per year and most often surfaces during late middle age.

I never found out for sure how Andi had contracted Creutzfeldt-Jakob disease. She could have been exposed to food in Africa that was contaminated with Creutzfeldt-Jakob disease prions or developed the disorder spontaneously.

Unfortunately for Andi, Creutzfeldt-Jakob disease is a one of the most rapidly progressive degenerative diseases of the brain. Patients can show symptoms within weeks. The time course of Creutzfeldt-Jakob disease is quite variable, but fatality often occurs within weeks to months. I drew cerebral spinal fluid and sent it to the laboratory for prion protein testing. Unfortunately, by the time the laboratory results had returned, Andi was already gone.

CASE 17
CARL FALLS DOWN AND FEELS BETTER

I was working at a Veteran's Administration Medical Center one holiday weekend when I received an urgent call from one of the locked mental health units. The charge nurse requested that I come immediately to the ward where a patient was having a grand mal seizure. I was the only clinician on the scene and so I was nominated to deal with this situation.

On the way, the nurse informed me that the patient was a 27-year-old man named Carl who had been admitted to the hospital three weeks ago with debilitating, suicidal unipolar **Major Depressive Disorder, Recurrent Type, Severe** (DSM-5 296.33, ICD-10 F33.2). It was Carl's fourth such admission in the last three years and this time he was not responding to antidepressant treatment. Carl had a comorbid diagnosis of epilepsy that had been active since childhood. He also had a history of noncompliance that included failure to take his prescribed antiseizure medication.

I ran down the corridors and entered the ward, where I observed Carl on the floor in the last moments of a grand mal seizure. Initially, Carl was unresponsive. His skin was flushed and he was perspiring. His pulse, was rapid at 200 beats per minute (normal=60-100 bpm), and his blood pressure was high at 200/100 mm of mercury (normal<120/80 mm Hg). When I bent over to ask him how he felt, Carl looked up dreamily and slowly said, "I feel fine, I guess."

A moment later Carl sat bolt upright with a smile on his face, looked at me, and shouted in my ear.

CHALLENGE

Your challenge is to tell me what the patient said. If you can determine what Carl shouted at me and the reason he said it, then propose a treatment plan to follow-up the episode.

SOLUTION

Carl's depression was relieved by his **grand mal seizure** (ICD-10 G40.6). Carl sat up and shouted into my face: "I feel great! I'm completely over my depression! I'm ready to go home!"

Other Diagnostic Considerations

There is a complex relationship between seizure disorders and the symptoms of unipolar and bipolar depression. Depressive symptoms are more likely in epilepsy, organic brain injury, and stroke than in the general population. The association of epilepsy with changes in the brain, particularly the left frontal lobe, is one possible explanation for the increased diagnosis of depressive disorders seen in these patients. Taking phenytoin and other sedating anticonvulsants can worsen an already depressed mood, whereas some anticonvulsants (such as carbamazepine/Tegretol) have antidepressant effects in Bipolar Disorder.

CLINICAL NOTES

Although seizure disorders are most often treated by neurologists, seizures can also play an important role in the treatment of mental disorders. In Carl's case, his elevated blood pressure and pulse resolved after the seizure, as expected. When he was cognitively clear, Carl admitted that he had not been taking his antiseizure medication, phenytoin (Dilantin). After an unremarkable Diagnostic Examination, I restarted Carl's phenytoin and waited until he had achieved his usual therapeutic blood level before sending sent him home to his family.

It is known that experiencing a grand mal seizure can reduce the symptoms of unipolar Major Depressive Disorder or Bipolar Disorder, or even bring them into remission, presumably through the same mechanism by which electroconvulsive therapy (ECT) is effective. In the 1930s, Manfred Sackel discovered that insulin coma improved the symptoms of patients then diagnosed as Schizophrenic. Other chemical seizure-inducing agents were subsequently used, including camphor oil, pentylenetetrazol (Metrazol), and flurothyl (Indoklon). In the late 1930s, Ugo Cerletti and others demonstrated that a brief electrical pulse applied to the scalp could produce convulsions with the same therapeutic response as chemical seizures, and ECT was born. Modern ECT makes use of hospitalization, anesthesia, muscular relaxation, breathing support, and better control of the electrical stimulus in order to increase safety and efficacy.

The seizure produced by ECT is so small as to be almost unnoticeable. Nowadays, an electroencephalograph (EEG) is used to confirm that a seizure has been produced after the ECT stimulation. Before the electroencephalograph was used, the observation of minor tonic-clonic movements confirmed the presence of a seizure. When I was in training, I was taught to look for an upturning large toe as the single sign that a seizure had been produced.

There is only space to mention some of the possible explanations for the antidepressant effects of seizures and ECT. For example, one of the effects of seizures and ECT is to increase the availability of norepinephrine. During the course of a seizure, norepinephrine reuptake is partially blocked, the noradrenergic enzyme tyrosine hydroxylase is secreted, and massive amounts of norepinephrine are released. Increased blood pressure, pulse, and perspiration are some of the bodily signs of this release. After a seizure, beta-1 adrenergic receptors are downregulated and presynaptic norepinephrine alpha-2 receptors are upregulated to control norepinephrine action. Increases in available norepinephrine are also thought to underlie the antidepressant effects of psychiatric medications like duloxetine (Cymbalta), high dose venlafaxine (Effexor), desipramine (Norpramin), imipramine (Tofranil), and amitriptyline (Elavil). ECT also causes an up-regulation of serotonin 5HT-2 receptors and upregulates GABA receptors.

Other theories explaining the antidepressant effects of seizures and ECT have to do with post-convulsion cortisol release, the release of endogenous anticonvulsants, brain cell kindling, and post-tetanic potentiation of nerve cell physiology and microanatomy.

Naturally occurring seizures and ECT increase the seizure threshold like the mood-stabilizing medications used to treat Bipolar Disorder. In fact, mood stabilizers like carbamazepine (Tegretol, Equetro), lamotrigine (Lamictal), and valproate (Depakote), are used to treat both seizure disorders and Bipolar Disorder, and research shows that lithium salts (Eskalith, Lithobid) may also have anticonvulsant effects. Therefore, it is not surprising that both seizures and ECT can improve the course of Bipolar Disorder with manic, depressed, or mixed moods.

CASE 18
MISSY BARELY MOVES

Missy May was a 19-year-old girl who was brought to the hospital by her parents. Missy's father began our discussion:

"Doctor, for years Marjorie and I have struggled with our daughter, Missy May. Most of the time she had a terrible temper and she has destroyed a lot of our things just for the fun of it. Things just got worse until a year ago, when she got wilder. She told us she was hearing the voice of God telling her to smash all our living room furniture."

"Don't get the wrong idea, doctor," Missy's mother interrupted. "Missy could be the sweetest girl you ever saw. I mean, it's a real blessing to have such a beautiful daughter—everybody always comments. As a child, she would sit and talk and tell jokes for hours nonstop, but as she grew older, she just got more and more hyper."

"Yes," continued the father. "We took her all over with no luck until we found Dr. H. You see, all the young doctors tried the newest, most expensive drugs, but Dr. H is a very mature, white-haired physician. He knew of an old medication that he had used for years. Within six months of starting his magic drug, Missy's temper and behavioral problems were cured and she got sweet again. She was perfectly happy sitting in the living room all day, watching all her favorite shows, never yelling or complaining. She began to eat very slowly and she lost a lot of unnecessary weight. She was sweet and beautiful again. It was like a miracle.

"Marjorie and I were really grateful to Dr. H and his magic medicine. Missy still heard voices from God but we didn't care because we had our loving daughter back. However, Dr. H told us that our daughter would never be normal as long as she heard those voices. He kept increasing the medication and she got quieter but no better. Now she just seems strange and she's been falling down a lot. We're worried that she might hurt herself falling down. We still love Dr. H for what he did for our family but we wanted to get another opinion so we brought her to the hospital. We didn't know what else to do. We haven't told Dr. H where she is."

Neither of Missy May's parents could tell me the name of Dr. H's magic medicine or its dose. I called and left messages for Dr. H but my telephone calls were not returned.

I sent Missy May's parents away to perform her Diagnostic Examination. Missy was a tall, rail-thin young woman with carefully applied makeup. Unlike her wild description, she appeared quite calm and quiet. Her face barely moved when she spoke. In fact, she barely moved at all.

"I never go outside the house anymore," she said in a baby-like whisper, "so I don't get any exercise. I never used to need hardly any sleep but since I started taking Dr. H's medicine, I sleep more than 10 hours every day."

Missy May denied any physical symptoms of decreased or increased appetite, insomnia, agitation, indecisiveness, or poor concentration, restlessness, feeling keyed-up, edginess, muscle tension, or her mind going blank. However, she complained that her legs were stiff in the morning and she had difficulty walking. "I am very slowed down in my body," she said, "and I just seem to fall right over all the time.

"I still have weeks where I feel irritated and angry," Missy continued. "I have energy but it's just too hard to complain or throw tantrums. Most of the time I feel so unmotivated that I just don't care about my life, anymore." Missy denied feeling sad, hopeless, anxious, or guilty. She said, "I still get hungry but I just don't eat very much these days."

When I asked if she felt worthless or like a bad person, Missy giggled softly. "How could I be a bad person if God talks to me? I have a very special rôle in the coming of heaven." I admitted that she had a point. She denied thoughts of death or suicide.

In the *attention* portion of her Cognitive Examination, Missy's thoughts were slowed and her test responses were sluggish. She was Oriented to place and date but not time. She demonstrated good Basic Verbal Comprehension but she failed a test of Vigilance.

In *language* assessment, Missy's voice was almost inaudible. Her speech was slow and she would occasionally stop mid-sentence, as if she had difficulty getting the answer out. If she was silent for too long, she appeared to be frustrated and she would look up at the ceiling and slowly shake her head from side to side. When I asked her to write her answers, she complied in a microscopic script that trailed off before completing the answer. Further cognitive testing was impossible because of her slowed thinking and difficulty speaking.

I was again surprised when Missy got up to leave. It took her some time to rise from the chair. When she was finally standing, her back remained bent forward. She walked with her feet so close together that she seemed about to topple over. She took short steps and her new shoes scuffed the floor when she walked.

CHALLENGE

At first, it seems that we have very limited information about Missy May. The parents cannot tell us their daughter's prior diagnosis and we cannot find out what medicine she has been taking. With her treatment history in mind, we must draw our solution from what we *can* see in her mental status examination. Consider her behavior, mood, speech, and cognition and try to answer these questions: 1) what was the original source of Missy May's symptoms, 2) what was Dr. H's "magic" medicine that seemed to relieve her behavioral problems without eliminating her auditory hallucinations and, 3) what treatment would you recommend?

SOLUTION

Missy is experiencing **Bipolar I Disorder, Most Recent Episode Manic, with Psychotic Features** (DSM-5 296.44, ICD-10 F31.2) and **Neuroleptic-Induced Parkinsonism** (DSM-5 332.1, ICD-10 G21.11).

Missy met the following criteria for a **Manic Episode**:

A. The following have been present most of the day nearly every day:
Increased goal-directed activity or energy. Missy's mother told us that, "As a child, she would sit and talk and tell jokes for hours nonstop, but as she grew older, she just got more and more hyper."
Plus at least one of these:
    a. **Elevated mood.**
    b. **Expansive mood.**
    c. **Irritable mood.** Missy's parents noted that "most of the time she had a terrible temper" and she said "I still have weeks where I feel irritated and angry."

These symptoms last at least one week or any duration if hospitalization is necessary. Missy's condition had been present for years and it was now so severe that she required hospitalization.

B. At least three of the following symptoms (four if the mood is only irritable):
    1. **Inflated self-esteem or grandiosity.** (*Grandiosity*): Missy heard voices from God and felt that she had "a very special rôle in the coming of heaven." The notion that God had singled her out to do battle with the furniture is also grandiose.
    2. **A decreased need for sleep (needs <3 hours).** Missy said "I never used to need hardly any sleep."
    3. **Talking more than usual or interrupting others (pressured speech).** Her mother noted that Missy "would sit and talk and tell jokes for hours nonstop."
    4. **Rapid or racing thoughts.**
    5. **Distractibility.** Missy had *attention* impairment, but there was no way to tell if it was a result of her pathology or sedation from her medication.
    6. **Increased goal-directed activity or psychomotor agitation.** (*Psychomotor agitation*): Missy's mother said that "she just got more and more hyper."
    7. **Excessive involvement in activities that have a high potential for painful consequences (costly or risky impulsive actions).** Missy's mother said that "she has destroyed a lot of our things just for the fun of it."

The evidence suggests that Missy May was given a high potency antipsychotic medication at increasing doses in an attempt to bring her bipolar symptoms to remission. This was later confirmed. As a result of high antipsychotic doses, Missy May showed signs of **parkinsonism**, including paucity of movement (hypokinesia); slowness of movement (bradykinesia) while walking, rising from her chair, and eating; movement hesitation; hunched posture; minimal movement of the face (mask-like facies); shuffling gait; and a tendency to fall. When I performed a brief neurological examination, I also found lead pipe rigidity and cogwheeling tonus in her muscles and joints, additional signs of parkinsonism. However, Missy was not suffering from Parkinson's disease (DSM-5 332.0, ICD-10 G20). Instead, all the symptoms of her iatrogenic **drug-induced secondary parkinsonism** resulted from high doses of an antipsychotic medicine.

Other Diagnostic Considerations

Dr. H initially gave Missy an erroneous diagnosis of Schizophrenia based on her prominent auditory hallucinations and delusions. For example, Missy believed that she heard the voice of God and that she played "a very special rôle in the coming of heaven." However, these hallucinations and delusions were caused by Bipolar Disorder, not Schizophrenia.

After increasing her antipsychotic, Dr. H believed that Missy had begun to show negative symptoms of Schizophrenia such as *flat affect, alogia, and avolition.* However, these changes were caused by her drug-induced parkinsonism. For example, her "flat affect" was really an inability to move her facial muscles caused by parkinsonism. Her "alogia," or lack of speech, was an inability to move her vocal chords due to parkinsonism. And her "avolition," or lack of action, was really a result of stiffness and an inability to move her body muscles caused by parkinsonism.

Missy's mood episodes should have also pointed Dr. H away from his incorrect diagnosis. DSM-5 Criterion D for Schizophrenia states that Schizophrenia cannot be diagnosed in the presence of Bipolar Disorder. Persistently irritable mood is one of the criteria for the diagnosis of Bipolar Disorder and she showed other symptoms of bipolar mania. Her ego-syntonic, hyperreligious hallucinations and delusions were more characteristic of Bipolar Disorder than Schizophrenia.

Some clinicians think of Major Depressive Disorder when they hear of Missy's anhedonia, weight loss, hypersomnia, and slowed thoughts and movements (psychomotor depression). However, Missy denied sadness and any physical symptoms of decreased or increased appetite, insomnia, agitation, indecisiveness, or poor concentration. Her slowness, lack of activity, and hypersomnia were the result of sedation and parkinsonism caused by high doses of antipsychotic medicine.

Organic brain injury can cause irritability, motor fatigue, slowing, and psychosis, but organic injury alone would not account for Missy's other symptoms. If she had shown focal neurological symptoms, I would have requested a computerized tomography (CT) scan or magnetic resonance imaging (MRI) to rule out organic brain injury.

Cognitive Testing

Missy's slowed speech and thoughts and impaired Vigilance resulted from sedation caused by her high antipsychotic medicine dose.

CLINICAL NOTES

I finally heard from Dr. H, who told me he had given Missy a first-generation, high-potency antipsychotic medicine—these medications are associated with increased likelihood of movement disorder side effects, including parkinsonism. Initially, Dr. H felt that he had been successfully treating Missy's problem because, as he raised the antipsychotic dose, she appeared more placid and quiet. Her parents were pleased that Missy May became so docile after she had been so wild. However, as Dr. H further increased Missy's antipsychotic dose in an attempt to eliminate her hallucinations and delusions, Missy May was left with parkinsonian symptoms at the age of 19. This is a terrible diagnosis to miss if a patient like this ever comes to you.

Dr. H's treatment failed because it was based on the wrong diagnosis. Although antipsychotic medications are a good treatment for Schizophrenia, they seldom eliminate the symptoms of Bipolar Disorder, which is optimally treated by mood stabilizing medications (such as lithium salts, carbamazepine/Tegretol, valproate/Depakote, etc.).

Missy's parkinsonian symptoms gradually faded after her antipsychotic was taken away. Off medications, Missy May began to exhibit more manic symptoms of angry mood, pressured speech, racing thoughts, distractibility, and an intense preoccupation with religious rituals that she stayed up late at night to perform. When Missy was started on a mood stabilizing medication at a therapeutic dose, her bipolar symptoms diminished. She continued hearing voices, but she told me that they were now so faint that she did not bother to listen to them. Finally, another mood stabilizing medication was added and her voices vanished forever.

CASE 19
MARTY IS A TV STAR

I walked into the dayroom of a Northern California hospital late one afternoon to interview a man who had just been admitted to the ward. I glanced at his chart and learned that his name was Marty Roberts and that he was a 24-year-old, married warehouse worker.

I started the conversation. "Hello, Mr. Roberts. How did you happen to come to the hospital, today?"

"Hello, Doc. I came here in a car," Mr. Roberts replied brightly.

"Yes and how did it happen that you came here in a car?" I continued.

"I guess it was because they put me in a car and drove me here," said Mr. Roberts.

I decided to drop this line of questioning. "What were you doing today before you came here, Mr. Roberts?" I asked.

"I was at the baseball stadium with my wife and 18-month-old daughter. I love her very much."

"And did anything happen at the baseball stadium today that was upsetting to you?" I queried.

"Yes, what happened at the baseball stadium today was that I got in a fight with my wife. I got into a fight with my wife because she's always on me about my job. She is always on me about my job because she thinks I do not make enough money for her. She thinks I don't make enough money because she wants to go out all the time and spend money but I think she should stay home and help her mother take care of the baby."

"I see. Why does your wife want to go out and spend money instead of staying home and taking care of the baby?" I asked.

"Everybody says she got married too young. She married too young because she got pregnant with our baby. After she had our baby, she was too young to take care of it," Mr. Roberts explained.

"Was there anything in particular that your wife said that made you upset, today?" I asked.

"Yes, doc. I got upset today because my wife thinks that I do not make enough money at my job. When my wife thinks I don't make enough money at my job, she says she's going to leave me. When she says that, it really breaks me up. It breaks me up so much that her mother tells her she shouldn't say that to me but she says it anyway. I really wish she wouldn't say that to me but her mother says she got married too young."

There seemed to be something vaguely familiar about Mr. Roberts' conversation style but I could not place it at the time.

In his Diagnostic Examination, Mr. Roberts reported normal sleep, weight, exercise, and nutrition and denied accelerated heart rate, chest pain, chills, hot flushes, difficulty concentrating, distractibility, dizziness, edginess, feeling keyed-up, exaggerated startle response, excess sweating, fatigue, hypervigilance, hypoactivity, hyperactivity, insomnia, hypersomnia, lightheadedness, mind going blank, muscle tension, nausea, numbness or tingling, pounding heart, restlessness, shaking, tremor, shortness of breath, weight changes, or past traumatic episodes.

Mr. Roberts denied affective symptoms such as feeling super happy, sad, irritable, or angry. He said that he enjoyed his life and his activities like he always did. Mr. Roberts denied suicidal or violent thoughts or intentions, denied hallucinations, and showed no evidence of delusions or formal thought disorder.

On his Cognitive Examination, Mr. Roberts performed normally on tests of *attention* and *language*.

However, in *memory* tests, Mr. Roberts could only repeat three of seven words on a test of Digit Span. He could only recall three of Four Presidents and he could only remember three of the six words in a test of Cued Delayed Memory. Mr. Roberts could only remember three items in tests of Category Recall and Free Recall from a Story.

In *abstract thinking* tests, Mr. Roberts was unable to do Simple Arithmetic in his head. His Proverb Interpretation was concrete. For example, he interpreted the proverb, "Don't cry over spilt milk," by saying, "You spilt it. Just clean it up." When asked to interpret "Rome was not built in a day," he replied, "It took a long time to build Rome." Mr. Roberts also failed tests of Set Analysis and Judgment.

In tests of *sequential thinking,* Mr. Roberts could complete only three of the four steps on a Four-Step Sequential Command. He easily repeated the three Luria Sequential Movements after they were demonstrated. However, he could only repeat three steps of the six or nine-part rhythm sequences in a test of Rhythm Reproduction.

At that point, there was a small commotion in the dayroom. Several patients were watching and pointing at the television screen where the news report was showing a scoreboard high above the nearby baseball stadium. A little dot was moving on the scoreboard. As the camera zoomed in, I was able to see a young man holding onto a tiny baby suspended far above the crowd. With surprise, I realized that the man was my patient, Mr. Roberts.

I turned back to my patient and said, "I just saw you on the news. You were at the baseball game standing on top of the scoreboard with a baby."

"Yes doc. I was on the top of the scoreboard with my daughter."

"Why did you climb up there in the first place?" I wondered.

"Well, doc. The reason that I climbed up there in the first place was my wife said she was going to leave me. I can't stand it when she says she's going to leave me, so I climbed up there. I thought that if I climbed up there maybe she wouldn't leave me."

I was puzzled by Mr. Roberts' behavior, but when I considered his presentation and I saw his old chart, I understood.

CHALLENGE

From the limited information available, try to deduce what is happening with Mr. Roberts.

SOLUTION

Mr. Roberts' has mild **Intellectual Disability** (DSM-5 319, ICD-10 F70):

A. **Intellectual deficits in *memory* and learning, *abstract thinking*, reasoning and planning, confirmed by both clinical assessment and standardized intelligence testing.** (*Cognitive deficits*): Mr. Roberts Cognitive Examination showed deficits in *memory, abstract thinking*, and *sequential thinking*. When I saw Mr. Roberts' old charts, they contained standardized IQ testing done at age 17 that showed significant cognitive deficits.

B. **Failure to meet developmental and sociocultural standards for personal independence and social responsibility in one or more activities of daily life, such as communication, social participation, and independent living across school, work, home, and social environments.** (*Social responsibility*): Climbing to the top of a high scoreboard with your infant daughter is not responsible. (*Communication*): Mr. Roberts had difficulty explaining his thoughts and actions in our interview. His decision to take his child up to the top of a stadium scoreboard to communicate his frustration to his wife showed poor communication skills. (*Home living*): Mr. Roberts had difficulty dealing with his irresponsible wife and her mother at home. Mr. Roberts' marriage relationship was stressful. He seemed bewildered by his wife's threats to leave him and was unable to get her to participate in caring for his child.

C. **The deficits begin in childhood.** Mr. Roberts' old charts contained psychological testing performed at age 17.

Other Diagnostic Considerations

Poor cognition, poor social insight, impulsive reactions, and poor judgment can result from most mental disorders. However, Mr. Roberts exhibited none of the hallucinations, delusions, or disorganized behavior of Schizophrenia.

He denied the sadness or anhedonia of Major Depressive Disorder as well as the physical symptoms of weight changes, sleep problems, psychomotor changes, or fatigue. Mr. Roberts also denied the "super happy," expansive, or irritable emotions of manic Bipolar Disorder and the physical symptoms of insomnia, distractibility, or increased activity needed for that diagnosis.

Mr. Roberts denied the fear of Panic Disorder as well as the physical symptoms of palpitations, pounding heart, accelerated heart rate, excess sweating, trembling, shaking, shortness of breath, chest pain, nausea, dizziness, lightheadedness, numbness, tingling, chills, and hot flushes. He denied the anxiety and worried thoughts of Generalized Anxiety Disorder and the physical symptoms of restlessness, edginess, feeling keyed-up, being easily fatigued, mind going blank, muscle tension, and sleep disturbance. He also denied past traumatic episodes or physiological symptoms of Posttraumatic Stress Disorder such as hypervigilance, exaggerated startle response, sleep problems, recurrent dreams, or flashbacks

Cognitive Testing

Most adults can hold about seven items simultaneously in their working memory (see Chapter 8). However, on his Cognitive Examination, Mr. Roberts demonstrated that he could only hold about three items at once in working memory. For example, he could only remember three items in tests of Digit Span, Four Presidents, Cued Delayed Memory, a Four-Step Sequential Command, and Rhythm Reproduction.

Abstract thinking requires the ability to hold many items in working memory at once so they can be compared simultaneously. Without the ability to hold more than three items in working memory, Mr. Roberts could not perform even basic abstract tasks like Simple Arithmetic. For example, Proverb Interpretation requires the patient to make generalizations from many details found in specific examples. Without normal *abstract thinking* ability, Mr. Roberts could not hold enough information in his head at once to make the generalizations, and so his interpretations were concrete. The inability to hold more than a few items in working memory also affects the capacity to judge future consequences from current actions and Mr. Roberts failed tests of Judgment and Insight. These failures help account for his poor judgment in real life.

Where there is insufficient space for *abstract thinking*, there may still be enough for *sequential thinking*, where single thoughts are analyzed one after the other in linear fashion. Sequential information processing can be performed with only three items in simultaneous memory (the previous thought, the present thought, and the anticipated next thought). Mr. Roberts demonstrated that his working memory could hold about three items at once. A preference for *sequential thinking* often manifests as linear speech patterns.

Mr. Roberts's speech demonstrated a linear pattern where the end of each sentence formed the beginning of the next. This speech style is often seen in individuals who are unable to hold more than a few items at a time in their working memory. I have seen this linear speech style in patients suffering from Intellectual Disability, Schizophrenia, organic brain injury, and Delirium. Mr. Roberts' Proverb Interpretations were concrete. I have also seen concrete proverb interpretations in patients suffering from Intellectual Disability, Schizophrenia, Traumatic Brain Disease, and other brain diseases.

CLINICAL NOTES

When I saw Mr. Roberts medical records, I found that he had been assigned a social caseworker years before. When I interviewed her, I found that Mr. Roberts had done well and held down a simple warehouse job until eighteen months ago. At this time, he married a woman in the same Social Services program when she told him that she was pregnant with his child. They moved into her mother's home and were lost to Social Services follow-up at that time.

Mr. Roberts had been able to function well under minimal stress as a single man living alone with the support of a caseworker. However, without this support, he was overwhelmed by his new living arrangements and his new responsibilities as a husband and father. On top of this, his wife's threats to leave him were bewildering. When he had another fight with his wife at the stadium, he showed poor judgment with disastrous consequences.

Unfortunately, I had no opportunity to help Mr. Roberts. Shortly after I finished his assessment, officers of the law arrived at the ward and escorted him from the building to a waiting patrol car. I looked out the window and watched until it had disappeared from sight in the growing dusk.

CASE 20
A FAMOUS APARTMENT MANAGER

On a cold, winter morning, I admitted Mr. C, a 59-year-old, unmarried male apartment manager, to the hospital psychiatric service. He was in a state of extreme agitation—laughing, coughing, and shouting, "I am famous! I am famous!"

Mr. C was so distractible that it was difficult for him to speak more than a few words coherently before going off on a tangent. He was so agitated that he went darting around the room in every direction. It was difficult to interrupt his flow of pressured speech, but Mr. C managed to tell me that he had not slept in the last two weeks. He denied using alcohol or street drugs. He had no prior history of psychiatric treatment of any kind. I walked him to the psychiatric ward and wrote orders for his treatment.

Over the days that I visited him, Mr. C's symptoms slowly cleared and he was able to tell me more of the story that preceded his admission. Prior to this episode, he led a very stable and predictable life, managing a handful of apartments. Everything had started three weeks ago, he said, when he caught a bad cold. This infection left him congested, with a wracking cough.

Mr. C controlled his cough with a 12-hour over-the-counter cough medicine that he discontinued after one week. As his congestion cleared, he got out of bed because he could no longer sleep. He found himself so motivated that he started painting four of the apartments he managed. However, he was too easily distracted to finish any of this work. He spent much of the day talking with his tenants—particularly a freshman college student named Lucy who was many years his junior.

Mr. C told me that Lucy had fallen madly in love with him and wanted to romance and marry him. He said that she had proposed to him many times but he thought their marriage was premature. Mr. C said that she was studying to be a newspaper reporter and that she was going to write an exciting biography about him and his accomplishments. In this way, they would both become famous and they could live together as a married couple on the fortune that the book would surely generate.

I was able to contact the freshman student and I spoke to her over the telephone. Lucy told me that her apartment manager was a weird old man who kept knocking on her door and trying to start conversations. She told me that Mr. C would talk to her for hours at a time if she couldn't find some excuse to get away. She also said that Mr. C gave her many compliments, including comments about her body that she found uncomfortable. She found these encounters so unpleasant that she had taken to staying locked in her bedroom as much as possible.

In his Cognitive Examination tests of *attention*, Mr. C was alert but distractible and he failed the test of Vigilance.

Mr. C did well on tests of *language*, but his Quality of Speech was loud, rapid, and pressured.

In the *memory* section, Mr. C failed Digit Span, Free Recall from a Story, and both Uncued and Cued Delayed Memory.

In his *abstract thinking* assessment, Mr. C did well on Simple Arithmetic. He failed Proverb Interpretation by answering with irrelevant sayings and proverbs. For example, when asked to interpret "Don't cry over spilt milk," he answered, "Tomorrow will be a brighter day."

In tests of *sequential thinking*, Mr. C failed Serial Sevens subtraction and the Arithmetic Story Problem (although he had no problems with Simple Arithmetic). He also failed the Rhythm Reproduction task.

CHALLENGE

Your challenge is to discover, with this limited information, what was wrong with Mr. C and what triggered his condition.

SOLUTION

Mr. C has **Bipolar I Disorder, Most Recent Episode Manic, with Psychotic Features** (DSM-5 296.44, ICD-10 F31.2):

A. The following have been present most of the day nearly every day:

Increased goal-directed activity or energy. Mr. C began working many projects at once and he was agitated in his examination.

Plus at least one of these:
   a. Elevated mood. Mr. C laughed inappropriately and cried, "I am famous! I am famous!"
   b. Expansive mood.

c. **Irritable mood.**

These symptoms last at least one week or any duration if hospitalization is necessary. Mr. C's condition had been apparent for two weeks and it was now so severe that hospitalization was necessary.

B. **At least three of the following symptoms (four if the mood is only irritable):**
1. **Inflated self-esteem or grandiosity.** (*Inflated self-esteem*): Mr. C showed unjustified self-esteem by believing that he was so interesting and important that a book deserved to be written about him. (*Grandiosity*): It was grandiose to believe that his personal history was so remarkable that it would cause a freshman student's first book to earn a "fortune" that could support "a married couple." It was also grandiose to believe that "Lucy had fallen madly in love with him," had "proposed to him many times," and "wanted to romance and marry him." It was grandiose to expect that he could paint four apartments at the same time.
2. **A decreased need for sleep (needs <3 hours).** Mr. C told me "that he had not slept in the last two weeks."
3. **Talking more than usual or interrupting others (pressured speech).** (*Talkative*): Instead of doing his job, Mr. C "spent much of the day talking with his tenants." (*Pressured*): "It was difficult to interrupt his flow of pressured speech." On his Cognitive Examination, Mr. C's "speech was loud, rapid and pressured."
4. **Rapid or racing thoughts.** Rapid speech demonstrates flight of ideas.
5. **Distractibility.** Mr. C. was too easily distracted to finish any of the four apartments that he started painting. Mr. C's cognitive testing results also demonstrated distractibility (see below).
6. **Increased goal-directed activity or psychomotor agitation.** (*Goal-directed activity*): Mr. C started painting four apartments at once. He became more personal with the freshman student. (*Psychomotor agitation*): Mr. C "was so agitated that he went darting around the room in every direction."
7. **Excessive involvement in activities that have a high potential for painful consequences (costly or risky impulsive actions).** Mr. C's dalliance with the freshman student could have had painful consequences.

Mr. C's episode was manic, not hypomanic, because his symptoms were severe enough to cause marked impairment in work and social functioning. He was psychotic because he was experiencing delusions—his beliefs that his tenant had fallen in love with him, wanted to romance and marry him, had proposed to him, wanted to write his biography, and expected them to become famous and live off the proceeds were grandiose delusions.

Other Diagnostic Considerations

Psychosis can also be found in Schizophrenia, Schizophreniform Disorder, Schizoaffective Disorder, Brief Psychotic Disorder, severe Major Depressive Disorder, Acute and Posttraumatic Stress Disorders, Schizotypal Personality Disorder, other personality disorders under stress, Major Neurocognitive Disorder, Delirium, Traumatic Brain Disease, Substance Intoxication and Withdrawal, overdose of any drug, toxins, or other medical illnesses affecting the brain. However, Schizophrenia, Brief Psychotic Disorder, Major Depressive Disorder, Acute Stress Disorder, Schizotypal Personality Disorder, and several other personality disorders contain exclusion criteria that do not allow their diagnosis if the patient's symptoms can be explained by Bipolar Disorder. Furthermore, other mental disorders do not exhibit the same physical symptoms as Bipolar Disorder, such as combined insomnia, hyperverbosity, racing thoughts, distractibility, and hyperactivity.

Cognitive Testing

The pattern of Mr. C's Cognitive Examination is not diagnostic but it resembles the performance of other bipolar patients I have tested. On his Cognitive Examination, Mr. C failed tests of Vigilance, Free Recall from a Story, both Uncued and Cued Delayed Memory, Serial Sevens, the Arithmetic Story Problem, and Rhythm Reproduction—all these tests require several items to be held in working memory to complete the task. When distracting thoughts enter working memory, they displace the information necessary to complete the test. I have also seen bipolar patients attempt to interpret proverbs by repeating sayings and other proverbs.

CLINICAL NOTES

It is important to determine what triggered Mr. C's first Manic Episode, so that the problem can be removed if possible. The onset of this episode coincided with his consumption of an over-the-counter cough medicine containing the opiate dextromethorphan. He had first started dextromethorphan in response to his cough and had continued to take it in high doses even as his viral infection waned, because of the salutary manic effects he experienced.

Most non-narcotic cough nostrums contain relatively benign ingredients that are only slightly effective. However, 12-hour cough syrups and lozenges often contain dextromethorphan, an opiate that has antitussive effects but produces no significant analgesic or addictive effects. Dextromethorphan is an isomer of the codeine analog methorphan and it is nearly as effective as codeine for the treatment of cough. In addition to its narcotic activity, dextromethorphan is an NMDA-receptor antagonist and it inhibits serotonin reuptake. Like meperidine (Demerol), I have frequently seen dextromethorphan trigger Manic Episodes in susceptible individuals suffering from Bipolar Disorder. A Manic Episode cannot be diagnosed if the symptoms result only from the ingestion of a substance. However, Mr. C's mania continued for two additional weeks after he had stopped taking his narcotic cough syrup.

There are several other potential triggers for Mr. C's mania. Manic and depressed Bipolar Disorder episodes are frequently triggered by the time of year, often around dates when day length is at its shortest or longest. The onset of a viral infection can also trigger bipolar Manic Episodes. Studies have shown that many bipolar hospitalizations are preceded by viral infections.

When I gave Mr. C a mood-stabilizing medication (lithium or an anticonvulsant), his bipolar symptoms remitted rapidly and he was able to return to his usual life and job. When he was lucid again, he felt embarrassed about his manic behavior. Lucy, the freshman college student, felt very relieved that her apartment manager was back to normal.

CASE 21
GEORGE AND ANNA CAN'T MOVE AND LUCY CAN'T STOP

This is a case involving three individuals seen in different hospitals.

Mr. George was a 57-year-old, unmarried plumber who had originally presented to a Veterans' Administration hospital for symptoms of Chronic Obstructive Pulmonary Disorder. As Mr. George's COPD was stabilized with steroid medications, his behavior began to deteriorate. Initially, Mr. George became quiet, and then he stopped speaking altogether. When his food was returned uneaten, one of the nurses fed him by hand. When the medical staff cleared him, I received a request to consult on Mr. George's condition.

When I arrived on the ward, I found Mr. George sitting up stiffly in bed. His body was rigid and he resisted my efforts to move him. His eyes were closed and he did not speak or respond to me. When I raised Mr. George's arm into the air, it stayed where I placed it instead of falling down to the bed limply. I checked back with Mr. George several times during the day and it appeared that he had not moved from his position. I called Mr. George's physician and wrote an opinion in the chart.

The second patient, Mrs. Lucy, was a 47-year-old black woman who had been admitted to the medical ward of a Midwest community hospital for the treatment of pneumonia. As she recovered from her infection, Mrs. Lucy began to leave her bed and pace back and forth in front of the mirror in her room. As she gazed into the mirror, she spoke to her image, making bizarre faces and strange passes with her hands. At night, staff would find her pacing briskly up and down the corridor until they led her back to her room. I received a request from her internal medicine doctors to evaluate her on the ward.

When I entered her room, I found Mrs. Lucy pacing. She was very thin and she had worn through the bottoms of her hospital slippers from her activity. Underneath, her feet were raw and blistered.

"Good morning, Mrs. Lucy," I said, sitting down on the end of her bed.

"Good morning, Mrs. Lucy," the patient replied, sitting down next to me.

Throughout her evaluation, Mrs. Lucy repeated all the words I said to her but she would not answer my questions. When I moved, she tried to mimic my movements. When I asked her to open her eyes or mouth, she closed them. I called Mrs. Lucy's physician and wrote an opinion in the chart.

The third patient, Miss Anna, was a 21-year-old woman admitted to the large Neurology wing of a well-funded private teaching hospital. From the chart, I learned that Miss Anna had been unresponsive when she was first brought to the Neurology Wing. Only a minimal history was recorded. Five weeks had gone by before a psychiatry consultation was called.

When I arrived at her bedside, I saw an attractive young girl dressed only in a thin paper hospital gown. She lay flat in her bed, covered by a single sheet, and a feeding tube was placed in her nostril. During my examination, Anna lay quietly in the bed, unresponsive to my speech or touch. The patient's limbs were unresisting and floppy when moved. She did not withdraw her hand in response to cold, vibration, pressure, or mild pain. The nurses on the ward told me that her body remained limp and immobile when they changed her gown and bedclothes daily. They had never seen her move voluntarily and her position in bed never changed.

Miss Anna had received an aggressive evaluation on the Neurology Ward. She had received computerized tomography (CT) and magnetic resonance imaging (MRI) scans, a lumbar puncture with collection of cerebrospinal fluid, and an electroencephalogram (EEG) with throat electrodes. Her case had been the subject of several departmental conferences wherein successive attending neurologists had reported their findings.

Because Miss Anna was so unresisting and compliant, she had become a model teaching patient assigned for medical students to perform their first complete neurological examination. Every few weeks, a new rotation of medical students would arrive to poke, pinch, prick, and pound on her body. Overall, I had some concern with the medical ethics of this situation. Medical students would spend hours in her room late at night without any supervision. In passing her room, I had found her undraped on one occasion.

As attending physicians, residents, and students cycled on and off the neurology service, their notes had all indicated that Anna's evaluation was "inconclusive." I called the attending physician and wrote my opinion in the chart.

CHALLENGE

What do these three patients have in common? What would you do for their treatment?

SOLUTION

All three patients are suffering from **Catatonia**, a complex condition that can present in different ways. Catatonia is not a diagnosis—it is a condition that can manifest in Schizophrenia, unipolar Major Depressive Disorder, Bipolar Disorder, Conversion Disorder, hepatic encephalopathy, and other conditions.

Mr. George met the following criteria for **Catatonia**, a clinical picture dominated by at least three of the following:
1. **Stupor (does not react to surrounding environment).**
2. **Catalepsy (the body remains in the position into which it was been placed).**
3. **Waxy flexibility (wax-like resistance to being moved).** "When I raised Mr. George's arm into the air, it stayed where I placed it instead of falling down to the bed limply."
4. **Mutism (little or no vocalization).** "Initially, Mr. George became quiet, and then he stopped speaking altogether." Also, during my examination, "he did not speak or respond to me."
5. **Negativism (ignores or resists instructions and movement).** "I found Mr. George sitting up rigidly in bed. He resisted my efforts to move him."
6. **Posturing (voluntarily assumes posture).**
7. **Mannerisms (odd or bizarre nonfunctional movements).**
8. **Stereotypies (frequent, repetitive movements).**
9. **Agitation.**
10. **Grimacing.**
11. **Echolalia (repeats examiner's words).**
12. **Echopraxia (repeats examiner's movements).**

I gave Mr. George a diagnosis of **Catatonia of unknown origin** (DSM-5 293.89, ICD-10 F06.1) and I recommended a transfer to the psychiatric ward and further search for past medical records. Mr. George's medical staff was happy with my recommendations. Before Mr. George was transferred to the psychiatric ward, I arranged for an amobarbital (Amytal) interview. This is a traditional part of Catatonia evaluations. As the barbiturate amobarbital was administered intravenously by an anesthesiologist, Mr. George returned to consciousness and began speaking and moving normally. When I asked why he had been so quiet, Mr. George replied, "I was told by the Lord God Jesus Christ to remain absolutely still until I had a sign from him. As his representative on earth, I was commanded not to move in order to ensure peace among nations and in heaven."

There is no agreement about why the so-called "amobarbital interview" raises patients from a catatonic state. Based on his comments to me, Mr. George was responding to a powerful psychotic delusion. In such cases, the barbiturate may relax patient's vigilance or lower their inhibitions to allow them to disregard the delusion. The interview can also be done with injectable lorazepam (Ativan), which can be given more safely in a wider range of doses.

Once on the psychiatric ward, Mr. George began to demonstrate expansive and irritable mood, hyperreligious grandiosity, pressured speech, insomnia, distractibility, and flight of ideas, confirming the diagnosis of a Manic Episode. Old charts were found containing a history of prior Manic Episodes. At that time, Mr. George was given the diagnosis of **Bipolar I Disorder, Most Recent Episode Manic, Severe** (DSM-5 296.43, ICD-10 F31.13) **with Catatonia** (DSM-5 293.89, F06.1). He cleared rapidly on a mood-stabilizing medication (lithium or an anticonvulsant) and he was discharged to outpatient follow-up.

In addition to rigid, immovable posture and waxy flexibility, there is a hyperactive form of Catatonia, demonstrated by the second patient. Mrs. Lucy showed the following criteria for **Catatonia,** a clinical picture dominated by at least three of the following:
1. **Stupor (does not react to surrounding environment).**
2. **Catalepsy (the body remains in the position into which it was been placed).**
3. **Waxy flexibility (wax-like resistance to being moved).**
4. **Mutism (little or no vocalization).**
5. **Negativism (ignores or resists instructions and movement).** Mrs. Lucy showed negativism by closing her eyes and mouth when I asked her to open them.
6. **Posturing (voluntarily assumes posture).**

7. **Mannerisms (odd or bizarre nonfunctional movements).** As Lucy gazed into her mirror, she made "strange passes with her hands."
8. **Stereotypies (frequent, repetitive movements).**
9. **Agitation.** After her infection subsided, Lucy left her bed and "began to pace back and forth in front of the mirror in her room." "At night, staff would find her pacing briskly up and down the corridor." She was so active that she had worn through her slippers and "her feet were raw and blistered."
10. **Grimacing.** As Lucy gazed into her mirror, she made "bizarre faces."
11. **Echolalia (repeats examiner's words).** Mrs. Lucy "repeated back the words I said to her."
12. **Echopraxia (repeats examiner's movements).** "When I moved, she tried to mimic my movements."

Again, my consult note gave a diagnosis of **Catatonia of unknown origin** (DSM-5 293.89, ICD-10 F06.1) and I recommended both a transfer to the psychiatric ward and further search for past medical records. Mrs. Lucy's physicians were also happy with my recommendations. They transferred her to their small psychiatric ward, which managed to locate prior psychiatric records containing the diagnosis of **Schizophrenia** (DSM-5 295.90, ICD-10 F20.9) **with Catatonia** (DSM-5 293.89, F06.1). After resuming her former low-dose antipsychotic treatment, Mrs. Lucy was able to return to her board and care home.

The third patient, Miss Anna, demonstrated a passive, stuporous picture of **Catatonia,** a clinical picture dominated by at least three of the following:

1. **Stupor (does not react to surrounding environment).** Miss Anna "had been unresponsive when she was first brought to the Neurology Wing." While there, she "lay quietly in the bed, unresponsive to my speech or touch." Anna's arms and legs "were unresisting and floppy when moved. She did not withdraw her hand in response to cold, vibration, pressure, or mild pain. The nurses on the ward told me that her body remained limp and immobile when they changed her gown and bedclothes daily. They had never seen her move voluntarily and her position in bed never changed."
2. **Catalepsy (the body remains in the position into which it was been placed).**
3. **Waxy flexibility (wax-like resistance to being moved).**
4. **Mutism (little or no vocalization).** Miss Anna never spoke.
5. **Negativism (ignores or resists instructions and movement).** Miss Anna never responded to verbal instructions or physical attempts to guide her movements. She did not react to pain or other sensory stimuli during her neurological examination.
6. **Posturing (voluntarily assumes posture).**
7. **Mannerisms (odd or bizarre nonfunctional movements).**
8. **Stereotypies (frequent, repetitive movements).**
9. **Agitation.**
10. **Grimacing.**
11. **Echolalia (repeats examiner's words).**
12. **Echopraxia (repeats examiner's movements).**

Like the other patients, I gave Anna a diagnosis of **Catatonia** of unknown origin (DSM-5 293.89, ICD-10 F06.1) and again I recommended a transfer to the psychiatric ward and further search for past medical records. Unfortunately, Miss Anna's attending neurologist did not like my diagnosis or recommendations. He told me that he and his colleagues were sure that Miss Anna had a complex neurological problem and were hopeful that further diligent medical examination and evaluation would soon solve it. Meanwhile she was to remain on the Neurology Ward without treatment.

Other Diagnostic Considerations

Medical conditions that can produce Catatonia include brain cancer, head trauma, encephalitis, hepatic encephalopathy, hypercalcemia, iatrogenic parkinsonism, and neuroleptic malignant syndrome. The workup for physical causes may include brain scans and lumbar puncture. Laboratory tests of liver function, serum calcium, and blood ammonia levels can help identify metabolic disease, whereas elevated serum creatine phosphokinase (CPK), white blood cell count, and serum transaminases can provide evidence of neuroleptic malignant syndrome. The results of Miss Anna's laboratory tests were all normal.

CLINICAL NOTES

Catatonia was originally thought to be a passive response of the nervous system. Psychiatry founding fathers Kraepelin and Bleuler then characterized Catatonia as a subset of Schizophrenia. However, studies have shown that fewer than ten percent of catatonic patients have an underlying diagnosis of Schizophrenia. Fifty percent or more are found to have Bipolar I Disorder with a manic, depressed, or mixed mood.

With the correct diagnosis and treatment, Mr. George and Mrs. Lucy recovered quickly and were able to return to their normal lives. However, Miss Anna did not fare so well.

Miss Anna's workup ended suddenly when her family visited from their small rural community. After they saw Anna in her hospital bed, they demanded her immediate release from the hospital. In a flash, her limp body was strapped into a wheelchair and trundled to the door of the hospital, where a small, battered white car was waiting. There her family—a weather-beaten father, a substantial mother, and a burley son—carried her to the car and placed her in the back seat. As they drove noisily from the hospital parking lot, I watched through the back window of their automobile as Anna screamed and flailed her arms. After they were gone from sight, I stood alone in the cold air until my duties called me back into the hospital, again.

CASE 22
THEY'RE KILLING ALL THE CATS!

I was attending an early morning staff meeting on a hospital psychiatric ward when a staff member from the adjacent ward burst through the door, screaming, "They're killing all the cats!"

I dashed out into the courtyard where I beheld a strange sight. About a dozen patients, most of them young women in nightgowns, were circled around a green dumpster, crying. Two patients were lying down on the wet asphalt in the path of a trash collection truck, which was trying to back up to the dumpster. The trash truck's rear hooks were extended, preparing to pick up the massive dumpster and crush its contents into the trash truck's current load of fresh garbage. The truck driver stood outside the cab of his truck, shouting at the young charge nurse, who was standing across from him with her arms crossed and her jaw set.

When I walked up and looked into the dumpster, I could hardly believe my eyes. Inside the dumpster were three soiled and crying patients and half a dozen ragged cats scurrying around, trying to avoid capture. As soon as a patient caught a cat and threw it out of the dumpster, it would hop up and jump right back in again.

I recognized the scruffy cats as strays that chronically skulked around the hospital grounds waiting for milk and food handouts put out by the patients. There had been some criticism regarding this practice, but staff members of the ward defended it as being "humane" and "therapeutic." This private ward was known as a location where patients with personality disorders could be placed, due to the close supervision and community structure.

Standing at the edge of the group, half out of the doorway, was a tall, painfully thin male patient named Louie. His white skin was almost translucent and his face was framed by shoulder-length hair died jet-black. His eyebrows were arched and his dark, sightless eyes were wide open, giving him a rather Munchian appearance. He was the one who had sounded the cat alarm by stepping into a nursing meeting and calmly saying, "I thought you might like to know that they're crushing all the cats."

Many staff considered Louie a special case and devoted more time and energy to him than their other patients. This was not the first time that a conflict had arisen while Louie was on the ward, although with his quiet, introspective demeanor, he never appeared to foment trouble directly.

I had evaluated Louie prior to his current hospital stay, after another failed suicide attempt to cut his wrists. He already had a long hospital record that showed he was a regular visitor on this ward. The chart said that he was completely blind and had to be led around the hospital by other patients and staff because he could not walk even a few steps on his own.

When I had evaluated him, Louie described a history of abandonment fears manifested in intense and unstable interpersonal relationships, where he alternately idealized and devalued his relationship partners. He endorsed habits of impulsive eating and substance abuse, and he said that he was ambivalent about his gender preference. Louie claimed to have brief, intense episodes of sadness, anger and anxiety; chronic feelings of emptiness; and frequent displays of anger. Louie's wrists and inner arms bore hundreds of angry, red scars where he habitually cut himself with a razor blade. He showed no evidence of hallucinations or delusions and he denied episodes of sadness, anhedonia, euphoria, or irritability lasting a week or more.

I administered the Personality Inventory Scale from the *Mental Status Examination for Personality Disorders* (see Chapter 8).

On his Cognitive Examination tests of *attention*, Louie was alert and Oriented but he missed two out of eight target numbers read aloud to him on a Vigilance test.

Louie showed no problems in tests of *language*.

In *memory* testing, Louie could only remember four of seven digits on a Digit Span Test, ten items of clothing on a Category Recall test, and three out of six words after five minutes on a Cued Delayed Memory test.

In tests of *abstract thinking*, Louie scored only five of eight points on Set Analysis. The Greek Cross drawing test was not performed because of his blindness.

In tests of *sequential thinking*, Louie failed a test of Serial Sevens subtraction and the Rhythm Reproduction test.

As I left the ward, Louie was at the far end of a long corridor, about twenty meters away. I could see him well outlined against a sunny window, whereas I was in comparative shadow. On a whim, I silently waved goodbye and he waved back.

CHALLENGE

Your task is to give the pale man your best diagnosis, based on the limited facts. If you like, you may also like to try to predict what happened to the cats.

SOLUTION

Louie has **Borderline Personality Disorder** (DSM-5 301.83, ICD-10 F60.3):
Five or more of the following criteria:
1. **Chronic feelings of emptiness.** Louie endorsed "chronic feelings of emptiness."
2. **Fears abandonment.** "Louie described a history of abandonment fears."
3. **Chronic, intense anger.** Louie admitted to "frequent displays of anger."
4. **Unstable interpersonal relationships characterized by idealization and devaluation.** Louie experienced "intense and unstable interpersonal relationships, where he alternately idealized and devalued his relationship partners."
5. **Unstable identity.** Louie "was ambivalent about his gender preference."
6. **Impulsivity.**
7. **Frequent suicidality or self-mutilation.** (*Suicidal behavior*): Louie was hospitalized for "another failed suicide attempt to cut his wrists." (*Self-mutilation*): Louis' wrists and inner arms "bore hundreds of angry, red scars where he habitually cut himself with a razor blade."
8. **Rapid and dramatic mood changes.** Louie said he had "brief, intense episodes of sadness, anger, and anxiety."
9. **Brief episodes of paranoia or dissociation.**

The Personality Inventory Scales confirmed Louie's diagnosis of Borderline Personality Disorder.

Other Diagnostic Considerations

Louie's presentation resembles a mood disorder, but he denied prolonged episodes of sadness, anhedonia, euphoria, or irritability necessary to diagnose unipolar Major Depressive Disorder, Dysthymia, or depressed Bipolar Disorder.

A combination of clinical skill, education, and experience are needed to accurately identify personality disorders. The general diagnostic criteria for a personality disorder are 1) aberrant relationships and interpersonal behavior; 2) abnormal ways of perceiving and interpreting self, other people, and events; 3) emotional responses that are abnormal in range, intensity, changeability, and appropriateness; and 4) poor impulse control. Louie gave evidence of all these maladaptive ways of thinking and acting.

Cognitive Testing

Louie's Cognitive Examination showed mild to moderate deficits in areas of *attention*, *memory*, *abstract thinking*, and *sequential thinking*. This broad distribution of deficits suggests three possibilities: 1) that Louie just does not do well on tests, 2) that Louie simply was not trying very hard at his testing, or 3) that there were deficits upstream in *attention* and *memory* that colored the subsequent tests, which depend on intact *attention* and *memory* function. Previous studies have found similar *attention* and *memory* deficits in populations of individuals with Borderline Personality Disorder (see Chapter 8).

CLINICAL NOTES

There were no crushed cats and there never had been any. Every morning the feral animals rooted through the dumpster for food and every morning they hopped safely out of the dumpster when the trash truck started to lift it overhead. The pale blind man had instigated the paranoia, although no one asked how he was able to see the cats being trapped.

Patients with Borderline Personality Disorder are well known for provoking emotions, controversy, and strife on inpatient hospital wards. Borderline patients suffer from chronic feelings of painful emptiness. Drama, emergencies, suicide attempts, rage episodes, and fomenting trouble increase noradrenergic release and endorphin activation, helping individuals with Borderline Personality Disorder wake up, pay attention to the world, and feel more normal. Louie's habit of cutting himself with a razor blade is a common practice among borderline personality disordered patients—they claim that it is calming and reduces anger and depression (perhaps by activating natural opiate endorphin pathways). See *Mental Status Examination for Personality Disorders* for more details.

Louie's Blindness

The supposedly blind man's sight must have been sharp indeed in order to see me waving in the dark corridor. I tested his ability to see over the succeeding months by quickly raising and lowering my eyebrows whenever I met him on the ward. He responded to my "eyebrow flag" by quickly raising and lowering *his* eyebrows. This unconscious response is a hard-wired social behavior communicating recognition in all primates. When he repeatedly raised his eyebrows in response to mine, I knew that he was seeing me.

I diagnosed Louie's feigned blindness as **Factitious Disorder Imposed on Self** (DSM-5 300.19, ICD-10 F68.10). Factitious disorder is the intentional production of symptoms motivated by the desire to assume the sick rôle. Alternative diagnoses for false blindness include Conversion Disorder (DSM-5 300.11, ICD-10 F44) and Malingering (DSM-5 V65.2, ICD-10 Z76.5). In Conversion Disorder, an apparently medical symptom occurs unintentionally in response to psychological factors or stress in the absence of any medical explanation. In Malingering, feigned symptoms are produced intentionally for material gain, such as acquiring money or avoiding work—it is often present in Antisocial Personality Disorder.

Studies have shown that individuals with Factitious Disorder usually leave treatment after being confronted. The staff said that they had a good therapeutic relationship with the pale man and they said that he was improving with treatment. I saw no reason to stir things up myself, so I did not confront him about his "blindness." I suspected that some members of his treatment team had already realized that he could see.

CASE 23
GLORIA'S FRIENDS

Gloria's parents asked me to see her in the hospital after a suicide attempt. Laboratory tests showed cocaine in her blood. The record said that she freely admitted to the Emergency Room doctor that she had sniffed cocaine frequently for one month. I found Gloria's parents getting coffee in the waiting area.

"Good morning," I began. "When did Gloria begin having problems?"

Gloria's mother replied. "About two months ago, Gloria began to say that she was always tired and she started staying in her room all the time. My husband thought she just needed a vacation but she didn't want to go to Europe. Instead, she started getting up very early and making noise so nobody could sleep. She stopped eating at the family dinner table, lost weight, and stopped participating in family activities. She stopped seeing all her old friends, even girls with whom she had grown up.

"One month ago, Gloria started staying out every night without telling us where she was going. When she came back, she always smelled like she had been drinking. We fought with her about this but she would lock herself in her room and would not come out even if we yelled at her. Her grades went downhill but she didn't seem to care. We never expected anything like this."

"Do either of you ever use cocaine?" I asked.

"We used to use cocaine about once a month at parties and Gloria saw us doing it three months ago. We went to see a counselor the very next day. My husband and I went to regular individual and family therapy sessions. We stopped using cocaine and we even stopped drinking. But it was already too late. Gloria would never see a therapist or come to family therapy with us but we went by ourselves, anyway."

Gloria's father added, "You're the first doctor she's seen about this."

When I went into her hospital room, I saw an attractive girl of about seventeen, with long, dark brown hair and stylish but rumpled clothes, sitting on the edge of the bed. Her fingernails and toenails were well-manicured but her make-up from the previous evening was smeared across her face. Even under these conditions, she had a sense of grace.

"Hello Gloria," I ventured. "They told me that you tried to kill yourself last night by jumping out a window."

"I don't remember anything from last night," Gloria said, with a sullen expression.

"And I heard that you had been taking some cocaine?"

"Yeah," Gloria rejoined. "Everybody knows that I do cocaine whenever I can get it. Sometimes I think everybody in town knows what a complete loser I am."

"Where did you go last night?"

"I went out partying with my friends."

"Do these friends have names?"

"I really don't know all their names. One guy is named Ron. I just meet them at this club I always go to. I have a good fake identification and they always buy me drinks so I'll hang around with them. And they always bring cocaine."

"When did you first use cocaine?" I queried.

"It was when I went to a party with my parents three months ago. I was grounded and they knew I would just go out if they left me at home, so they took me along to the party. There was cocaine sitting around on little silver trays and my parents were snuffing it up just like everybody else. So, I tried some when nobody was looking. For the first time in years, I felt good. Usually I feel like hell all the time, especially in the morning, even if something good happens. However, it's kept my weight down—I'm down from 127 pounds to 120."

Gloria declined to say anything else and she would not take part in my cognitive testing. I left her sitting on the bed in her hospital room.

CHALLENGE

Based on this patchwork of information, what is Gloria's diagnosis? How would you approach this patient? What would you offer as treatment?

SOLUTION

Gloria suffers from unipolar **Major Depressive Disorder, Single Episode, Severe, with Melancholic Features, Severe** (DSM-5 296.23, ICD-10 F33.2), and **Mild Cocaine Use Disorder** (DSM-5 305.60, F14.10).

Gloria met the following criteria for a **Major Depressive Episode:**
At least five of the following symptoms nearly every day for at least two weeks:
1. **A sad, depressed mood (can be irritable in children and adolescents).** Gloria said that she usually felt "like hell all the time."
2. **A loss of interest or pleasure in most activities (anhedonia).** Two months ago, one month before she began going out to use cocaine, Gloria "stayed in her room all the time," refused a trip to Europe, "stopped participating in family activities," and "stopped seeing all her old friends."
3. **A significant change in appetite or weight (e.g., a change of more than 5% of body weight per month).** One month before she began going out to use cocaine, Gloria "stopped eating at the family dinner table" and "lost weight." Gloria said, "I'm down from 127 pounds to 120." Seven pounds is more than 5% of her previous body weight, although we do not know how much weight loss is attributable to depression versus cocaine use.
4. **Insomnia or hypersomnia.** One month before she began going out to use cocaine, Gloria "started getting up very early."
5. **Psychomotor depression or agitation.**
6. **Fatigue or low energy.** One month before she began going out to use cocaine, "Gloria started saying she was always tired."
7. **Thoughts of guilt or worthlessness.** Gloria said, "Sometimes I think everybody in town knows what a complete loser I am."
8. **Difficulty concentrating or making decisions.**
9. **Recurrent thoughts of death, suicide, or a suicidal attempt or plan.** (*Suicide attempt*): Gloria was in the hospital for trying to kill herself "by jumping out a window."

The symptoms must cause a significant impairment in school, work, home, or social life; and they must include either depressed mood or anhedonia.

Gloria also satisfied criteria for **Melancholic Features**, thought by many to reflect *unipolar* major depression:
A. **Either of the following, occurring during the most severe period of the current episode:**
   1. **Loss of pleasure in all or almost all activities (anhedonia).** One month before she began going out and getting cocaine, Gloria ceased interest in travel, family activities, and her old friends in favor of staying in her room.
   2. **Lack of reactivity to usually pleasurable stimuli—does not feel much better, even temporarily, when something good happens.** Gloria said that she felt like hell, "even if something good happens."
B. **Three or more of the following**:
   1. **Distinct quality of depressed mood characterized by despondent, morose, despair, or empty mood.** Gloria said, "Usually I feel like hell." Her manner was despondent.
   2. **Depression regularly worse in the morning.** Gloria said she felt bad, "especially in the morning."
   3. **Early morning awakening at least two hours before the usual time of awakening.** One month before she began going out for cocaine, Gloria's parents noted that "she started getting up very early."
   4. **Marked psychomotor depression or agitation**.
   5. **Significant anorexia or weight loss.** One month before going out for cocaine, Gloria "stopped eating at the family dinner table" and she lost more than 5% of her previous body weight.
   6. **Excessive or inappropriate guilt.** Gloria said, "Sometimes I think everybody in town knows what a complete loser I am."

Additionally, Gloria's use of cocaine fulfilled the following criteria for **Cocaine Use Disorder:**
At least two of the following occurring within a 12-month period:
1. **The patient takes a substance in larger amounts for a longer period than intended.**
2. **The patient tries or wants to reduce substance use.**
3. **The patient spends considerable time obtaining, using, and recovering from the substance effects.**
4. **The patient feels strong urges or cravings to use the substance.**
5. **Substance use causes impairment in school, work, family, or social function.** One month ago, after Gloria started going out and using cocaine, "her grades went downhill, but she didn't seem to care."
6. **Use continues despite social problems attributable to the substance.**
7. **School, work, home, or social activities are curtailed because of the substance.**

8. **Use continues despite physical danger attributable to the substance.** Going to bars alone and staying out all night with anonymous older men who gave her cocaine could easily have been physically hazardous. Driving home under the influence also poses a serious physical hazard.
9. **Use continues despite physical or psychological problems attributable to the substance.** Gloria continued to use cocaine despite her perception that it made her look like "a complete loser." Also, Gloria's parents were yelling at her and going to individual and family therapy as a result of her continued cocaine use. However, it is not clear if her school problems and social avoidance were a direct result of depression, cocaine, or a combination of the two.
10. **Tolerance—increased amounts are needed and/or the effects of the substance decrease.**
11. **Withdrawal—characteristic withdrawal symptoms and/or substances are taken to avoid withdrawal.**
The disorder is characterized as Mild when 2-3 symptoms are present.

Other Diagnostic Considerations

Clinicians disagree about whether depression causes cocainism or cocaine causes depression. Usually these arguments center around which disorder came first or which was responsible for the bulk of the patient's symptoms. The time course of Gloria's symptoms indicates that she began having depressive symptoms a month before she began using cocaine. If I believed that Gloria's depression resulted from her drug use, her diagnosis would be Cocaine-Induced Depressive Disorder (DSM-5 292.84, ICD-10 F14.14).

The presence of many melancholic depressive symptoms are consistent with unipolar depression, which is usually quite treatable with appropriate psychotherapy and antidepressants. If Gloria was using cocaine to curb symptoms of depression, I hoped that treating her depression would help curb her interest in cocaine abuse.

CLINICAL NOTES

I wanted to develop a treatment for Gloria that would be effective for both Major Depressive Disorder and Cocaine Abuse. I also asked Gloria to go to 12-step meetings, and she agreed. We discussed her cocaine abuse, emotions, and interpersonal relationships in weekly sessions of individual Interpersonal Psychotherapy.

I chose bupropion (Wellbutrin) as an antidepressant because both bupropion and cocaine bind to the dopamine transporter protein in the corpus striatum and the norepinephrine transporter protein in the cerebral cortex. Cocaine also binds to the serotonin transporter protein and the serotonin Type 3 (5HT-3) receptor. I hoped that bupropion's similarities to cocaine might help relieve Gloria's cocaine cravings.

About 30-40% of all suicides are committed by individuals experiencing depression from unipolar Major Depressive Disorder, depressed Bipolar Disorder, Persistent Depressive Disorder, or a personality disorder. Over 50% of suicides involve drugs and alcohol. I kept close watch over Gloria's medications and asked about suicide during every session.

Fortunately, our double treatment approach was successful. Gloria kept her therapy appointments, attended meetings, returned to her school efforts, and remained euthymic and sober. She kept in touch with two depressed (but not cocaine-abusing) girlfriends she had met in the hospital and discussed her situation with them daily. Gloria's treatment was strengthened by her new friends who understood depression and by her participation in her 12-step program. After declaring that her male "cocaine friends" were "losers" and "just using me," she stopped associating with them.

Gloria's family moved away after two years. I was encouraged by a brief conversation we had at our last session.

"It will be a big change when we stop our appointments," I said. "How are you feeling, now, Gloria?"

"I feel good," Gloria replied. "It's completely different from cocaine, though. I don't feel high or even very up. I just feel like me, except not depressed. I remember feeling this way when I was a child. I think that if I had known I could feel like this again, I would never have started using cocaine in the first place."

CASE 24
SUZIE MOVES OUT

On New Year's Day, I received a call from Suzie's father.

"Doctor," Mr. Thompson said, "I need you to see my daughter in the hospital. Suzie wasn't doing well in college. In October, she left school and came back home. She was really skinny. I expected we would get closer but Suzie just locked herself in her room. She wouldn't even come down to eat. After a week, when I came home from work one evening, she wasn't in the house, and there was no letter or anything to tell me where she was or why she had left. When I didn't get a call, I searched everywhere with the help of the police and all my friends, but we couldn't find her. Finally, I gave up looking and figured that she would call me when she ran out of money. Yesterday, I was driving around the back of my bank to park and I saw her sitting in a little alcove around a boarded-up door they never use. I made her get in the car and I took her to the hospital."

I saw 22-year-old Suzie on the psychiatric ward of a major private hospital. Her chart said that she had signed into the hospital weighing 100 pounds (down from her usual weight of 125) and that she denied having a menstrual period for the last three months. Her chart showed no prior history of mental or emotional treatment, and the Emergency Room staff had drawn laboratory tests that cleared her of general medical disorders. Urine drug and alcohol screens were negative.

When I interviewed Suzie, she told me that she had taken up residence in this doorway a few days after leaving her home and had spent the last three months living there. Suzie said that she sat motionless in the bank doorway all day long despite the cold and inclement weather, drinking water from a nearby park fountain at night, and occasionally eating food she found in nearby garbage cans. She used the public restrooms at the park late at night, but if she could not hold her urine during the day, she would just discharge it in her pants. When I asked her what she did all day, sitting there in that tiny space, she smiled and said, "I daydream. Just daydream."

Suzie spoke very softly during her interview and stayed curled up in her chair, barely moving. Her affect was bright and effusive. Suzie would occasionally laugh as if at some personal joke, even when the topic was serious or sad. She denied feeling depressed, hopeless, anxious, irritable, or angry. When I asked her how she *did* feel, she smiled and said, "Dreamy. Just dreamy."

Suzie denied any thoughts of violence to herself or others. When asked if she heard any voices or saw any visions, she turned her head and looked at me coyly, with a slight smile on her face. When she muttered under her breath and tracked unseen objects around the room, she appeared to be responding to unseen stimuli.

When I asked about her weight, Suzie's face clouded and she seemed ready to cry. "I just can't get rid of this awful fat, no matter what I do."

"What fat do you mean?" I asked, looking at her emaciated frame.

"This horrible fat," Suzie replied. She slowly drew her pajama top up to her breasts and revealed folds of skin hanging around the area where her waist used to be. "I just hate this fat," she said sorrowfully.

I completed a brief neurological examination that was unremarkable.

In Cognitive Examination tests of *attention,* Suzie failed the Vigilance test.

In *language* testing, Suzie failed Object Part Naming because she could not name the parts of a watch or pen. Her Quality of Speech was rapid and tangential, showed a tendency to stray from the point. She demonstrated blocking or derailment, spending long moments in pauses between words where she appeared to be lost in thought.

In her *memory* evaluation, Suzie failed Digit Span and the Four Presidents test, and she could not remember any of the six target words in a test of Cued Delayed Memory.

Suzie failed all the tests of *abstract thinking*. In response to the proverb, "Never cry over spilt milk," she smiled and gave the irrelevant reply, "Don't be discouraged if it's raining. Tomorrow will be sunny." To the proverb "A barking dog never bites," she giggled and said, "I like doggies." Suzie could not perform Set Analysis and when she was read a test of Judgment, she burst into giggles. Her Greek Cross drawing looked like a scribble.

After failing the Serial Sevens subtraction test of *sequential thinking*, Suzie declined further testing.

To the nurses' chagrin, I wrote no orders for sleeping medications. When I returned early the next morning, I was told that Suzie had neither eaten nor slept. Instead, she had wandered around the ward all night in her pajamas, singing softly to herself. Now, she waited patiently for her interview. When I sat down across from her, she smiled and said, "I can read your mind."

"Oh?" I smiled. "If you can read my mind, then what am I thinking now?"

Her face lit up, and she seemed delighted. "I know what it is," she said, smiling. "You're thinking that you're in love with me."

CHALLENGE

What is going on with Suzie? Those of you who have treated many such cases before may find this easy—some others with different experience may not. Based on this evaluation, what diagnosis would you give, how would you confirm your diagnosis, and what treatment would you offer?

SOLUTION

Suzie is experiencing **Bipolar I Disorder, Most Recent Episode Manic, with Psychotic Features** (DSM-5 296.44, ICD-10 F31.2) and **Anorexia Nervosa, Restricting Type** (DSM-5 307.1, ICD-10 F50.01):

Suzie's initial symptoms confirmed that she was having a **Psychotic Episode** of unknown origin:
1. **Delusions**. Suzie thought that she could read my mind but she could not. Also, despite her "emaciated frame," Suzie thought that she was fat.
2. **Hallucinations**. Suzie "muttered under her breath and tracked unseen objects around the room," appearing to be "responding to unseen stimuli." When asked what she did all day, she said, "I daydream. Just daydream."
3. **Disorganized speech—such as frequent derailment or incoherence**. (*Derailment*): "She spent long moments in pauses between words where she appeared to be lost in thought," illustrating "blocking or derailment."
4. **Grossly disorganized or catatonic behavior**.
5. **Negative symptoms such as flat affect, alogia (muteness or minimal speech), or avolition (lack of motivation)**. (*Avolition*): Suzie demonstrated avolition by sitting "motionless in the bank doorway all day long" without moving or visiting the restroom, "despite the cold and inclement weather."

Suzie also met the following criteria for a **Manic Episode**:
A. **The following have been present most of the day nearly every day:**
Increased goal-directed activity or energy. Susie wandered through the park at night and stayed up walking all night in the hospital.
Plus at least one of these:
    a. **Elevated mood.** "Suzie would occasionally laugh as if at some personal joke, even when the topic was serious or sad."
    b. **Expansive mood.** Suzie's "affect was bright and effusive."
    c. **Irritable mood.**
These symptoms last at least one week or any duration if hospitalization is necessary. Suzie's condition had been persistent for two months and it was now so severe that she required hospitalization.
B. **At least three of the following symptoms (four if the mood is only irritable):**
    1. **Inflated self-esteem or grandiosity.** (*Grandiosity*): Suzie thought that she had the power to read my mind.
    2. **A decreased need for sleep (needs <3 hours).** Instead of sleeping, Suzie "wandered around the ward all night in her pajamas, singing softly to herself."
    3. **Talking more than usual or interrupting others (pressured speech).**
    4. **Rapid or racing thoughts.**
    5. **Distractibility.** Suzie's tangential, blocked speech, her daydreaming, and her performance on the Cognitive Examination all indicated distractibility (see below).
    6. **Increased goal-directed activity or psychomotor agitation.** (*Psychomotor agitation*): Walking all night is evidence of psychomotor agitation.
    7. **Excessive involvement in activities that have a high potential for painful consequences (costly or risky impulsive actions).**

Suzie also met the following criteria for **Anorexia Nervosa, Restricting Type**:
Restriction of energy intake causing significantly low body weight. Suzie "signed into the hospital weighing 100 pounds (down from her usual weight of 125);" a body mass of only 80% of her usual expected weight.
Intense fear of gaining weight or becoming fat, or persistent behavior that interferes with weight gain. Suzie was very upset about her perceived excessive weight and "fat," despite the fact that she was "emaciated."

Disturbed perception of body weight/shape, excessive importance attached to body weight/shape, or denial of the seriousness of low body weight. (*Disturbed perception*): Suzie perceived her "emaciated frame" with "folds of skin hanging around the area where her waist used to be" as larded with fat.

Anorexia can be diagnosed in the presence of other mental disorders, and Restricting Type or Binge-Eating/Purging Type should be specified. In this case, Anorexia Nervosa was present in the context of a psychotic bipolar episode and may have been caused by it or may have developed on its own.

Other Diagnostic Considerations

Bipolar Disorder, Schizophrenia, Schizophreniform Disorder, Schizoaffective Disorder, Brief Psychotic Disorder, severe Major Depressive Disorder, Acute and Posttraumatic Stress Disorders, Schizotypal Personality Disorder, Substance Use Disorders, and brain diseases can all cause psychosis. As her psychosis resolved, Suzie's grandiosity, insomnia, distractibility, and anorexia persisted, and she demonstrated a full complement of bipolar symptoms.

Anorexia Nervosa is sometimes confused with Bulimia Nervosa. In DSM-5, Bulimia Nervosa cannot be diagnosed if the patient meets the criteria for Anorexia Nervosa. To make the diagnosis of Bulimia Nervosa, a patient must have recurrent episodes of binge eating with recurrent compensatory behaviors (self-induced vomiting; abuse of laxatives, diuretics, or enemas; fasting; or excessive exercise) at least twice a week for three months.

Cognitive Testing

Blocking, derailment, and tangential speech all result when the thread of conscious thought is interrupted by distractions. Tests of Vigilance, Digit Span, Cued Delayed Memory, and Serial Sevens Subtraction all require the testee to hold several items in working memory at the same time, and are therefore vulnerable to distractibility. Distractibility is a diagnostic criterion for a Manic Episode. In the Proverbs Interpretation test I have often seen individuals with Bipolar Disorder make incorrect interpretations consisting of proverbs, sayings, and other irrelevant material.

CLINICAL NOTES

I initially placed Suzie on a low dose of an atypical antipsychotic to treat her psychosis. After a few days, Suzie's psychosis began to clear and her bipolar symptoms remained. At this time, I placed Suzie on a mood–stabilizing medication (lithium salts, carbamazepine/Tegretol, valproate/Depakote, etc.). When her bipolar symptoms began to resolve, I withdrew the unneeded antipsychotic medicine. After she was clear, we began psychoeducation therapy to help her understand her illness, medications, and the importance of maintaining regular sleep, meals, and exercise.

I have frequently seen eating disorders in conjunction with Bipolar Disorder. In some cases, the weight loss is a consequence of staying up days without sleeping, a manic failure to eat, obsessive hyperfocus on thinness, or a grandiose need for the body to be perfect. In many of these cases, bringing the Bipolar Disorder under control provided relief from the eating disorder. In less fortunate patients, the eating disorder persisted after the bipolar symptoms resolved, leaving clinicians to treat the eating disorder on its own.

Fortunately, Suzie's body perception and fear of fatness normalized as her manic symptoms remitted with mood-stabilizing medication. Soon she was discharged into outpatient treatment and her father's care.

CHAPTER 5
THE MENTAL STATUS EXAMINATION IN THE CLINIC

Clinics may be associated with hospitals and university medical centers or they may be freestanding public and private institutions. They usually provide clinicians with a steady diet of patients—some with new diagnostic challenges, others with long-standing diagnoses and stable treatment plans, and still others with incorrect diagnoses and histories of ineffective, inappropriate treatments. The successful clinic-based clinician must be an effective member of a team consisting of other clinicians, support staff, administrators, and the patient population.

CASE 25
IS FATHER LOSING HIS MIND?

Mr. Green was a 69-year-old man who was brought by his daughter Jill to see me at an Alzheimer's Disease Clinic in a large, university teaching hospital. Jill had made an urgent appointment after a disturbing incident the night before, when she could not arouse her father from sleep. When she was finally able to wake him, he had remained in a slowed, disoriented state for several hours. After he finally arose from bed, he stumbled and he seemed to lack coordination.

Jill filled me in on the background details. Mr. Green had been living alone since his wife had died six months ago. His daily routine included an early morning walk, conversing with neighbors, grocery shopping at a market down the block, and watching his favorite television in the evenings. He enjoyed visiting a local seniors' center once a week. For years, he had consumed a glass of wine two or three times a week. His daughter visited every two weeks for dinner and conversation, during which time she took care of any chores that were difficult for Mr. Green to perform alone. She assured me that her father had been alert and mentally active at her visit two weeks ago.

Mr. Green had seen his primary care physician just 10 days before seeing me. At that time, his physical examination and basic laboratory tests were normal.

Mr. Green was being treated with the beta-blocker propranolol (Inderal) 20 mg daily for hypertension, the benzodiazepine diazepam (Valium) 2.5 mg daily for anxiety, and the benzodiazepine-like zolpidem (Ambien) 10 mg nightly for sleep. Mr. Green had recently been troubled with allergies and was taking an over-the-counter cold preparation containing 25 mg of the antihistamine diphenhydramine (Benadryl) twice daily. The last chart note mentioned that the patient appeared somewhat slowed and less sharp than usual, and consequently Mr. Green's primary physician had requested a consultation from a neurologist in his medical group.

Mr. Green had seen the neurologist one week prior to seeing me. At that time he had complained of feeling slowed down. His neurological examination was unremarkable. A computerized tomography (CT) scan and a magnetic resonance imaging (MRI) scan done at that time were normal. The neurologist prescribed the nonsedating antidepressant fluoxetine (Prozac), 20 mg daily. She told Mr. Green that if he wasn't feeling better in six weeks to call for a prescription of mirtazapine (Remeron) 15 mg daily, which she said was good for both depression and anxiety.

My brief neurological examination was also normal.

In our Diagnostic Examination, Mr. Green appeared lackadaisical. He said that he was sleeping very well and that his appetite was good. He denied attention problems, sadness, anxiety, or anger. He harbored no suicidal or violent thoughts and he denied auditory or visual hallucinations.

In his Cognitive Examination of *attention*, Mr. Green failed tests of Orientation and Vigilance.

Mr. Green's *language* testing was normal, but his responses were slow.

In *memory* testing, Mr. Green could only remember two of the seven numbers read to him on the Digit Span test. He was not able to recall the most recent Four Presidents and he could only recall eight items of clothing in 30 seconds in the Category Recall test. Mr. Green could only remember two of six words after one minute on a test of Cued Delayed Memory.

In *abstract thinking* tests, Mr. Green gave up Simple Arithmetic after 30 seconds. His drawing of a Greek Cross was poorly proportioned, earning a score of only two out of eight points. He declined to do Proverb Interpretation, Set Analysis, or Judgment tasks.

In *sequential thinking* tasks, Mr. Green could perform only three steps of a Four-Step Sequential Command and gave up completely after failing a test of Serial Sevens subtraction.

On the Folstein Mini-Mental Status Examination, Mr. Green exhibited significant cognitive impairment, with an overall score of 12 out of 30. His scores on individual sections of the Folstein Mini-Mental Examination resembled his performance on his Cognitive Examination.

CHALLENGE

In an ideal clinical world, we would defer our decision-making until we had contacted both the primary physician and the neurologist. However, with no more information than you have, see if you can determine the cause of Mr. Green's problems.

SOLUTION

Mr. Green is suffering from iatrogenic sedation from multiple sedative medications. He qualifies for the diagnosis of **Propranolol, Diphenhydramine, Alcohol, Zolpidem, and Diazepam Intoxication** (DSM-5 292.89, ICD-10 F13.929).

Mr. Green met the following criteria for **Sedative, Hypnotic, and Anxiolytic Intoxication**:

A. **Recent ingestion of a sedative, hypnotic, or anxiolytic**. (*Sedative*): The propranolol (Inderal) Mr. Green took for his blood pressure is sedating and this effect is amplified in seniors. The diphenhydramine (Benadryl) contained in his over-the-counter cold medicine, has powerful sedative effects in many patients. Mr. Green "consumed a glass of wine two or three times a week"— the criteria for Alcohol Intoxication are the same as those for Sedative Intoxication. In addition, alcohol may prolong the half-life of other sedatives. (*Hypnotic*): Zolpidem (Ambien) is a sedative that is marketed as a hypnotic for sleep. Initially, zolpidem may have been a reasonable choice for this elder man because it is gone from the body in less than nine hours. However, fluoxetine (Prozac) can lengthen zolpidem's half-life by almost 20%. (*Anxiolytic*): Diazepam (Valium) is a sedative that is marketed for anxiety. Although it was given in small doses, it is eliminated so slowly that it can accumulate in the bloodstream. It has a typical half-life in seniors of 50-90 hours. The sedative effects of all these medications are additive, giving Mr. Green a very large sedative effect.

B. **Clinically significant maladaptive behavioral or psychological changes that developed during, or shortly after, sedative, hypnotic, or anxiolytic use**. Initially, Mr. Green could not be aroused, and then he was disoriented for hours.

C. **One (or more) of the following signs, developing during, or shortly after, sedative, hypnotic, or anxiolytic use:**
  1. **Slurred speech.**
  2. **Incoordination.** In the initial incident, Mr. Green "seemed to lack coordination."
  3. **Unsteady gait.**
  4. **Nystagmus.**
  5. **Impairment in *attention* or *memory*.** In cognitive testing, Mr. Green failed *attention* tests of Orientation and Vigilance. He also failed *memory* tests of Digit Span, recall of Four Presidents, Category Recall, and Cued Delayed Memory.
  6. **Stupor or coma.** Initially, Mr. Green's daughter "could not arouse her father from sleep." Then "he had remained in a slowed, disoriented state for several hours."

D. **The symptoms are not due to another medical condition or another mental disorder**. Mr. Green had been seen by his primary care physician and a neurologist who found no physical problems. "A computerized tomography (CT) scan and a magnetic resonance imaging (MRI) scan...were normal."

When coding Substance-Related Disorders, use the specific names of the substances (propranolol, diphenhydramine, alcohol, zolpidem, and diazepam) rather than the general categories Sedatives, Hypnotics, and Anxiolytics.

Other Diagnostic Considerations

The appearance of impaired consciousness in an elder suggests Delirium, which is an emergency condition. If you had given Mr. Green the diagnosis of Delirium and recommended a trip to the Emergency Room, you would have erred in a safe direction and protected Mr. Green. However, the diagnosis of Delirium requires that the changes in consciousness and cognition occur within hours to days, whereas Mr. Green had begun to appear slowed down at his primary care appointment 10 days ago. Infection, metabolic imbalance, covert cancer, and other causes of Delirium are less likely considering that Mr. Green had just been cleared by two other physicians who performed examinations, scans, and laboratory tests.

The neurologist made an erroneous diagnosis of unipolar Major Depressive Disorder, Single Depressive Episode, based on Mr. Green's psychomotor depression. However, Mr. Green did not exhibit the two prerequisites for unipolar Major Depressive Disorder—he denied dysphoria and he enjoyed his usual, active, and sociable daily routine, ruling out anhedonia. Most importantly, the neurologist failed to rule out a medical cause of the patient's condition (sedating medications), which excludes the diagnosis of Major Depressive Disorder altogether.

In elders who have an abnormal Folstein Mini-Mental Status Examination, many clinicians think of Alzheimer's Disease. However, Alzheimer's Disease appears gradually and persistently and neither the primary physician nor the neurologist had reported any cognitive decline just two weeks earlier. Furthermore, Mr. Green's daughter denied noticing any such decline until the day before she brought her father to my office.

Cerebrovascular Disease can present suddenly, but the diagnosis requires the presence of strokes, deficits in *sequential thinking*, and evidence of Vascular Disease from the history, physical examination, and/or imaging studies. Mr. Green did not have a history of small declines and recoveries over time that is usually seen in cerebrovascular disease. There were no observable deficits on either the neurologist's examination or my brief examination and Mr. Green's recent CT and MRI scans showed no evidence of infarcts.

A single stroke could explain Mr. Green's symptoms, but he showed none of the impairment in *language* such as aphasias (see Chapter 2) that are often seen after a stroke. Furthermore, his neurological examinations were normal and his scans showed no evidence of a recent stroke. Although there is no way to rule out a very small stroke, the presence of so many sedating drugs is sufficient to explain all his symptoms.

Cognitive Testing

The key to understanding Mr. Green's condition was his poor Level of Consciousness with slowed and confused thinking. Mr. Green's Cognitive Examination showed significant deficits in *attention* and *memory* that caused poor *abstract thinking* and *sequential thinking*, rather than a focal pattern that could be associated with a localized deficit or injury.

CLINICAL NOTES

Mr. Green was taking three prescription sedatives. Over-the-counter antihistaminic and anticholinergic allergy medications are also notorious for lowering the level of consciousness in elders. The combination of all these sedatives plus an alcoholic drink was enough to push Mr. Green into a stupor that was revealed when his daughter unsuccessfully tried to rouse him. There was no evidence of a mental or emotional disorder.

The neurologist invited Mr. Green to call for a prescription of mirtazapine (Remeron) if he wasn't feeling better. Mirtazapine is a tetracyclic antidepressant with serotonin, norepinephrine, and strongly sedating antihistamine properties, which would only have exacerbated Mr. Green's sedation.

Mr. Green may have also been experiencing a condition called "sundowning." Sundowning is a decrease in the level of consciousness and attention that some elders experience around dusk and early in the morning when light levels and sensory stimulation are at a minimum. This phenomenon can be combated by opening blinds in the morning, installing brighter lights, and encouraging seniors to schedule their daily activities like waking, meals, exercise, and bedtime at the same times every day. Orientation can often be improved by installing large wall calendars and clocks, and playing news and talk shows on radio and television, to help provide clues to the date and passage of time during the day.

Mr. Green's sedated condition placed him at risk for a fall. Fall-related injuries are the most common cause of accidental death in those over the age of 65. Falls account for over 600,000 deaths per year, worldwide.

Elders often see many physicians and they tend to collect multiple medications. During my tenure at the Alzheimer's Disease Clinic, I found that over half of my patients' cognition returned to normal or near-normal after their excessive, overlapping medications were slowly discontinued. In Mr. Green's case, after tapering his diazepam, zolpidem, fluoxetine, and his over-the-counter antihistaminic cold medicine, Mr. Green began to look and act like his usual self, again.

CASE 26
PAT'S PROBLEMS COME BACK

I saw Pat at a community outpatient mental health clinic. This clinic was notable for serving a high proportion of homeless and treatment-naïve persons and a large number of caseworkers were employed to meet the clients' needs. Medical treatment was challenging because of the clients' hesitancy to accept care, their ignorance of available services, and the simple difficulty of locating and transporting patients to their appointments.

Pat presented a number of challenges in diagnosis and treatment. He frequently could not be found for his appointments and the notes in his medical chart were made by many different clinicians. Pat himself was a poor historian—he was chronically homeless, refused placement in board and care homes, and wandered through the streets during all hours of the day and night. Nevertheless, he insisted that he had finished high school in a prestigious private academy and that his family members were wealthy. He could not state the reason why he had not gone on to higher education and he said he could no longer recall the telephone numbers or addresses of his family members. Most of the clinic staff scoffed at his high-sounding statements.

Pat came with an old diagnosis of **Schizophrenia** (DSM-5 295.90, ICD-10 F20.9), although there was no longer any diagnostic information in his medical chart to reveal why that diagnosis had been made. One note in his chart mentioned a teenage hospitalization for a severe motor vehicle accident, and I ordered past records from that hospital.

Pat's caseworker's notes suggested the diagnosis of **Intermittent Explosive Disorder** (DSM-5 312.34, ICD-10 F63.81). Pat had a history of aggressive episodes, which sometimes resulted in incarcerations for assault or violence. Other times, Pat would seem to disappear for days or weeks. During these interruptions, Pat was out of contact with the clinic, so he had no continuous care.

The clinic's Director of Social Services told me that Pat suffered from mental impairment as a result of chronic **Severe Alcohol Use Disorder** (DSM-5 303.90, ICD-10 F10.20), although this was not listed in his chart. When I tested Pat with a hand-held Breathalyzer, he was not intoxicated, and several urine screening tests were negative for alcohol or drugs of abuse.

Pat's interactions with female staff were frequently inappropriate—too personal, too sexual, or just uninterpretable. He only recognized the Social Services director and me—he treated other people as if they were new acquaintances. Pat's conversation was peculiarly perseverative. Each time he came to the clinic, he would talk incessantly about some topic, repeating the same sentences over and over. On his next visit, he would have forgotten about the previous topic and he would perseverate about something else.

Pat had persistent fears about medications and physicians. He refused injections and he had an aversion to taking oral medicine. He presented on several occasions with visual hallucinations, usually of faces that he saw in the clinic clock. Once he came to the clinic with the complaint that unseen insects were biting him.

In his Diagnostic Examination, Pat appeared disheveled and poorly groomed. His hygiene was poor and his clothes smelled of stale beer. When asked about his sleeping habits, he said, "When I get tired, I lie down and sleep wherever I am."

Pat exhibited an obvious tremor but he denied any physical problems including pounding heart, shortness of breath, dizziness, sweating, or chest pain. He denied problems with attention, hyperactivity, or impulsivity. Pat's affect was labile, vacillating between elation, paranoia, and rage during the course of his appointments. He denied sadness, anxiety, or irritability. He also denied suicidal ideation, and I could not find any history of suicidal intentions, plans, or attempts.

In his Cognitive Examination of *attention,* Pat failed Orientation. His responses were distractible, confused, and he treated his evaluation as if it were a big joke, laughing and making side remarks.

In the *language* section, Pat failed tests of Verbal Registration and Immediate Repetition, and Object and Part Naming, but he understood and complied with a written command to "Close Your Eyes." Pat's Quality of Speech was halting and hoarse and required considerable effort. His speech style was spare, and he mainly used nouns and verbs with few modifying words.

Pat complained about the poor state of his *memory*—he was only able to repeat four of seven numbers in a test of Digit Span. Pat failed to recall Four Presidents or remember any words in Uncued or Cued Delayed Memory tests.

The only other tests that Pat would try were the *abstract thinking* test of Simple Arithmetic and the *sequential thinking* test of Serial Sevens substitution—he failed both.

Pat's treatment options were limited. He was too cognitively impaired and too unreliable to take part in psychotherapy. Pat refused to take depot injections and he was unreliable in his ability to take oral medications. He often lost his prescriptions or emptied the bottle in a state of confusion. In an attempt to provide control for alcohol withdrawal, poor attention, labile moods, and explosive behavior, I prescribed clonidine patches (Catapres TTS). These were applied to Pat's arm and changed by his caseworker weekly. This regimen proved to be remarkably effective for six months. Pat's follow-ups were more regular and he appeared at his appointments well-groomed and better dressed. During this time, Pat's emotions were less labile, according to his caseworker, and he was not incarcerated. Pat was able to participate in clinic programs and his life quality improved significantly.

After six months, his caseworker changed and Pat's mental health returned to its former, impaired state. He and his caseworker confirmed that he was taking the same medication that had been helpful before. When he came to the clinic, he had new complaints of severe stomachache and headache, particularly after taking his medication.

CHALLENGE

See if you can determine Pat's diagnosis. Then, try to imagine why his successful medication regimen failed. Many explanations are possible—try to find one that fits all the information presented here.

SOLUTION

Pat suffered from **Major Neurocognitive Disorder with Behavioral Disturbance** (DSM-5 294.11 ICD-10 F02.81) due to an **Unspecified Neurocognitive Disorder** (DSM-5 799.59, ICD-10 R41.9). When records from his early hospitalization were found and downloaded, they confirmed the diagnosis of **Traumatic Brain Injury** (ICD-10 S06.2X9S),

Pat met the following criteria for **Major Neurocognitive Disorder**:

- **A significant quantifiable decline in *attention, language, memory, abstract thinking, sequential thinking*, or social function.** (*Attention*): Pat failed Orientation. (*Language*): Pat had Broca's aphasia. See below. (*Memory*): Pat often forgot to take oral medications and he forgot many clinic appointments. On his Cognitive Examination, Pat failed *memory* tests of Digit Span, Four Presidents, Uncued Delayed Memory, and Cued Delayed Memory. (*Abstract thinking*): Pat also failed Simple Arithmetic, a test of *abstract thinking*. (*Sequential thinking*): Pat failed Serial Sevens, a test of *sequential thinking*. (*Social function*): "Pat only recognized the Social Services director and me—he treated other people as if they were new acquaintances." The inability to recognize faces is called *prosopagnosia*.
- **These deficits interfere with the patient's ability to be independent in his or her everyday activities (e.g., paying bills or managing medications).** Pat lived on the street—he could not hold a job or manage his own health care without help.

Other Diagnostic Considerations

Pat's diagnosis of Schizophrenia was incorrect—although he reported hallucinations and his speech was disorganized, these were due to his past Traumatic Brain Injury compounded by his lifestyle and possible substance use. Schizophrenia cannot be diagnosed if symptoms are due to a another medical disorder such as Traumatic Brain Injury.

Pat's caseworker noted his intermittent explosive episodes involving abusive language, assault, and violence. However, the diagnosis of Intermittent Explosive Disorder cannot be made in the presence of a another medical condition such as Traumatic Brain Injury.

The clinic's Director of Social Services implied that Pat suffered from Alcohol Use Disorder. Pat certainly failed to fulfill the usual rôle obligations of work and home life and he had recurrent legal problems with arrests for assault and violence. However, Pat's breathalyzer and his urine drug and alcohol screening tests were always negative.

Cognitive Testing

Pat's Cognitive Examination revealed deficits in areas of *attention, memory, abstract thinking,* and *sequential thinking*, but his most important and revealing deficits were in the area of *language*. Pat suffered from Broca's aphasia. His verbal and written comprehension was intact but his oral repetition and naming were impaired. His speech was halting, hoarse (dysarthric), and made up mostly of nouns and verbs in a telegraphic style. Broca's aphasia is typically caused by an injury in Broca's area of the brain, in the anterior language cortex, perisylvian cortex, and insula.

CLINICAL NOTES

When records from his early hospitalization were downloaded, we learned that Pat had functioned well until his late teens when he was hit by a bus and suffered closed head Traumatic Brain Injury. After his accident, Pat dropped out of sight until he appeared at out clinic. In addition to Broca's aphasia and cognitive impairment, Pat demonstrated many behaviors that are often associated with the sequelae of Traumatic Brain Injury, including inappropriate affect, labile mood, restlessness, impulsivity, perseverative thought, poor abstract thinking, and poor social judgment. I have often heard patients with organic brain deficits tell me of seeing faces in clocks and feeling insects crawl on their skin. Pat had numerous other risk factors for organicity, including head injuries from fights, malnutrition, past medication overdoses, and unproven substance use.

I prescribed an "alpha-agonist" (clonidine/Catapres) to Pat. Alpha-agonists are frequently used in treating high blood pressure and Attention-Deficit Hyperactivity Disorder. By reducing the amount of norepinephrine released from the brainstem (*locus ceruleus*), they can improve attention, reduce hyperactivity, diminish rage, and decrease impulsivity. Alpha-agonists may also have mood stabilization effects. The use of a patch delivery system, where medication under an adhesive patch gradually travels through the skin into the bloodstream, was ideal for Pat because he disliked and was unreliable at taking oral medications and the patch could be managed by his caseworker, who visited him and changed the patch weekly.

Helping patients comply with their medication, psychotherapy, and social treatment is essential to achieve remission of mental and emotional symptoms. In outpatient clinics, an unscheduled change or discontinuation of medication is often followed by a patient's sudden relapse. Medication changes also occur when patients run out of medications unexpectedly, cannot remember to take their medications, divide their doses to make their prescriptions last longer, stop or start cigarette smoking, change their diet, or change the time and method of dosing. Unfortunately, clinicians are seldom informed about these changes.

Pat's first caseworker met with him weekly and helped him take off old patches and put the new patches on his arms. During this time, he was able to maintain steady state medication levels and his health improved. When Pat was assigned a new caseworker, she merely handed the patches to him each week and told him to use them. Poor Pat forgot what to do and he was eating his weekly patches instead of applying them to the skin of his arms as directed. This accounted for his decompensation and his severe stomachache and headache.

After educating his caseworker about Pat's pharmacological treatment, Pat resumed using his patches correctly and quickly returned to his former, improved mental status.

CASE 27
WHAT HAPPENED TO SARAH?

Sarah was a middle-aged patient who was assigned to the public clinic where I worked. Sarah was receiving public services under the diagnosis of **Schizophrenia** (DSM-5 295.90, ICD-10 F20.9) and mild **Intellectual Disability** (DSM-5 319, ICD-10 F70). She was living at a boarding home and remained stable on a relatively high dose of an antipsychotic plus an anticholinergic (benztropine/Cogentin) for potential antipsychotic-induced movement disorders. She was also receiving a benzodiazepine sedative (lorazepam/Ativan) for anxiety and insomnia. Staff generally considered her to be a "chronic case" who was not expected to do any better. Surprisingly, I was unable to find any diagnostic work-up in her voluminous chart.

Sarah was very sociable and she had many friends among the clinic staff and other clinic patients. She engaged them in long, animated conversations where she did most of the talking. She acted younger than her age and tried to engage male staff members in sexual flirtations.

In her Diagnostic Examination, Sarah was distractible, disinhibited, and activated, frequently rising from her chair and walking around my office despite the sedative properties of her medications. She had an almost unending list of questions to ask me about toxic substances in the air and she lectured me about their consequences for her health. Sarah complained that she only slept an hour or two per night but she did not seem too worried about it. She carelessly endorsed all of the physical symptoms in my examination, including pounding heart, dizziness, lightheadedness, excessive sweating, chest pain, feelings of detachment, nausea, stomachache, shortness of breath, tingling fingers and face, trembling and shaking, chills and hot flushes, easy fatigability, muscle tension, poor focus, and feeling keyed-up and edgy. "Most of the time I just feel like jumping out of my skin," she confided.

Sarah said that she was distractible but denied other characteristics of inattention. However, she endorsed all the criteria for Attention-Deficit/Hyperactivity Disorder, Predominantly Hyperactive-Impulsive Type. She denied sadness and repeated several jokes at the expense of certain clinic staff. Sometimes she laughed for no apparent reason. However, her optimistic outlook was punctuated with bursts of anger addressing the uncaring nature of persons outside the interview. She had seen so many mental health professionals that she denied hearing voices before being asked.

On her Cognitive Examination, Sarah was alert but quite distractible. In tests of *attention*, Sarah knew the year and month but she could not tell me the correct date or time. When asked to hold up her hand on a test of Basic Verbal Comprehension, sometimes she held it up and sometimes she did not. She failed a test of Vigilance.

In the *language* section, Sarah's Quality of Speech was notable for being loud, voluble, and tending to veer off topic. She declined to perform any more tests.

I was not satisfied with Sarah's behavior or diagnosis. Over many months, I gradually reduced her dose of antipsychotic, anticholinergic, and benzodiazepine sedative. She became even more activated but there was no significant change in her other symptoms.

CHALLENGE

Like many long-standing public clinic patients, Sarah came with very little in the way of history or records to justify her diagnosis and treatment. She had no family or friends who could provide information about her history, and the members of the clinic seemed to have already agreed on a clinical formulation to explain her condition. However, I was not convinced of her diagnosis. See if you can determine what was really going on with Sarah.

SOLUTION

Sarah has chronic, untreated **Bipolar I Disorder, Most Recent Episode Manic, Severe** (DSM-5 296.43, ICD-10 F31.13):

A. The following have been present most of the day nearly every day:
Increased goal-directed activity or energy. Sarah was agitated during the day and stayed up most of the night.
Plus at least one of these:
    a. Elevated mood. "Sometimes she laughed for no apparent reason."
    b. Expansive mood. Sarah's manner was joking and her outlook was "optimistic."
    c. Irritable mood. Her mood was "punctuated with bursts of anger."
These symptoms last at least one week or any duration if hospitalization is necessary.
B. At least three of the following symptoms (four if the mood is only irritable):

1. **Inflated self-esteem or grandiosity.** (*Self-esteem*): Sarah treated clinic staff like peers—she was remarkably self-assured. (*Grandiosity*): She lectured her doctor on topics of environmental medicine.
2. **A decreased need for sleep (needs <3 hours).** "She only slept an hour or two per night, but she did not seem too worried about it."
3. **Talking more than usual or interrupting others (pressured speech).** (*More talkative*): Sarah was "voluble" and engaged others "in long, animated conversations." (*Pressured*): Her pressured speech was evidenced in conversations where "she did all of the talking."
4. **Rapid or racing thoughts.**
5. **Distractibility.** Sarah seemed distractible in her examination, and her speech tended to "veer off topic." She did poorly on cognitive tests of *attention*.
6. **Increased goal-directed activity or psychomotor agitation.**
7. **Excessive involvement in activities that have a high potential for painful consequences (costly or risky impulsive actions).** (*Socially*): Sarah engaged others "in long, animated conversations." (*Sexually*): Sarah "tried to engage male staff members in sexual flirtations." (*Psychomotor agitation*): Sarah demonstrated psychomotor agitation by "frequently rising from her chair and walking around my office" and by her statement that she felt "like jumping out of my skin."

Sarah's symptoms severely impair her potential to go to school, work, or maintain normal family relationships. These manic symptoms have been present for years.

Other Diagnostic Considerations

There are many people like Sarah who carry incorrect diagnoses of Schizophrenia when they actually suffer from Bipolar Disorder, brain diseases, and other problems. These individuals do not receive the treatment they need and the inappropriate schizophrenic medications and management often make their conditions worse. A diagnosis of Schizophrenia requires the presence of delusions, hallucinations, disorganized speech (with frequent blocking or incoherence), grossly disorganized or catatonic behavior, or negative symptoms (flat affect, mutism, or lack of motivation). Sarah showed none of these. Sarah's concern about air pollution was within cultural norms. Sarah also seemed too socially engaged for a diagnosis of Schizophrenia. Schizophrenia cannot be diagnosed in the presence of Bipolar Manic, Mixed, or Depressed Episodes.

Sarah's erroneous diagnosis of mild Intellectual Disability was predicated on staff observations of her poor function. She failed to meet sociocultural standards for personal independence and social responsibility because of her untreated Bipolar Disorder, not because of a developmental disability. Her cognitive problems were caused by her Bipolar Disorder and her sedating antipsychotic, anticholinergic, and anxiolytic medications, not intellectual disability. There was no evidence that her deficits had begun in childhood and there was no early standardized testing in Sarah's chart. Even if testing had been done, the distractibility and other cognitive deficits present in active Bipolar Disorder can confound the results of intelligence testing and norms for individuals with Bipolar Disorder are not available.

Although Sarah endorsed all the criteria for Attention-Deficit/Hyperactivity Disorder, Predominantly Hyperactive-Impulsive Type, this was not her correct diagnosis. Cognitive problems, not hyperactivity or impulsivity, were the cause of her inability to live independently and her impairment in school, work, and family life. Moreover, Attention-Deficit/Hyperactivity Disorder cannot be diagnosed if symptoms are better accounted for by another diagnosis such as Bipolar Disorder. Bipolar Disorder explains all of Sarah's symptoms, whereas Attention-Deficit/Hyperactivity Disorder Predominantly Hyperactive-Impulsive Type only explains some of her symptoms.

Cognitive Testing

Because *attention* is required for all mental tasks, Sarah's poor *attention* best explains the cognitive deficits that caused her to receive the incorrect diagnosis of mild Intellectual Disability. Her distractibility probably resulted from her Bipolar Disorder compounded by three sedative medications.

CLINICAL NOTES

The worst consequence of Sarah's misdiagnosis was that she had received inappropriate treatment that prevented her recovery. For the most part, her mania had been treated for years with sedatives—high-dose antipsychotics, benztropine, (Cogentin) and lorazepam (Ativan). When the unnecessary sedatives were discontinued and Sarah received a mood-stabilizing medicine (such as lithium salts, carbamazepine/Tegretol, or valproate/Depakote), her cognition and behavior improved dramatically.

In her new condition, Sarah was able to remember her own history back to adolescence. Sarah had been born into a middle-class Texas family and had a relatively normal childhood. Far from being developmentally disabled, she went to an affluent private high school and graduated with honors (which we were able to confirm by calling her high school). Upon graduation, Sarah matriculated at a large private Texas university, where she did well until her sophomore year when she had her first psychiatric break.

At this time, Sarah's parents died suddenly and she inherited a significant sum of money. Sarah left school and began traveling around the West, staying in expensive hotels, drinking, and spending large sums of money on her and several boyfriends. Finally, she ran out of money and found herself with nowhere to live. This was the last thing she remembered until she surfaced in our clinic about five years later. She moved quickly into state mental health services and had been there ever since.

Bipolar disorder is still underdiagnosed. Unfortunately, Sarah's case is not unique. Over the following months, as our clinic staff became sensitive to these issues, we found that several other members of our "chronic Schizophrenic" population had also been misdiagnosed.

CASE 28
JIM'S ROOMMATE DIES

Jim was a 39-year-old man with a 20-year history of **Schizophrenia** (DSM-5 295.90, ICD-10 F20.9). He was first brought to my clinic office by his caseworker with a complaint of auditory hallucinations.

In his Diagnostic Examination, I noticed that Jim had very little facial expression. He sat a little farther away from me than most patients and he looked away from me as we talked. Jim said he was sleeping well on his current medication and gaining weight from eating the starchy meals at his board and care home. Jim denied physical symptoms of anxiety and endorsed none of the criteria for attentional disorders. He said he was a little depressed because he was out of cigarettes and he wished that he knew more girls. Jim denied crying or sadness, however, and said that he was not hopeless, anxious, or irritable.

Jim said that his usual day consisted of breakfast, brushing his teeth, walking to the nearby convenience store to get coffee, and coming home for lunch. In the afternoons, he either went back to the convenience store for more coffee or a beer, or stayed in his board and care home watching television. He described these details with some satisfaction and said that he enjoyed most of his days. He said that the highlight of his days was smoking cigarettes and drinking an occasional beer.

When I asked Jim about hearing voices, he agreed with no surprise. "Doctor," he said, "for years I've been hearing voices broadcast into my head from the top floor of a building called Franklin's Tower, located in downtown Chicago. Lately the voices have been getting louder."

"Exactly what do you hear, Jim?" I asked him.

Jim replied, "It's some kind of code or signal repeating over and over in a foreign language."

"What are they saying?" I asked.

"How do I know what they are saying, doctor?" Jim answered in a calm voice. "I told you it's in a foreign language. I don't speak any foreign languages."

I apologized for my thickness and pushed on with the interview. "Well, why do you think they picked *you* to broadcast to?"

Jim looked into my eyes for the first time. "I wish I knew. I think they made a mistake when they picked me to broadcast to. I can't even understand the words. I've asked all my doctors what was going on but nobody ever tells me anything."

I replied, "I think that you have a disease called Schizophrenia, Jim. I've known other individuals with Schizophrenia who heard strange things like this."

"Really? Is that what is going on?" Jim replied. "I always wondered what it was. Thank you very much. I feel better now. Nobody ever tells me anything."

On his Cognitive Examination, Jim made no errors on tests of *attention* or *language*, although his Quality of Speech was devoid of any emotional tone.

In the *memory* section, Jim could recall only one president.

In his assessment of *abstract thinking*, Jim made errors in Simple Arithmetic and his Proverb Interpretation was concrete. In response to, "Don't cry over spilt milk," he said, "It's spilt, don't cry." To "Rome wasn't built in a day," he replied, "It took a long time to build Rome, I think." Jim did not understand the instructions for Set Analysis and persisted in telling me how each pair of items was similar, not different. His drawing of a Greek Cross was irregular and he said, "I haven't had to draw anything since fourth grade."

Jim performed well in tests of *sequential thinking*. His inability to do Simple Arithmetic invalidated tests of Serial Sevens subtraction and the Arithmetic Story Problem.

I followed Jim for the next two years. He received a low dose of atypical antipsychotic and he did well.

One day, Jim was brought to the clinic by two young trainees and the head of Social Services, who seemed to be comforting the other two until I arrived. They sent Jim into my office and waited out in the hall to speak to me.

The first trainee was very worried. "We don't know what to do. Everybody is in shock. I don't know what to do and so I got with my friend, but neither one of us knows what to do. It was so unexpected.

"Jim's roommate, Bob, came in late last night and hung himself from the ceiling while Jim was sleeping. When Jim awoke, the first thing he saw was his roommate hanging dead in their room. Jim called the board and care operator and reported the suicide in his room. He hasn't talked much all day and we can't get him to talk about it."

"Our supervisor wondered if you need to give him more medications. Some other caseworkers suggested you could give him sedatives to calm him down. Do you think he should go to the hospital?"

CHALLENGE

What is your sense of Jim and his diagnosis? Imagine that Jim is waiting in your office. What would you do?

SOLUTION

Jim carries the correct diagnosis of **Schizophrenia** (DSM-5 295.90, ICD-10 F20.9):

At least two of the following usually present during a one-month period (at least one must be 1, 2, or 3):
1. **Hallucinations.** Jim heard voices.
2. **Delusions.** Jim believed foreign individuals were broadcasting voices into his head from a building in downtown Chicago.
3. **Disorganized speech (with frequent stopping, derailment or incoherence).**
4. **Disorganized or catatonic behavior (immobility, stereotypies, posturing, mannerisms).**
5. **Negative symptoms—diminished expression of emotion (flat affect), diminished words or content in speech (alogia), or failure to engage or persist in activities (avolition).** (*Flat affect*): Jim "had very little facial expression" and his "speech was devoid of any emotional tone."

There has been significant impairment in self-care, school, work, family, or social function since the onset of the disturbance. Jim was not able to go to school or work independently with the hallucinations, delusions, and cognitive impairment caused by his Schizophrenia.

Other Diagnostic Considerations

Some clinicians might have considered other disorders in the psychotic category. However, Jim did not meet the criteria for Schizophreniform Disorder because his disease has been present for more than six months. He did not meet the criteria for Brief Psychotic Disorder, because his disorder has been present for more than one month. He could not be given the diagnosis of Delusional Disorder, because his hallucinations met the criteria for Schizophrenia. Jim could not be given the diagnosis of Schizoaffective Disorder, because there was no Manic or Major Depressive Episode. Although he demonstrated flat affect and did not engage in close, intimate relationships, Jim did not have Schizotypal Personality Disorder because there was no evidence of suspicion, paranoia, ideas of reference, sensory illusions, odd appearance, or behavior that began early in life and continued consistently throughout his lifetime. He showed none of the symptoms of Catatonia such as motor immobility, catalepsy, excessive motor activity, posturing, resistance to instructions, mutism, posturing, mannerisms, grimacing, or repeating others' words or behaviors.

Jim exhibited shallow interpersonal behavior typical of Schizophrenia. Although he was always polite and appropriate in his conversations with me, he exuded no social warmth. Jim avoided eye contact with me and he did not communicate his emotions in his face, voice, or actions. He maintained a greater social distance than other patients. He had very little personal involvement with his roommates, even when one of them hung himself in their shared room. Even his delusions and hallucinations were impersonal and distant.

Cognitive Testing

Jim's Cognitive Examination showed poor *abstract thinking* with concrete Proverb Interpretation. However, he did well on *sequential thinking* tasks where he did not have to perform arithmetic or hold multiple items in memory at the same time. These test results and his style of speech suggest a linear, sequential thinking style.

CLINICAL NOTES

It is not always necessary to give patients more medicine every time something goes wrong. Sometimes it is more important to understand their reactions and help them process their concerns in their own way. Individuals with Schizophrenia express little social warmth or attachment but they can still use help processing their feelings logically and sensibly. Oftentimes it is possible to do this while maintaining the low level of expressed emotion that is comfortable for many schizophrenic patients.

When I entered my office, Jim was sitting down. I said, "Hello, Jim. I heard there was something happening at your board and care home, today."

Jim thought carefully and said, "I think I see the doctor today."

This was a safe conclusion, because I was the doctor and he was seeing me. "Yes, I think you *do* see the doctor today. Did anything else happen this morning, Jim?"

Jim looked away and then stared out the window, saying, "Do you mean did anything happen with Bob? Yeah, he's my roommate."

"Yes. Did anything happen with Bob your roommate? What exactly did happen with Bob, anyway?"

"Well, doctor, they said my roommate Bob died during the night. That's all I know. Nobody ever tells me anything."

"So what did you think when you woke up this morning?" I asked.

"When I woke up this morning, I thought, 'Bob's not here. Maybe Bob's in the washroom. I'll yell out for him.' So, I yelled out 'Bob!' in case he was in the washroom. But he wasn't in the washroom."

"So you yelled out for him but he wasn't there. What did you think when you yelled out for him and he wasn't there?"

"Well, I was surprised when I yelled out for him and he wasn't there. I thought he might be in the washroom but he wasn't there. Then I saw him hanging. So, I told the board and care operator. I didn't want to get in trouble."

I said, "That was good that you told the board and care operator. I'm glad you didn't get in trouble. What do you think will happen with Bob now, Jim?"

Jim smiled. "Nothing's going to happen with him, doctor. He's dead. You know that."

"Yes, indeed. Nothing is going to happen with him," I admitted. "I heard that you and Bob were roommates for several years. Tell me, what did you think of Bob?"

"OK. I guess I thought of him as OK. He was better than the roommate I had before. But my other roommate never borrowed my cigarettes. Bob always used to borrow my cigarettes. And my money. He would borrow them but he never gave them back."

I said, "If he never gave them back, that sounds more like stealing than borrowing to me."

"Yeah. It sounds more like stealing than borrowing to me, too. But I didn't want to get in trouble, so I just let him do it."

"How will your life be different with Bob gone, Jim?"

Jim thought a moment. "Well, now I have the room to myself for a while. That will be different. I guess they'll get me a new roommate."

"And what are you feeling about Bob now that he's gone?" I queried.

Jim was suddenly thrust deep into thought. "I'm not feeling much about Bob now that he's gone. I'm feeling that he won't be stealing my cigarettes, any more. That's good."

"Yes, I agree. That *is* good that he won't be stealing your cigarettes, anymore. You know, Jim, I often think it's nice that, when something happens, then it's over and it doesn't have to bother us any more."

"Yeah," said Jim. "It doesn't have to bother us any more and you don't have to think about it any more."

"Yes, I agree," I replied. "You *don't* have to think about it any more. That's good."

Jim replied, "Yeah, that's good. Are we almost done?"

"Yeah, Jim, we're done. You can go whenever you want. What do you want me to tell your caseworkers?"

"I guess I want you to tell my caseworkers that I'm OK and I can go back to the board and care and walk to the convenience store."

"OK, Jim. I'll tell them that you're OK and you can go to the convenience store."

Life went on for Jim after that. There were no repercussions from his roommate's suicide, and Jim's caseworkers were happy that Jim seemed back to normal.

This incident opened a door to closer communication with Jim. About a year later, Jim had a conversation with me about death.

"Doctor?" Jim said, "Do you remember when my roommate died? I wanted to ask you a question about death. I've asked everybody but nobody ever tells me anything. I heard on television that life is like a snowflake. Do you think that life is like a snowflake that just floats down and then it is gone? Or do you think there is something after that?"

"Well, Jim," I replied, "what do *you* think?"

"Well, I wish that there was something after that. But I really think that there isn't anything after that."

"Well, if life is just like a snowflake that floats down and then it is gone, then it's a hell of a ride."

"Yeah," Jim replied. "It's a hell of a ride."

Patients with Schizophrenia often have flat affect and do not seem to react much to others' communication or social contact. Their linear speech patterns require more attention to follow than other patients' speech. However, when I consider their frankness and logic, my Schizophrenic patients often surprise me with how much they have to say.

CASE 29
MR. SNOW HAS BAD LUCK

Mr. Snow came to my clinic office late in the day for his initial appointment and a request for disability services. He was 35 years of age and he denied any personal or family history of physical, mental, or emotional illness. His chart showed that he had a rapid pulse of 105 beats per minute (normal=60-100 bpm) and an elevated blood pressure of 150/80 mm of mercury (normal<120/80 mm Hg). The caseworker who brought him stayed out in the hall.

Mr. Snow made a dramatic case for disability status. He said, "Doctor, I am having a run of very bad luck. Three months ago, I was the vice-president of a major Internet search engine corporation but I was let go for trivial reasons. My employers didn't care that I have two children and a wife, and I really need the money. I tried to borrow money from my friends but they would only give me a few dollars and when I went back to them for more, they all turned me away."

"Where are your wife and children now?" I asked.

"We lost our house to creditors," Mr. Snow moaned. "My wife and children are staying with her mother but if I don't get money fast, they will be out on the street. All my savings are gone and I need a lot of money right away."

"Why aren't you able to work at this time, Mr. Snow?" I queried.

"Oh, I'm unable to do anything right now because I have a bad self-image. Besides, it is not even worth looking for work because the only job I could get wouldn't give me enough money. All I can do now is run some errands for these friends of mine. But they don't give me what I really need."

"But I'm still not sure why you are not *able* to work at this time," I said.

"Oh, I'm on medical leave from work. They were paying for my medical treatment but now they won't give me a dime. That's why I need to get my disability money, fast."

Mr. Snow's dress was more expensive than most other clients' at the clinic. He wore a white branded polo shirt and a nice pair of white woolen trousers that matched his shock of white hair. On his feet were worn-out canvas tennis shoes without socks. It was a cool day but he was perspiring.

In his Diagnostic Examination, Mr. Snow was agitated and he moved from his seat on several occasions. A fine tremor was visible in his fingers. He told me, "I've only been sleeping one or two hours at night and I'm exhausted. I'm hungry all the time but all I can eat is a few candy bars all day." Mr. Snow said he was easily distracted and had difficulty relaxing. Mr. Snow endorsed feelings of sadness but denied experiencing hopelessness, emptiness, or boredom. He did not seem to be elated or expansive.

Mr. Snow was irritable during his examination. "I don't see why I have to go through this humiliation just to get money that's coming to me. I mean, it's my money, isn't it? Do you think I will be able to get my money today?" he asked anxiously.

On his Cognitive Examination, Mr. Snow passed all tests of *attention* and *language*, although his Quality of Speech was overly loud.

In *memory* assessment, when I asked him to name the last Four Presidents to test his distant memory, Mr. Snow replied, "How should I know? They're all a bunch of crooks, anyway."

In *abstract thinking* tests, Mr. Snow failed Proverb Interpretation. In response to the proverb, "Don't cry over spilt milk," he snapped, "No one can force you to change your life." His interpretation of the proverb, "Rome wasn't built in a day," was "Everything takes longer when people will not give you what you need." When I asked him to interpret an extra proverb, "Never throw pearls before swine" he said, "If you leave money or jewelry lying around, don't be surprised if somebody takes them. They probably need the money." Being asked what he should do if he found himself in a burning theater irritated Mr. Snow. "Run out of that place before you get burned up," he answered.

When queried on his *sequential thinking,* Mr. Snow said, "I refuse to do any more of these stupid tests. Can't we hurry this along?"

CHALLENGE

Mr. Snow had no accessible medical records and he would not give me a telephone number to contact his wife or his primary physician. Based on the information you have, what diagnoses would you consider for Mr. Snow and which treatment approaches might be helpful? Will you sign the letter giving him disability status?

SOLUTION

I first suspected that Mr. Snow suffered from a drug problem when I noted that his pulse and blood pressure were elevated, that he was agitated, that he was sweating, and that he suffered from a tremor. Before I recorded a final diagnosis, Mr. Snow's caseworker knocked on my door and I asked Mr. Snow to wait in the hall while I spoke with her alone.

"I wanted to tell you Mr. Snow's real story," she began. "A year ago, he was the vice president of a big corporation—he had a large, expensive home, a nice wife, and two beautiful children. Mr. Snow drank socially and sniffed cocaine at parties with his friends until a friend introduced him to smoking crack cocaine. Over the next few months, Mr. Snow gradually devoted his life to the task of obtaining and using as much crack cocaine as he could get. He stopped going to work and frequented a crack house until it became his second home. Mr. Snow increased his use of alcohol as a sedative to counter the overstimulation of the cocaine. He stopped visiting his home and cut off communication with his wife and children, who had no idea what was going on.

"Mr. Snow continued to use larger amounts of cocaine, in search of the strong highs he had first experienced. To support his now-expensive habit, Mr. Snow gradually withdrew all his family's savings from the bank and refinanced his house. He called his relatives with vague stories, asking for money to support his children. When all that money was gone, Mr. Snow returned to work and pleaded with his coworkers to give him large 'loans' so he 'could just get back on his feet.' He even took what little cash he could get from secretaries, receptionists, and housekeeping staff.

When Mr. Snow had depleted his family and coworkers, he went to his employers, revealed he had a drug problem, and begged for their help. Initially, Mr. Snow's employers were supportive. They offered him paid time off and gave him money for drug treatment programs that he immediately spent on more cocaine. Finally, his employers placed him on indefinite leave. At that time, he turned to carrying drugs in exchange for cocaine. His wife and children arrived home one day to find themselves evicted without any warning and they were out on the street until his wife's parents took them in. During this time, his wife and children never heard a word from him."

With this information, I gave Mr. Snow the diagnoses of **Cocaine Intoxication** (DSM-5 292.89, ICD-10 14.229), **Cocaine Withdrawal** (DSM 292.0, ICD-10 F14.23), and **Severe Cocaine Use Disorder** (DSM-5 304.20, ICD-10 F14.20).

During his interview, Mr. Snow demonstrated **Stimulant Intoxication**:
A. **Recent use of amphetamine, cocaine, or another stimulant.**
B. **Clinically significant problematic behavioral or psychological changes (e.g. euphoria or affective blunting; changes in sociability; hypervigilance; interpersonal sensitivity; anxiety, tension, or anger; stereotyped behaviors; impaired judgment; or impaired school, work, home, or social functioning) developed after use of a stimulant.** (*Sociability*): Mr. Snow was irritable and imperious during his examination and he described how he had ill-used his friends and associates. (*Anxiety, tension, or anger*): Mr. Snow acted tense and angry during his examination. (*Impaired judgment*): It shows poor judgment to try to browbeat drug money from a physician while denying that you have any medical problems. (*Social or occupational functioning*): Mr. Snow had lost his job, his home, his family, and his friends.
C. **Two (or more) of the following developing after use of the stimulant:**
   1. **Rapid or slowed heart rate.** Mr. Snow "had a rapid pulse of 105 beats per minute (normal=60-100 bpm)."
   2. **Pupillary dilation.**
   3. **Increased or decreased blood pressure.** Mr. Snow had an elevated blood pressure of 150/80 mm of mercury (normal <120/80 mm Hg)."
   4. **Perspiration or chills.** Although "it was a cool day," Mr. Snow "was perspiring."
   5. **Nausea or vomiting.**
   6. **Weight loss.**
   7. **Psychomotor agitation or retardation.** "Mr. Snow was agitated and he moved from his seat on several occasions."
   8. **Muscular weakness, respiratory depression, chest pain, or cardiac arrhythmias.**
   9. **Confusion, seizures, dyskinesias, dystonias, or coma.**

Mr. Snow also demonstrated **Stimulant Withdrawal**:

A. Cessation of (or reduction in) prolonged amphetamine-type substance, cocaine, or other stimulant use. Mr. Snow's frantic need to get money for drugs showed that he was running out of his supply.
B. Within a few hours to several days after cessation or reduction:
   Dysphoric mood. Mr. Snow "endorsed feelings of sadness."
   Plus two (or more) of the following physiological changes, developing:
   1. **Fatigue.** Mr. Snow said, "I'm exhausted."
   2. **Vivid, unpleasant dreams.**
   3. **Insomnia or hypersomnia.** Mr. Snow commented that, "I've only been sleeping one or two hours at night."
   4. **Increased appetite.** Mr. Snow noted that "I'm hungry all the time."
   5. **Psychomotor depression or agitation.** In his Diagnostic Examination, "Mr. Snow was agitated and he moved from his seat on several occasions."
C. These symptoms cause clinically significant distress or impairment in school, work, home, social, or other important areas of functioning. These symptoms, withdrawal cravings, and the need to get more cocaine caused Mr. Snow to lose his job, home, family, and friends.

Overall, Mr. Snow showed the these symptoms of **Stimulant Use Disorder**:
At least two of the following occurring within a 12-month period:
   1. **The patient takes a substance in larger amounts for a longer period than intended.** Mr. Snow wanted "a lot of money right away" and his attempts to get money from employers and friends indicate that he needed cocaine in large quantities to "support his now-expensive habit."
   2. **The patient tries or wants to reduce substance use.**
   3. **The patient spends considerable time obtaining, using, and recovering from the substance effects.** Over the past three months, Mr. Snow "gradually devoted his life to the task of obtaining and using as much crack cocaine as he could get" and he employed many strategies for milking money from his employers, coworkers, friends, and family—these took up a considerable amount of his time and effort.
   4. **The patient feels strong urges or cravings to use the substance.** Mr. Snow demonstrated strong urges to get and use cocaine.
   5. **Substance use causes impairment in school, work, home, or social function.** These symptoms, withdrawal cravings, and the need to get more cocaine caused Mr. Snow to lose his job, home, family, and friends.
   6. **Use continues despite social problems attributable to the substance.** Mr. Snow was homeless because of his cocaine disorder.
   7. **School, work, home, or social activities are curtailed because of the substance.** Mr. Snow "stopped going to work," "stopped visiting his home," "cut off communication with his wife and children," and lost his house to creditors in his need to acquire and use cocaine. His whole world revolved around getting and using cocaine.
   8. **Use continues despite physical danger attributable to the substance.**
   9. **Use continues despite physical or psychological problems attributable to the substance.** Mr. Snow continued to use cocaine despite insomnia, fatigue, psychomotor agitation, distractibility, sadness, anxiety, and rage that were driven by cocaine.
   10. **Tolerance—increased amounts are needed and/or the effects of the substance decrease.** The caseworker told me that "Mr. Snow continued to use larger amounts of cocaine, in search of the strong highs he had first experienced."
   11. **Withdrawal—characteristic withdrawal symptoms and/or substances are taken to avoid withdrawal.**. Mr. Snow showed withdrawal symptoms (see above) and he was desperately trying to obtain more cocaine to "support his now-expensive habit."
The disorder is characterized as Severe when six or more symptoms are present.

Other Diagnostic Considerations

Mr. Snow had a drug problem—elevated pulse and blood pressure, agitation, excessive sweating, tremor, insomnia, appetite changes, distractibility, and irritability would be expected if he were using stimulants or going through substance withdrawal. If you considered Substance Use disorders, then you are prepared to help Mr. Snow.

Some clinicians might consider giving Mr. Snow a diagnosis of Bipolar I Disorder, Most Recent Episode Manic, because of his angry mood, grandiosity, distractibility, insomnia, agitation, and impulsive behavior. A case could also be made for the diagnosis of Generalized Anxiety Disorder because of his persistent worries, irritability, restless sleep, poor focus, and keyed-up appearance. Furthermore, Mr. Snow showed several symptoms of Panic Attack, including racing heart, excessive perspiration, and tremor. He also exhibited distractibility, agitation, difficulty relaxing, and excessive speech, which are symptoms of Attention-Deficit/Hyperactivity Disorder. However, cocaine can mimic all these symptoms and other diagnoses are excluded when the symptoms can be explained by substance use.

Some of Mr. Snow's beliefs and behavior resemble those found in Narcissistic Personality Disorder, such as grandiosity, entitlement, lack of empathy, exploitiveness, and arrogance. He also evidenced some symptoms of Antisocial Personality Disorder, including irritability, lying and conning others, impulsivity, lack of concern for the safety of himself and others, failure to support himself, lack of guilt and remorse, and grounds for arrest (see *Mental Status Examination for Personality Disorders*, Chapter 8). However, these symptoms can be produced or exacerbated by Substance Use Disorders and any personality diagnoses should be deferred until he is free from the effects of cocaine.

Mr. Snow should be reevaluated when he is free from cocaine effects to see if he has another diagnosis.

Cognitive Testing

Mr. Snow's Cognitive Examination was unscorable because he refused most of the tests and simply used the testing situation as a platform to air his irritability and drug-seeking mission.

CLINICAL NOTES

Like many addicts, Mr. Snow did not explain that he had a substance use problem—it is up to the clinician to be alert to the possibility of substance use. Depending on your patient population, you may see many individuals coming to you in activated withdrawal looking for some way that you can help them continue their habit. The experience produced by smoking crack cocaine provides a particularly strong motivation for its continued use.

When I returned to my office, Mr. Snow addressed me crossly. "Can I get my money, now? My children are hungry."

"This disability money is for patients who have mental disorders," I explained patiently. "Do you have a mental disorder, Mr. Snow?"

"No, of course not. But you know how it works. You and me are in on the scam. You just sign the papers and I get the money. One of my friends told me."

"Well, abuse of and dependence on cocaine can be considered a mental disorder. Do you think you qualify for either of those?" I asked.

"No!" Mr. Snow shouted. "I didn't come in here to play games. I want the money! You *know* this is all a game. You make up some things and we both know it's just so I can get my money."

"I can't very well justify recommending you for disability status if you don't have any disability," I replied. "Can you think of *any* mental illness or substance problem that you might have that could be considered a disability? I'd be happy to recommend you to a no-cost detoxification center or drug treatment program."

Mr. Snow stood up. "I've been wasting my time!" he yelled. "I'm not like *these* people!" (He waved his arm wildly to designate the clinic). "I'm not crazy. I just want the *money*!

"Look," he fumed. "I need the money right away, so you make up some excuse and write it down and sign it so I can get my disability money. But if you won't play the game, I'm leaving!" Mr. Snow stared angrily at me for a moment and then stomped out of the clinic in a rage.

I dialed the Social Services supervisor and left a message about Mr. Snow's needy family, although I was sure that she knew about them already. After finishing with Mr. Snow's chart, I took a deep breath, drank down the remainder of my cold coffee, and went home.

CASE 30
MAUDIE SMILES

Maudie was brought in a wheelchair to see me at an Alzheimer's Center by her husband and their two adult daughters. Her previous psychiatrist had retired and her husband and two daughters wanted help with a clinical decision about pain control.

Maudie was a 69-year-old woman who had been diagnosed with severe **Alzheimer's Disease** (DSM-5 331.0, ICD-10 G30.9) and **malignant bone cancer** (ICD-10 C41.9). She lived at home with her husband, who cared for her. Because of the combined diseases, her motor behavior was quite limited. She could not walk or feed herself, and she was completely mute. However, her husband knew what she wanted and liked, and their life was stable.

Maudie's oncologist had advised the family that cancer of the bone was one of the most painful of diseases and he had provided the husband and family with hydromorphone hydrochloride (Dilaudid), a powerful opiate analgesic in a liquid form.

The family came to me because they were conflicted about how to use this pain medicine for Maudie, who could not communicate her needs. The youngest daughter wanted high-dose analgesia out of concern for her mother's comfort "in her dying months."

However, the older daughter was opposed to opiates, altogether. "I do not want my mother to die a drug addict," she told us.

The husband, who was the same age as his wife, was caught in the middle. He felt overwhelmed and confused. He did not want to offend either of his daughters but they scoffed at his contention that he could adjust the analgesic daily by observing his wife's behavior.

On examination, Maudie was alert and followed me with her eyes. Unlike most patients in pain, her face looked unusually relaxed and she wore a slight but peaceful smile on her face. Her blink and swallow reflexes were intact. She followed my commands to stare at my finger and to look up and down. She exhibited a barely perceptible grip in her right hand. Other than these minor movements, I could find no other voluntary movement. I could not elicit even rudimentary speech.

CHALLENGE

What more could you learn from Maudie's examination? How would you advise the family about Maudie's treatment decisions?

SOLUTION

My clinical problem was how to perform a mental status examination with a woman who could not converse. First, I sent the family back to the waiting room so I could evaluate Maudie in private. I could see that Maudie was alert and I wondered if she was oriented and cognizant inside. I explained to her that I would conduct an interview and I would like her to blink her eyes in response to my questions: two blinks for "yes" and one blink for "no."

By using this strategy, I conducted a more sophisticated interview with Maudie. What I discovered was that Maudie's cognitive impairment was much less severe than it had appeared in the context of her cancer. By blinking her eyes in response to my questions, I was able to perform a minimal Cognitive Examination. I tested her *attention* and found that she was aware of the place, date, and time. She also did well on a test of Vigilance where she blinked each time she heard me say "five" in a string of numbers. She did well on a *language* test where she selected the name of the parts of my pen from several choices. In a test of *memory*, Maudie could remember only one out of three objects after a one-minute delay. In a test of *abstract thinking,* she demonstrated the ability to do Simple Arithmetic.

When I discovered that Maudie was alert and could communicate, I realized that I could ask her about her pain. From her family's comments, I knew that she had not had any opiates for over 24 hours, so I inquired about the severity of her pain.

When I asked Maudie "Is your pain severe right now?" she blinked twice. When I asked, "Is your pain very, *very* severe now?" she blinked twice again. Again, I asked, "Are you in such severe pain that that you can barely stand it?" and again she blinked twice.

Then I began a discussion of what she wanted and needed in her treatment, just as I would with any other patient in my clinic office.

I said, "You know we have some very good pain medicines, including some new ones that might be able to take a lot of your pain away, maybe all of it." Maudie blinked twice to show that she understood.

"Would you like to try any of these pain medicines?" I asked.

Maudie blinked, "No."

I asked, "Is it because you think they wouldn't work?"

She replied, "No."

I asked, "Is it because you think your family wouldn't like you to take pain medicine?"

Maudie replied, "No."

"Is it because it would make you sleepy and sedated?" I queried.

She replied, "Yes."

"Is it because you want to be clear-headed so you can see all the things around you, your husband, and your children?"

Maudie blinked numerous times, and I imagined I saw a slight movement in her smile.

"Now, you should know that I have some new and really good pain medicines that relieve pain and are only a *little* sedating," I said. "Would you just like to give one of them a try?" I asked.

She blinked, "No."

"Are you sure you don't want to try one of them? I realize you are in a lot of pain, and I am sure I could find something less sedating than Dilaudid. If you do not want to try anything, blink once for no."

Again, Maudie blinked, "No."

"Would you like me to explain what you want to your family?"

Maudie blinked numerous times.

I spent some more time with Maudie, during which she told me that she was not depressed, anxious, or angry. I found that she enjoyed her life as long as she was not sedated.

I had assumed her peculiar smile was a result of a neurological deficit but I began to suspect that it was real.

Other Diagnostic Considerations

A minimum of communication with the patient was sufficient to clarify her diagnosis and improve her treatment. This case is a reminder that diagnoses and treatment decisions should never be based solely on past evaluations and the reports of family members.

Cognitive Testing

Even in her debilitated condition, it was possible to give Maudie a minimal Cognitive Examination that showed she had at some proficiency in areas of *attention, language, memory,* and *abstract thinking*. If the patient ever desired it, additional testing could further clarify the extent of her Neurocognitive Disorder.

CLINICAL NOTES

I called the family back into my clinic office. I reassured them that taking an opiate pain medication for a chronic disease was medically appropriate and I explained how this was different from the abuse of street drugs in the community. I told them about the good effects I had seen with opiate analgesics in other patients. Then, I shared my conversation with Maudie, explaining that she had refused pain medication. I told the family that I believed that she was able to understand the consequences of her decision and that she had the right to decide for herself if her mind was clear. I suggested that we delay opiates for a few more weeks.

The younger daughter was still concerned. "Aren't we *obligated* to give her medicine to take her pain away?" she asked. "If it were me, I couldn't put up with the pain and I would want the medicine."

I acknowledged the sincerity of her concern but I explained that it was our duty to respect her mother's wishes. I explained that, now that we had a way to speak with her, we could find out about the things she wanted and make sure she had them. This satisfied the younger daughter and she agreed.

The family did not express surprise that Maudie was cognizant. After the daughters had left my office, her husband confided that he had conversed with his wife before, using her grip to signal yes and no, but he had given up this practice when her motor control deteriorated. As her husband wheeled her out through my doorway, Maudie gave me her sweetest smile.

CASE 31
LAURA ITCHES

"I was sent to you by my dermatologist, Dr. Cutaneous," Laura told me when she had taken her seat in my clinic office. "I've been seeing him for three months now, trying to get control of my itching, but so far it hasn't worked. He has given me every medical test and study and everything comes back normal. My dermatologist prescribed cortisone pills and creams, antihistamines, and stuff to put on my skin to make it numb. He tells me that I have to stop scratching myself for the itching to go away but I just can't get myself to stop. It's as if my fingers have a life of their own."

Laura was a very thin, 30-year-old, unmarried accountant who was jittery and bounced around in her seat. Her eyes were very dark and watery.

"Where does this itching occur?" I asked.

"I feel like I am itching all over my body. Everywhere. Mostly I end up scratching and picking at my forearms, neck, and head because they are the easiest places to reach. It's worst when I'm trying to relax, like when I'm watching television."

Even as she spoke, Laura's hands were running up and down her arms, neck and trunk area, rubbing, picking, and sometimes scratching. There were long red tracks on her arms and neck, which contained both old and new excoriations.

Laura's pulse was elevated at 109 beats per minute (normal=60-100 bpm) and her blood pressure was high at 130/85 mm of mercury (normal<120/80 mm Hg). She seemed agitated and her hands were slightly tremulous. She told me that she had never been hospitalized and she had never before sought treatment from a mental health professional. She denied alcohol or drug abuse problems of any kind.

In her Diagnostic Examination, Laura said that she exercised three hours daily and took "an appetite suppressant called phentermine in order to keep my weight down." Laura complained of frequent nausea and insomnia but she denied palpitations, pounding heart, excessive sweating, shortness of breath, choking, chest pain, dizziness, lightheadedness, fainting, numbing or tingling, muscle tension, being easily fatigued, poor concentration, mind going blank, hypervigilance, exaggerated startle response, feeling dazed, derealization (feelings of unreality), depersonalization (feeling detached from oneself), or amnesia.

When asked about her emotions, Laura complained of mild anxiety but she denied sadness, hopelessness, irritability, or anger. Laura said that she enjoyed her life and her usual activities. I could detect no evidence of euphoria or expansive mood. Laura denied any obsessions or thoughts of suicide or violence and I could find no evidence of delusional thoughts or hallucinations in any sensory modality.

Although it is not necessary to test cognitive functions in a patient who complains of itching, I wanted to get more information about Laura's condition.

Laura did well on tests of *attention, memory,* and *sequential thinking.*

Laura's *language* tests were normal. However, her Quality of Speech was notable for rapidity and perseveration—she sometimes repeated what she had just said without appearing to notice.

Laura passed a test of Simple Arithmetic but failed the other tests of *abstract thinking*. For example, for the proverb, "Don't cry over spilt milk," she said, "Don't be upset about little things," missing the reference of the proverb to the past. The correct interpretation would have been, "Don't be upset about minor problems that happened in the past." For the proverb "Rome wasn't built in a day," she said "Persevere to reach your goals," which is too vague. In Set Analysis, Laura simply described the meanings of truth/justice, poverty/misery, and daisy/flower without explaining their relationship. Her Greek Cross drawing was poorly proportioned. On a test of Judgment, Laura said that if she were in a burning theater, she would tell the man sitting next to her and ask him to pass the information down the row, an incorrect answer that could leave most of the theatergoers perishing in flames. On a test of Insight, she said the reason people should tell the truth was "so your husband or boyfriend won't leave you," which was too limited in scope.

"There are lots of things going on with me," she continued, "but the only thing I'm worried about is the itching. I can't go to work and I won't go out like this. I avoid everyone I know. It's pretty ironic that I work so hard to stay thin and I end up staying at home all alone because of this itching."

Laura paused a moment before continuing. "I guess things are looking pretty bleak when they send you to the psychiatrist."

CHALLENGE

Poor Laura is in trouble, and she needs you to help her. Use all your skills as a diagnostician to find a solution that explains all her symptoms and complaints as well as the objective findings. Good luck!

SOLUTION

Although Laura denied drug abuse problems of any kind, she is experiencing **Phentermine Intoxication** (DSM-5 292.89, ICD-10 F15.229) and **Moderate Phentermine Use Disorder** (DSM-5 304.40, ICD-10 F15.2).

Laura met the following criteria for **Stimulant Intoxication**:

A. Recent use of a stimulant. "Laura said she was taking "an appetite suppressant called phentermine."
B. Clinically significant problematic behavioral or psychological changes (e.g. euphoria or affective blunting; changes in sociability; hypervigilance; interpersonal sensitivity; anxiety, tension, or anger; stereotyped behaviors; impaired judgment; or impaired school, work, home, or social functioning) developed after use of a stimulant. (*Sociability*): Laura had stopped going out socially. (*Anxiety*): Laura complained of anxiety. (*Tension*): Laura "was jittery and bounced around in her seat." "She seemed agitated and slightly tremulous." (*Impaired judgment*): Laura showed poor judgment in taking a substance that was causing significant physical, psychological, and social problems. Laura failed a test of Judgment on the *abstract thinking* section of her Cognitive Examination. (*Impaired function*): Laura had stopped going to work and socializing.
C. Two (or more) of the following developing after use of the stimulant:
   1. Rapid or slowed heart rate. "Laura's pulse was 109 beats per minute."
   2. Pupillary dilation. I realized later that the reason "her eyes were very dark" was because Laura's pupils were widely dilated.
   3. Increased or decreased blood pressure. Laura's blood pressure was high at 130/85 mm of mercury.
   4. Perspiration or chills.
   5. Nausea or vomiting. (*Nausea*): Laura complained of nausea.
   6. Weight loss. Laura was "very thin."
   7. Psychomotor agitation or retardation. (*Agitation*): "Laura was jittery and bounced around in her seat." "She seemed agitated and slightly tremulous."
   8. Muscular weakness, respiratory depression, chest pain, or cardiac arrhythmias.
   9. Confusion, seizures, dyskinesias, dystonias, or coma.

Overall, Laura showed these symptoms of **Stimulant Use Disorder**:
At least two of the following occurring within a 12-month period:
   1. The patient takes a substance in larger amounts for a longer period than intended. Weight loss medications are not intended for long-term use, according to their labeling. However, Laura may not have read the package labeling or been informed by her doctor.
   2. The patient tries or wants to reduce substance use.
   3. The patient spends considerable time obtaining, using, and recovering from the substance effects.
   4. The patient feels strong urges or cravings to use the substance.
   5. Substance use causes impairment in school, work, home, or social function. Laura was not going to work or socializing—she stayed at home by herself.
   6. Use continues despite social problems attributable to the substance. Laura wasn't going out and she said, "I avoid everyone I know."
   7. School, work, home, or social activities are curtailed because of the substance. The symptoms of Laura's phentermine use made her feel like "I can't go to work and I won't go out."
   8. Use continues despite physical danger attributable to the substance. It is not healthy to artificially elevate your heart rate or blood pressure—prolonged use of stimulants at high doses is associated with an increase risk of heart arrhythmias. However, Laura may not have realized that her heart rate and blood pressure were elevated, and she may not have been informed by her doctor or read the package insert explaining potential side effects of phentermine.
   9. Use continues despite physical or psychological problems attributable to the substance. Laura realized that she was experiencing physiological symptoms including itching, nausea, and agitation that should have alerted

her to possible physical problems. Laura was not thinking efficiently, as evidenced by her failure on cognitive tests of *abstract thinking*.

10. **Tolerance—increased amounts are needed and/or the effects of the substance decrease.**
11. **Withdrawal—characteristic withdrawal symptoms and/or substances are taken to avoid withdrawal.**

The disorder is characterized as Moderate when 4-5 more symptoms are present.

In coding substance-related disorders, the clinician should record the name of the specific substance used rather than the name of the drug class. Thus, Laura's diagnoses were Phentermine Intoxication and Phentermine Abuse.

Other Diagnostic Considerations

The first clues to Laura's condition were her elevated pulse and blood pressure, which suggested a physiological problem. Like most stimulants, phentermine is known for causing intense grooming, picking, and scratching at higher doses. Phentermine was also responsible for Laura's complaints of frequent nausea and insomnia.

Most clinicians think first of Excoriation (Skin-Picking) Disorder (DSM-5 698.4, ICD-10 L98.1) when they hear Laura's story. However, this diagnosis is ruled out if the skin picking is a result of the physiological effects of a substance like phentermine.

Many clinicians think of an anxiety disorder when they hear about Laura. She met Panic Attack criteria of rapid heart rate, tremor, and nausea. However, these symptoms did not peak within minutes and she showed no other physiological panic symptoms of palpitations, pounding heart, excessive sweating, shortness of breath, choking, chest pain, stomachache, dizziness, lightheadedness, fainting, numbness, tingling, derealization, depersonalization, fears of losing control, dying, or going crazy.

Laura exhibited Generalized Anxiety Disorder symptoms of mild anxiety, insomnia, and restlessness, but she did not have excessive anxiety and uncontrollable worried thoughts about activities such as work or school performance lasting at least six months. Moreover, she did not exhibit Generalized Anxiety Disorder symptoms of irritability, muscle tension, easy fatigability, poor concentration, or her mind going blank.

Bipolar mania sometimes presents with excessive anxiety and agitation but Laura did not exhibit irritability, expansive mood, or euphoria, and there was no evidence of grandiosity, a decreased need for sleep, pressured speech, racing thoughts, flight of ideas, distractibility, increased goal-directed activity, or impulsive actions with potentially painful consequences.

Laura's symptoms could have been caused by a variety of sympathomimetic stimulants, which can cause similar picking, agitation, insomnia, and elevated vital signs. However, Laura specifically mentioned taking phentermine and phentermine abuse explained all her symptoms.

Cognitive Testing

Laura's Cognitive Examination was abnormal. She did well on sections screening for functions of *attention*, *language*, *memory*, and *sequential thinking* but failed five of the six tests of *abstract thinking*. This failure in *abstract thinking* was caused by phentermine.

CLINICAL NOTES

Laura was abusing phentermine (Adipex, Obermine, Phentrol, Supramine, and others), a prescription stimulant that is widely used for weight control. You may not have heard of it because it receives little attention in the press. It is related to phendimetrazine, (Bontril, Prelu-2), benzphetamine (Didrex), and methamphetamine (Desoxyn, "speed"), which all share the potential for habituation and abuse. Like other stimulants, excessive use of phentermine can cause picking and scratching of the skin, resulting in characteristic lacerations over areas of the body that are within easy reach. At high doses, it is cardiotoxic, and heart arrhythmias, stroke, and even myocardial infarctions are concerns in patients with cardiovascular risk factors.

Like many substance abusers, Laura did not think that she was using phentermine inappropriately and she did not appear to connect her symptoms with the use of phentermine. She could have blamed her doctor for continuing to prescribe the medication or failing to inform her of its potential side effects. Nevertheless, it is Laura's responsibility to insure that what she puts into her body is helpful, not harmful, and that she is using medications appropriately.

Phentermine's ability to produce psychiatric symptoms makes it particularly relevant for the clinician. It is often associated with anxiety, irritability, and panic. As we saw in Laura, the nervous system stimulation caused by phentermine can cause impaired cognitive function. There are case histories of paranoia and frank psychosis following heavy use.

Phentermine has only short-term efficacy for weight reduction—the temporary appetite suppression it causes probably results from a sensation of nausea. Generic phentermine is widely available on the Internet and in the community for weight control or as an alternative to abusing methamphetamine. It is notable that generic phentermine is manufactured in yellow, black, or black and yellow capsules that resemble familiar forms of "speed," making it attractive for street drug sale.

I advised Laura to taper off her phentermine and use other means to lose weight. Within a few weeks, her itching and scratching had subsided and her wounds were healing.

CASE 32
ANNE'S BEAUTIFUL LONG, RED HAIR

Anne was a young-looking woman in her thirties, with a full head of thick, beautiful red hair that contrasted stylishly with her dark green velvet dress and hat. As she entered my clinic office, she looked up and voiced her main complaint.

"Doctor, you must help me!" Anne moaned. "I pull my hair. Underneath this wig, I am completely bald!

"I've pulled my hair ever since I was a teenager," Anne explained after she sat down. "It would get worse when I was under stress and then get better but it never went away completely.

"My habit used to be manageable. Sometimes I would unconsciously pull some hair out while I was at home alone watching television. I was usually able to confine my pulling to the weekends. Then tax time came. I am an accountant and the most stressful time of year for accountants is tax time. This year I began pulling my hair at work. I couldn't help it—I started to feel this awful urge and then I would have to pull. I would go to the Ladies' restroom and pull hair. After I pulled some hair, I always felt much better. Sometimes I would pull a little at my desk when I thought no one was watching.

"Well, tax-time came and went but I didn't stop pulling. I started to be worried that people in my office would notice all the torn-out hair in my wastebasket every day. Finally, I was in a meeting with my boss and I absent-mindedly pulled out a handful of hair and dropped it on the floor. My boss gave me this look that made me so embarrassed that I walked out the door and never came back. I never even cleaned out my desk.

"My husband doesn't even know that I walked out of my job. I let him think that I was fired for doing poor work. Now all I do is sit at home alone and pull out all my hair. Help!"

CHALLENGE

Anne has a serious condition that is keeping her from enjoying her life. Give a formal name to this hair-pulling and then decide how you would treat it. When you are ready, go on to the Solution.

SOLUTION

Anne has **Trichotillomania (Hair-Pulling Disorder)** (DSM-5 312.39, ICD-10 F63.2):
- A. **Repeated hair-pulling causing hair loss.** Anne's hair-pulling began in adolescence and she is now completely bald.
- B. **Repeated attempts to decrease or stop hair pulling.** Anne told us that "I was usually able to confine my pulling to the weekends." "This year I began pulling my hair at work. I couldn't help it."
- C. **The disorder causes clinically significant distress or impaired school, work, home, or social functioning.**
- A. **Recurrent pulling out of one's hair resulting in noticeable hair loss**. Anne had lost her job and she could not tell her husband about her problem.

Other Diagnostic Considerations

Patchy hair loss can also be caused by a fungal infection (tinea capitis), an autoimmune disorder (alopecia areata), or repeated tugging on the hair (traction alopecia). However, when a patient admits to obsessively pulling hair, Trichotillomania is the obvious diagnosis.

In the past, the definition of Trichotillomania emphasized an increasing sense of tension preceding the hair-pulling and a sense of pleasure, gratification, or relief when the hair was pulled out. These qualities parallel the rôle of compulsions in relieving the stress of obsessions, and resemble habits such as nail-biting and gambling that relieve the urge to act out the habit.

CLINICAL NOTES

We usually hear little about hair-pulling because trichotillomaniacs typically try to conceal their habits. However, if you go to a wig store you will find individuals buying wigs and hairpieces to cover bald spots they created by pulling out their hair. Typically the disorder waxes and wanes throughout the lifespan, increasing during periods of increased stress. Hair-pullers report tingling and itching of the scalp but rarely experience pain when the hair is pulled.

To many authors, Trichotillomania appears to resemble the impulsive habits of nail biting, thumb sucking, and similar acts of impulsive self-stimulation. Trichotillomania may occur on its own or together with other disorders such as unipolar Major Depressive Disorder, Bipolar Disorder, or Borderline Personality Disorder. When comorbid conditions are present, they should be treated along with the hair-pulling. Despite the term "mania" in the name, Trichotillomania is not a component of a Manic Episode.

Behavioral therapy offers several avenues of treatment for Trichotillomania. Stress-reduction exercises such as progressive body relaxation, breathing exercises, and meditation can help patients reduce the effects of life-stressors that drive the hair-pulling (see *Calm Your Mind,* Chapter 8). Asking the patient to write down the place and time where each episode occurred can help pinpoint essential environmental triggers. Some examples of trigger situations include watching television, reading, or eating alone. After they are recognized, environmental triggers can often be minimized or avoided.

Other behavioral therapy techniques include monitoring, charting, response prevention, and habit reversal. In monitoring and charting techniques, patients are asked to keep a record of all habit occurrences throughout the day. One common method is to prepare a chart with columns for date, time of day, trigger (condition before the habit behavior), affect, and coping methods used during the episode. The therapist and patient then discuss these findings in the course of their therapy session. Response prevention involves waiting for or triggering the habit and then blocking the hair-pulling behavior or delaying it as long as possible. In habit reversal, the hair-pulling is substituted for other behaviors (such as lightly snapping a rubber band on the wrist).

There is no clear agreement on the best pharmacological treatment for Trichotillomania. I have personally used fluvoxamine (Luvox) and pimozide (Orap) successfully in the treatment of patients with severe hair-pulling. Both medications have strong serotonin effects.

Research studies have not demonstrated the efficacy of traditional psychotherapy in Trichotillomania. However, it was a great relief for Anne finally to be able to talk with someone about her habit. Together with relaxation training, habit reversal techniques, and medication, Anne's hair-pulling gradually reduced in intensity to the point that she could control it again.

Gradually Anne's hair grew back and she was able to forgo wearing her wig. The last thing I heard, she was thinking of calling her previous employers and asking for her job back.

CASE 33
TERRY WORRIES ABOUT HIS GAME

I was working in the student health clinic of a large university when 19-year-old Terry came into my office.

"I've got bad worries about my game, Doc. I need help," Terry began.

"What sort of worries do you have about your game?" I asked.

"I'm only worried about losing my attention while I'm pitching," the boy said. "I get up there on the pitching mound, and when I hear the crowd, I zone out. I think about it all the time."

"Why don't you tell me everything that's happening that you consider a problem?" I invited.

"OK, Doc," Terry replied. "But it'll be a long list. First, the head coach tells me I do not keep my head on. I'll go out on the field without my cap or glove. Sometimes I forget and leave them in my locker. Sometimes I can't even find things I need for a big game. Coach says that it's because I can't get my stuff organized. I can't even get my life organized.

"My pitching coach is mad at me, too, because he thinks I don't listen to him because I don't follow his instructions, but I try to. What happens is that I start doing a practice drill, but when I start thinking about zoning out, I get distracted, and I never finish the drill. Then he gets mad at me and blames me for all the careless mistakes I make on the field. It's really tough."

"You haven't mentioned school—how do you like your classes?" I queried.

"Don't even go there," Terri whined. "I've been having problems in school ever since I was in kindergarten. I just can't keep focused on my schoolwork. Then I start having worried thoughts of having to read or study for tests and I get even more distracted."

In his Diagnostic Examination, Terry denied problems with sleep or fatigue. He said that he had no difficulty with restlessness, edginess, or muscle tension. He denied symptoms of a pounding heart, chest pain, dizziness, shortness of breath, choking, nausea, stomachache, tremor, or tingling in his fingers or face. He said that he had no problem sitting in class without fidgeting or waiting his turn to speak. He denied elation, sadness, hopelessness, irritability, or anger. He was not expansive, and he denied hallucinations, delusions, obsessions, compulsions, or thoughts of suicide or violence.

In his Cognitive Examination tests of *attention*, Terry was alert and oriented but he failed a test of Vigilance requiring him to respond whenever the numeral "5" was spoken.

In tests of *memory*, Terry failed Digit Span, Free Recall from a Story, and both Uncued and Cued Delayed Memory.

Terry did well on all tests of *abstract thinking*.

In tests of *sequential thinking*, Terry failed Serial Sevens subtraction and the Arithmetic Story Problem.

I also administered the Nonverbal Tests of Abstract and Sequential Thinking from Appendix VI and the Luria Figure Drawing Test from Appendix VII. He completed these tests without any errors.

"So, what do you think is wrong, Terry?" I asked at the end of his evaluation.

"Oh, I know what's wrong because I used to see a therapist back home. I suffer from poor self-esteem and something called Generalized Anxiety Disorder."

CHALLENGE

Do you think Terry suffers from poor self-esteem and Generalized Anxiety Disorder? What is wrong with Terry and what would you do about it?

SOLUTION

Terry has **Attention-Deficit/Hyperactivity Disorder, Predominantly Inattentive Presentation** (DSM-5 314.00, ICD-10 F90.0):

Six of the following Inattention or Hyperactivity/impulsivity symptoms (five for ages 17 and older):

1. Predominantly Inattentive Presentation:
   a. **Poor attention to details or makes careless mistakes.** Terry had problems getting his equipment sorted out and onto the practice field. Terry also said that his coach blamed him "for all the careless mistakes I make on the field."
   b. **Difficulty sustaining attention.** In practice, Terry said he gets "distracted and I never finish the drill." In his academic activities, Terry said that he "just can't keep focused on my schoolwork."

- **c. Problems listening to others.** Terry said that his pitching coach "thinks I don't listen to him."
- **d. Failure to follow instructions and finish projects because of poor task persistence.** Terry's pitching coach said that "I don't follow his instructions" because "I start doing a practice drill but when I start thinking about zoning out, I get distracted and I never finish the drill."
- **e. Difficulty organizing tasks and activities (including difficulty managing *sequential thinking* tasks).** . Terry's head coach said that Terry couldn't get his "stuff organized." Terry added, "I can't even get my life organized."
- **f. Dislike or reluctance to do assigned tasks that require sustained mental effort.**
- **g. Loses things necessary for tasks or activities.** Terry said that he forgot his sports equipment, that he left "them in my locker," and that he "can't even find things I need for a big game."
- **h. Distractible.** Terry says he becomes distracted or "zones out" "when I hear the crowd" and "when I start thinking about zoning out."
- **i. Forgetful in daily activities.** Terry forgot his sports supplies, left them in his locker, or could not find them at all.

These symptoms must have been present for at least six months and some symptoms must have been present before 12 years of age. Terry said, "I've been having problems in school ever since I was in kindergarten."

They interfere with school, work, home, or social function. Terry presented for treatment because of problems with sports and he is having problems with his schoolwork.

Some symptoms must be present in at least two settings. Terry's performance was impaired in both school and sports.

The symptoms do not result from oppositional behavior, defiance, hostility, or a failure to understand tasks or instructions. There is no evidence of these problems.

The symptoms do not occur during Schizophrenia and are not better explained by Bipolar Disorder, Major Depressive Disorder, an Anxiety Disorder, a Dissociative Disorder, a Personality Disorder, substance intoxication or withdrawal. There is no evidence of these disorders.

Other Diagnostic Considerations

Terry did not qualify for the diagnosis of Generalized Anxiety Disorder as his therapist suggested. Terry said, "I'm only worried about losing my attention while I'm pitching." In comparison, Generalized Anxiety Disorder requires excessive anxiety or uncontrollable worries lasting at least six months. It cannot be diagnosed if the patient is only worried about the symptoms of a psychiatric diagnosis. Moreover, Terry denied the physical symptoms required for a diagnosis of Generalized Anxiety Disorder, including restlessness, edginess, being easily fatigued, muscle tension, sleep disturbance, mind going blank, or irritability. Terry does have concentration problems, but these are explained by his Attention-Deficit/Hyperactivity Disorder and do not require another diagnosis to account for them.

Bipolar distractibility, hyperactivity, and impulsivity (with increased speech, pressured speech, interrupting others, racing thoughts, agitation, and impulsive actions) can easily be confused with Attention-deficit/Hyperactivity Disorder in children and young adults. This is unfortunate because some antidepressants and stimulants used for Attention-deficit/Hyperactivity Disorder can make Bipolar Disorder worse. However, Terry showed no prolonged episode of elevated, expansive, or irritable mood.

Cognitive Testing

Terry did poorly on Cognitive Examination tests that require *attention*. Tests that he failed (Vigilance, Digit Span, Free Recall from a Story, Uncued Delayed Memory, Cued Delayed Memory, Serial Sevens, and the Arithmetic Story Problem), all require that information be held in working memory, where it is vulnerable to loss by distraction.

CLINICAL NOTES

Like many adolescents and adults, Terry had the inattentive but not the hyperactive/impulsive component of the disease. He did not fidget, squirm, or leave his seat in class; he denied restlessness; he can wait his turn to speak; and he did not seem hyperactive ("on the go") or intrusive in my interview. In contrast to Terry, who became distracted while taking tests, impulsive individuals frequently rush through their examinations and turn in answers that are incomplete or poorly thought-out.

Attention-Deficit/Hyperactivity Disorder is most often seen in grade school and high school children, where it usually manifests as ineffective study behavior and poor grades. Terry's case provides an opportunity to study

Attention-Deficit/Hyperactivity Disorder in an older individual where symptoms manifest in the context of baseball games and sports training, as well as in school.

I offered Terry a medication to improve attention (such as a stimulant or an alpha-2 agonist). Then I called the University Disability Center and sent Terry there for special help organizing his study materials and learning study strategies that were effective for a student with poor attention. I requested preferential seating for Terry in the front of his classrooms and I requested that he be able to take untimed tests in a testing environment free from distractions. The last thing I heard, Terry was passing his courses, and his pitching was unbeatable.

CASE 34
IS JUNE DEMENTED?

Mike brought his 70-year-old mother June to the clinic with concerns about her mental capacity. He told me that June had been doing quite well living by herself until the last few weeks, when she began making decisions that showed poor judgment. In one case, a door-to-door salesperson had sold her an expensive roof treatment that she did not need because her roof was already in good shape. A few days later, another man had come to her home and sold her an expensive driveway-resurfacing job that was unnecessary. These home improvement jobs were never performed. June had paid in cash but she had neither receipts for her money, nor any addresses or telephone numbers to contact the roofing or driveway companies. Moreover, there were some valuable items missing from her home for which she could not account.

Although she seemed all right to her son, Mike wanted me to evaluate her judgment in order to determine whether there was any fundamental problem "buried deep" that had escaped his notice.

In her Diagnostic Examination, June was appropriately dressed for the situation and season and she looked her age. During her examination, she sat quietly in her chair, and she spoke slowly and clearly in a measured rhythm. June said that she enjoyed her life and listed several enjoyable activities in which she had recently participated.

June maintained that she slept seven to eight hours daily, that her appetite was good, and that her weight was stable. The only physical complaints she noted were arthritic pains in her hands and stiffness in her neck, shoulders, and back, but she characterized these problems as "minor." June said that she took no medicine or supplements.

June denied having cardiac palpitations, pounding heart, rapid heart rate, excessive sweating, tremor, shortness of breath, choking, chest pain, nausea, stomachache, dizziness, lightheadedness, fainting, numbness, tingling, derealization (feelings of unreality), depersonalization (feeling detached from oneself), or fears of losing control, dying, or going crazy. She denied feeling keyed-up, restless, edgy, tense, or easily fatigued. She denied exposure to a traumatic event that involved actual or threatened death or injury to self or others, and she said that her concentration was "as good as ever, I suppose." She denied having obsessions or compulsions.

June admitted feeling anxious and confused about "throwing away her money," but she denied daily emotions of elation, sadness, hopelessness, irritability, or emptiness. When I asked her about feelings of anger, she replied, "Just angry at myself, I guess, for being so stupid." There was no evidence of expansive mood. She denied having thought disorder, delusions, or hallucinations and she brushed aside the possibility of suicidal or violent thoughts.

On her Cognitive Examination June did well in all areas of *attention, language, memory, abstract thinking,* and *sequential thinking.* She easily named 14 types of clothing in 30 seconds on a test of Category Recall and recalled 17 items on a test of Free Recall from a Story. I could not administer the Luria Sequential Movement test because her arthritic hands were too stiff and painful.

Because her judgment was in question, I asked her two additional Judgment tests. When I asked her, "What would you do if you found a stamped letter on the sidewalk?" she correctly answered, "Put it in the mailbox." When I asked her, "What do you think of a woman who went into a shop and left her baby on the sidewalk," she answered, "That's not right. The woman should have taken the baby with her."

Anne Colby and Lawrence Kohlberg's book, *The Measurement of Moral Judgment,* (see Chapter 8), provides a system for exploring complexities of the judgment process with quantitative scoring. The patient is presented with a moral dilemma that has no correct answer and she is asked to discuss the various options open to the people in the story and their implications. I described one test situation to June in which a man's wife will die unless she receives medicine but the only pharmacist who has the medicine is unavailable. In response, June was able to discuss the possible options available to the man and how they would affect him, his wife, and the pharmacist.

CHALLENGE

There is a wealth of information in June's presentation if you know what to look for. Your challenge is to come up with a solution that explains June's behavior and then suggest a remedy. Here are some clues. The problem is surprisingly common and it is especially relevant to elders. It will help if you approach the problem with a psychosocial model.

SOLUTION

June is not demented and her judgment is intact. She has **no psychiatric diagnosis**.

Other Diagnostic Considerations

June's normal Cognitive Examination rules out a diagnosis of Mild or Major Neurocognitive Disorder. She has no evidenced of Alzheimer's Disease, Cerebrovascular Disease, or other brain disorders.

Because June admitted to feeling anxiety, some clinicians consider giving her an anxiety disorder. However, she had no palpitations, pounding heart, rapid heart rate, excessive sweating, tremor, shortness of breath, choking, chest pain, nausea, stomachache, dizziness, lightheadedness, fainting, numbness, tingling, derealization (feelings of unreality), depersonalization (feeling detached from oneself), or fears of losing control, dying, or going crazy that are diagnostic of Panic Disorder.

June exhibited none of the symptoms of irritability, sleep problems, restlessness, being keyed-up, edginess, muscle tension, being easily fatigued, poor concentration, or mind going blank necessary to diagnose Generalized Anxiety Disorder.

June denied being exposed to a traumatic event and so she could not be given a diagnosis of Acute or Posttraumatic Stress Disorder.

She had neither obsessions nor compulsions so June did not have Obsessive-Compulsive Disorder.

June denied depressed mood and anhedonia, providing evidence that she enjoyed her life and her activities—therefore, she could not be given a diagnosis of Major Depressive Disorder. She evidenced none of the excessive activity, irritable, expansive, or elevated mood necessary for the diagnosis of a Manic Episode.

June showed no evidence of inattentiveness, hyperactivity, or impulsivity required for a diagnosis of Attention-Deficit/Hyperactivity Disorder.

Cognitive Testing

June passed all tests of basic brain functions, including *attention*, *language*, *memory*, *abstract thinking*, and *sequential* thinking. She also did well on the additional tests of Judgment.

CLINICAL NOTES

I explained to June's son that his mother was the object of a swindle frequently perpetrated by confidence-artists who canvas small residential neighborhoods looking for homes owned by senior adults. One or more of these criminals will then visit the home with a convincing story about the necessity and value of the work that they proffer.

For example, two men in work clothes will visit the home of an elder who lives alone. They explain that they were in the neighborhood working on a neighbor's house when they noticed that the elder's roof or driveway was in dire need of repair. They emphasize how effective the proposed treatment will be and how it will add to the value of the property. They point out the prohibitive cost of repairs if the problem is not taken care of right away. Because they are already in the neighborhood, the swindlers offer to do the job for a ridiculously low price, as long as the deal is closed immediately and in cash. While one swindler makes the pitch and distracts the mark, his accomplice roams the house, opening drawers and taking money or jewelry that is not locked up. The swindlers leave as few records as possible, and if bills of sale or receipts are demanded, they are simply be stolen back by the accomplice before leaving.

The much-vaunted "treatment" is usually just used motor oil sprayed liberally on the surface of the roof or driveway. Its glistening sheen provides reassurance that a good job has been done until it seeps away or washes off in the rain. By this time, the swindlers are long gone. Sometimes, the work may not be done at all, as was June's experience.

The solution for problems like June's is warning and educating elders about frauds, con-artists, and swindlers that target older adults. Elders are vulnerable targets for swindles perpetrated in person, on the telephone, and over the Internet. Victims may not report swindles because they do not want to face the embarrassment of being "taken." Potential targets should be warned to take their time and discuss any unusual commerce with others. Business transactions should never be made in cash—in event of dissatisfaction, payment on checks can be stopped, and many credit cards will remove a charge that is found to be fraudulent.

CHAPTER 6
THE MENTAL STATUS EXAMINATION IN PRIVATE PRACTICE

Many clinicians feel that private practice provides the greatest professional challenge of all practice venues, as well as offering the most fulfillment gained from helping others. Private practice allows clinicians to assess, diagnose, and treat patients as they choose, while building long-lasting professional relationships. However, unlike other clinical environments, private practice clinicians are less likely to have access to a wide range of nearby colleagues and consultants to help them in their practice.

CASE 35
TED DOESN'T LIKE EMOTIONS

Ted was a 39-year-old physician, a star abdominal surgeon at a large Health Maintenance Organization, who came to see me at the recommendation of a mutual colleague.

"Wes, I don't really know why I'm here," Ted began. "I'm a bright, young, successful guy. I'm at the top of my field and I drive a red sports car. I like the hospital where I work and I spend most of my time there. I have a great condo. Everything's great in my life."

"Why *did* you come here to see me, Ted?" I asked.

"Well, I guess I have a bit of an anger problem," Ted explained. "I'm a big guy and if I look the slightest bit irritated, the staff around me gets upset."

"Has anything changed in your life, lately?" I queried.

Ted suddenly looked very sad. "Wes, old age must be setting in, because I get more tired and it's harder for me to concentrate every month. I used to keep myself so busy that my mind never had a chance to think about anything, but now my mind is full of a lot of distracting thoughts. I'm falling apart and I think it's because of *them*!"

"Because of what, Ted?" I inquired.

"The *emotions*!" Ted almost shouted at me. "For the first time in my life, I'm having *emotions* and they're ruining my life. Instead of keeping my mind focused on my work, I keep having guilty thoughts about how I feel about myself, people, and everything. Yesterday I had to leave my clinic and go to the bathroom to cry. Wes, you *have* to help me get rid of these damned *emotions*!"

"But most people have emotions of some kind, Ted," I said.

"Well I'm not most people, Wes, and I don't want them. They're messing up my life." Ted began to cry.

"Tell me more about this anger problem, Ted," I encouraged.

"I'm not a very patient guy," Ted related, "and I sometimes get frustrated with the nurses and other staff if they don't do their jobs right. In the operating room, I'm told that I scream and throw instruments. Last week there was a really loud argument in the operating room and a nurse reported me to the Chief of Surgery. He told me that if I couldn't get my anger under control, I would lose my position. You've got to give me something. My job is all I've got!"

As I began his Diagnostic Examination, I noticed that Ted's expensive sports clothes were disheveled and soiled. He moved slowly during the interview, avoided eye contact, and seemed interpersonally distant.

Ted denied any other history of emotional problems, hospitalization, or psychotherapy. He denied use of any prescribed medications, over-the-counter preparations, supplements, alcohol, or street drugs.

"How has your appetite been, lately, Ted?" I asked.

"Well, I'm not a big eater these days," he admitted sadly. "I eat all my meals in the hospital cafeteria pretty much seven days a week. They have very healthy meals, you know. Our cafeteria is supplied by the same company that makes airline food."

"Hmm. What about your sleep?" I continued.

"I never had any problems sleeping until lately. I'd work late every night, go home late, and I was always so tired I fell asleep immediately, sometimes with all my clothes on. But now, even though I'm exhausted all day, when I lay down, my mind is full of thoughts and emotions that keep me from getting to sleep for hours. Then I wake up really early and I'm back to the thoughts, again."

Ted endorsed recent irritability but he seemed puzzled when I asked him about feelings of sadness, hopelessness, anxiety, panic, loneliness, or emptiness. He denied social avoidance, obsessions, compulsions, past trauma, delusions, or hallucinations. When I asked him about suicidal feelings, he became angry, saying, "I resent that! Do you think that I'm crazy?" Ted said that he had received a recent physical examination from his internist which was normal.

On his Cognitive Examination, Ted did well in *attention, language, abstract thinking,* and *sequential thinking.*

In tests of *memory*, Ted recalled only four of seven spoken numbers on a Digit Span test of working memory. He did not remember any target items after three minutes in a test of Uncued Delayed Memory and he only remembered three of the six target words in a Cued Delayed Memory test.

After I had finished my evaluation, I asked, "What can we do here today to make your life better, Ted?"

Ted replied, "Wes, I have to get rid of these emotions. I'm willing to take whatever pill you think would help me. I'm willing to do almost anything to deal with this situation. Except psychotherapy, that is. I won't do any psychotherapy. That's for crazy people."

CHALLENGE

Ted's impulsive anger episodes are endangering his livelihood and lifestyle. What is Ted's diagnosis and what treatment would you offer?

SOLUTION

Ted is suffering from unipolar **Major Depressive Disorder, Single Episode, Moderate** (DSM-5 296.22, ICD-10 F32.1):

At least five of the following symptoms nearly every day for at least two weeks:
1. **A sad, depressed mood.** Ted was poor at identifying his emotions. Although he cried during his appointment and told me that he "had to leave my clinic and go to the bathroom to cry," he did not endorse any sad moods that occurred every day.
2. **A loss of interest or pleasure in most activities (anhedonia).** Ted could not describe any positive life activities or events—he worked seven days a week and ate airline food in the hospital cafeteria. After work, he would "go home late" and fall "asleep immediately, sometimes with all my clothes on."
3. **A significant change in appetite or weight (e.g., a change of more than 5% of body weight per month).** Ted said, "I'm not a big eater these days."
4. **Insomnia or hypersomnia.** Ted said, "My mind is full of thoughts and emotions that keep me from getting to sleep for hours."
5. **Psychomotor depression or agitation.** (*Psychomotor depression*): Ted "moved slowly during the interview" and his "speech was slowed."
6. **Fatigue or low energy.** Ted complained that he was "exhausted all day."
7. **Thoughts of guilt or worthlessness.** (*Guilt*): Ted said, "I keep having guilty thoughts about how I feel about myself, people, and everything."
8. **Difficulty concentrating or making decisions.** Ted "complained about his focus," saying "it's harder for me to concentrate" and "instead of keeping my mind focused on my work, I keep having thoughts about how I feel about myself, people, and everything." He showed *memory* impairment in a test of Digit Span and in both Uncued and Cued Delayed Memory tests.
9. **Recurrent thoughts of death, suicide, or a suicidal attempt or plan.** When I asked Ted about suicidal feelings, he became angry but he did not *deny* thoughts of suicidality. I am concerned when a patient evades or refuses to discuss the question of suicidality. I decided to watch Ted carefully for the possible emergence of suicidality during treatment.

The symptoms must cause a significant impairment in school, work, home, or social life; and they must include either depressed mood or anhedonia. Ted feared for the loss of his job and his reason for living.

Ted experienced **Melancholic Features** that many clinicians associate with *unipolar* Major Depression:
A. **Either of the following, occurring during the most severe period of the current episode**:
 1. **Loss of pleasure in all or almost all activities.** Ted could not describe any positive life activities or events.
 2. **Lack of reactivity to usually pleasurable stimuli**. Ted said he was depressed despite the fact that "everything's great in my life," "I'm a bright, young, successful guy," "I'm at the top of my field," "I drive a red sports car," "I like the hospital where I work," and "I have a great condo."
B. **Three (or more) of the following**:
 1. **Distinct quality of depressed mood characterized by despondent, morose, despair, or empty mood**. Ted indicated that the depressive feelings he was experiencing were unusually miserable.
 2. **Depression regularly worse in the morning.** "I wake up really early and I'm back to the thoughts, again."

3. **Early morning awakening.** Ted said, "I wake up really early."
4. **Marked psychomotor depression or agitation.** (*Psychomotor depression*): Ted "moved slowly during the interview" and his "speech was slowed."
5. **Significant anorexia or weight loss.** Ted said, "I'm not a big eater these days."
6. **Excessive or inappropriate guilt.** Ted said, "I keep having guilty thoughts."

Other Diagnostic Considerations

In addition to unipolar Major Depressive Disorder, depressive episodes mood can be found in Bipolar I Disorder, Most Recent Episode Depressed, Bipolar I Disorder with Mixed Mood, and Bipolar II Disorder. However, Ted showed none of the stigma of bipolar depression and had no history of Manic Episodes. Fortunately for Ted, unipolar Major Depressive Disorder usually responds readily to appropriate psychotherapy and antidepressants, whereas bipolar depression is often treatment-resistant.

Dysphoric mood can also be found in organic brain injury from trauma, stroke, toxicity, and drug abuse, but "Ted had received a recent evaluation from his internist and he denied the use of any substances."

Ted's personality resembles Obsessive-Compulsive Personality Disorder, in that he devotes his life to work, to the exclusion of socialization and entertainment. If he still has problems after his Major Depressive Disorder is controlled, he should be reevaluated for Obsessive-Compulsive Personality Disorder (see *Mental Status Examination for Personality Disorders*, Chapter 8).

Cognitive Testing

Ted failed tests of Digit Span, Uncued Delayed Memory, and Cued Delayed Memory. *Memory* problems are often seen in patients with unipolar Major Depressive Disorder.

CLINICAL NOTES

Ted's devotion to his work has helped him be a successful surgeon but his attitudes and behavior are a prescription for operating room resentment. His rigid devotion to work has reduced his social support and opportunities to relax, while increasing the life stress that may have triggered his unipolar Major Depressive Disorder. Furthermore, the heavy time commitment required for premedical and medical education followed by surgical residency and specialty surgical training combined to limit his interpersonal experience and impede his social maturation. Good social skills help us decide when to use subtlety instead of force, encouragement rather than criticism, and patience instead of persistence. Tantrums are a normal way to handle frustration in a child, but not in a 39-year-old man.

Ted tried to keep his mind too busy to think and feel—this is a common strategy patients use to block depression. Unfortunately, this strategy inevitably fails when negative thoughts become too strong to block. Such patients often exhibit a paradoxical lack of insight into their own emotions and Ted was genuinely puzzled when asked to describe feelings of sadness, hopelessness, anxiety, panic, loneliness, or emptiness.

I treated Ted with an SSRI antidepressant that patients describe as "emotionally deadening," because Ted was requesting a lower level of emotionality. I would have preferred that Ted accept psychotherapy in an attempt to come to terms with his emotions, but he flatly refused. He had had a life that he perceived as stable and successful without emotions and he wished to return to it. Nevertheless, I insisted on seeing him for 50-minute sessions weekly to help him learn to get the most from his medication. During that time, we discussed how he felt about the staff and patients at the hospital and what they might be thinking and feeling around him. Ted was not an ideal candidate for insight-oriented psychotherapy, but he had no trouble participating actively in these discussions. I had some hope that this "inoculation of insight" would help him develop a less autistic and more empathic interpersonal style.

Ted's depression symptoms waned at the end of six months, whereupon he discontinued his treatment. For five years, Ted continued doing well in his job and career with no return of his unipolar depressive break. I hope his positive experience in my care will help him give psychotherapy a chance if his depression ever returns.

CASE 36
MARILYN MAKES A COMEBACK

Marilyn M, a 66-year-old actress, came to my office with concerns about Alzheimer's Disease, aging, and her career.

"Doctor, I want to go back to my work in films," she said. "It's possible that I will soon be offered a good part in a film but I am afraid I won't be able to take it because I have grown too old.

"I was diagnosed with clinical depression long ago but I've been taking the same antidepressant for 35 years without a depressive episode," she noted.

"One of my problems is that I am very tired all day, every day. Sometimes I'm so tired that I just give up and go to bed, even in the middle of the day. How can I take on a film role if I have no energy?"

I shrugged my shoulders to say I did not know.

"Also, I have a terrible difficulty concentrating and remembering that I never had before," Marilyn bemoaned. "Sometimes I'll be in the middle of doing something and I get so confused. This is worse in the evening before I go to bed. The way things are now—I could never learn my lines.

"I went to a neurologist to see if I have Alzheimer's but he told me I don't. He told me that I am experiencing the normal course of aging and he told me to adjust to it. I couldn't bear it if I was never able to work again.

"Another thing, doctor. Although I watch what I eat, I can't seem to take off any weight no matter what I do. I diet and I exercise but I just can't lose any pounds. Part of it is because I'm constipated but that's just another old-person's condition. I'm thirsty all the time, too. I went to my family doctor to see if I had diabetes but she said I didn't. She told me I would feel better if I stopped smoking but I quit and I feel even worse.

"I have skin problems, too. My skin just flakes away and looks horrible. I also have problems with my eyes. I went to my eye doctor and he said my eyes were too dry. Now I take eye drops but they don't help much. If I try to have sex, it's terribly painful. Maybe that's just old age, too. My daughter said I'm too old to be thinking about sex, anyway."

In beginning her Diagnostic Examination, I noticed that Marilyn was dressed somewhat lightly for the cool spring day. She sat quietly in her chair and did not move her hands and arms very much.

Marilyn said that she slept too deeply and longer than she wanted. She denied physical symptoms of pounding or racing heart, restlessness, edginess, excessive sweating, trembling, shaking, muscle tension, chills, hot flushes, shortness of breath, choking, chest pain, nausea, stomachache, dizziness, lightheadedness, a sense of detachment, or poor concentration.

Marilyn denied feeling elated, sad, hopeless, anxious, fearful, irritable, angry, or empty. She admitted feeling discouraged but she said that she was active and enjoying her life. There was no evidence of expansive mood. She showed no evidence of delusions, formal thought disorder, or hallucinations. She endorsed no shyness, obsessive thoughts, compulsive behaviors, or history of a traumatic episode. She had never tried to commit suicide and she denied any current thoughts of suicide or violence.

On her Cognitive Examination, Marilyn's attention sometimes wandered, her thoughts were slowed, and her voice was somewhat hoarse. However, she did well on tests of *attention*, *language*, and *abstract thinking*.

In *memory* tests, Marilyn failed Free Recall from a Story. She could not remember any of the words on the test of Uncued Delayed Memory, but after rehearsal, she remembered all the words on the Cued Delayed Memory test.

In tests of *sequential thinking*, Marilyn could only subtract 7 from 100 five times on the Serial Sevens test. She declined further testing.

Marilyn continued her list of complaints. "It's embarrassing but I don't think my physical system is working right. My family doctor said I'm just getting depressed again but this does not feel like the depression that I had twenty years ago. Besides, I'm taking my antidepressant."

CHALLENGE

Marilyn has seen three clinicians before us without finding a solution to her problems. Could it be that they did not listen carefully to her story? Try to diagnose Marilyn's condition, find the underlying cause of her problems, and suggest a treatment.

SOLUTION

Marilyn is experiencing the sedation, fatigue, dryness, constipation, weight gain, physical and mental slowing, and body warmth caused by the **anticholinergic side effects** (ICD-10 Y51.3) of her old tricyclic antidepressant.

Other Diagnostic Considerations

Because of her past history of Major Depressive Disorder, it is tempting to attribute all her problems to depression. Similarly, knowing that she is an elder adult makes it easy to blame her problems on old age. The two previous clinicians based their conclusions on Marilyn's history, but they were wrong.

The diagnosis of a Major Depressive Episode requires the presence of depressed mood or anhedonia, but Marilyn denied sadness and made it clear that she was active and enjoyed her life. Without those symptoms, a diagnosis of Major Depressive Episode cannot be made, despite Marilyn's symptoms of weight gain, hypersomnia, psychomotor depression, fatigue, and difficulty concentrating. She may have had a history of Major Depressive Disorder but her symptoms were controlled by her antidepressant and the most appropriate diagnosis for her depression is **Major Depressive Disorder, Recurrent, in Full Remission** (DSM-5 296.36, ICD-10 F33.42).

Marilyn is worried about her career, her concentration, her memory, aging, Alzheimer's Disease, overweight, poor vision, painful sexual intercourse (dyspareunia), and becoming depressed again. However, she does not exhibit the restless sleep, restlessness, edginess, muscle tension, poor concentration, mind going blank, or irritability needed to diagnosis Generalized Anxiety Disorder.

Cognitive Testing

On her Cognitive Examination, Marilyn's thinking was slowed and distractible. She had difficulty remembering targets which were uncued (but not those that she was warned to remember) and she had difficulty in serial subtraction (although her simple arithmetic abilities were good). These results do not support any focal disability, but they are consistent with mild sedation.

CLINICAL NOTES

Medicines that block the neurotransmitter acetylcholine (called anticholinergics) cause physical symptoms of sedation, fatigue, sleepiness, mental and physical slowing, impaired concentration, weight gain, constipation, thirst, dry skin and mucous membranes, and body warmth. These effects match all of Marilyn's complaints. Among antidepressants, the older tricyclics such as amitriptyline (Elavil), clomipramine (Anafranil), and doxepin (Sinequan) have the strongest anticholinergic action (see *The Depression Answerbook,* Chapter 8). Cold medicines, antihistamine allergy medications, and many other prescription and over-the-counter medications also have strong anticholinergic effects.

Anticholinergic compounds are famous for causing cognitive impairment by slowing thought and decreasing patients' ability to follow ongoing stimuli in their surrounding environment. Marilyn said that her concentration problems were worse in the evening because that is when she took her antidepressant. The stimulating effects of nicotine had countered her antidepressant's sedating effect and the metabolic effects of smoking decreased blood levels of her tricyclic antidepressant. When Marilyn stopped smoking on her doctor's advice, she felt worse.

Because elders metabolize medications more slowly as they age, their medication blood levels increase over the years. This is how medication doses that were originally benign cause problems as patients grow older. In addition to higher drug levels, there is evidence that elder adults are more sensitive to the effects of anticholinergics and antihistamines. It is common to see elder patients who take many anticholinergic medications present for unnecessary Alzheimer's Disease evaluations. One geriatric physician told me that, "Most of my job is taking away medications, not giving them."

I replaced Marilyn's old antidepressant with a newer one that was devoid of anticholinergic symptoms and she recovered in all respects. She stopped criticizing herself for being old and she landed her movie role. You may even see her sometime if you watch late-night television.

CASE 37
HELP! I CAN'T TELL YOU WHAT'S WRONG

I was watching heat waves rise from the sidewalk when tall, blond Cindy walked into my office ten minutes late for our first appointment. She stumbled over a table as she entered the room, but I could not tell if she was clumsy or failed to see the obstacle. She sat down and began to speak.

"Doctor," she said. "My name is Cindy. I have a problem I need to talk about with you.

"Actually, my problem involves depression, but it's...it's very complicated. Only my doctor and I know about it and he has promised not to tell anyone. I'm not sure I want to let anyone else know about it. Also, I'm not really sure that it's a psychiatric problem and so I'm not sure that you will know anything about it. Maybe I shouldn't even be here in the first place." Cindy squirmed slightly in her chair.

"What *do* you feel comfortable talking about, today?" I inquired.

"Well, my cousin is disabled with depression," Cindy said. "And I wanted to ask you some questions about him, anyway. So maybe I could start there."

When I looked away for a moment, I saw Cindy surreptitiously rub the left side of her neck and face. She kept her hands in her lap but when she did move her arms, I could see a coarse tremor on her right side.

Cindy launched into a description of her depressed cousin's problems in a tone that seemed too cheerful for the quality of her cousin's sad story. In two instances, I was surprised to see Cindy softly laugh aloud. Finally, she said, "My depression problem isn't about my cousin. It's about me," and stopped.

In contrast to her reluctance to be interviewed, Cindy was quite cooperative on her Cognitive Examination. She failed the Vigilance test in the *attention* section.

Cindy did well on all tests of *language,* although her Speech Quality was monotonic and she spoke in bursts, as if she was trying to get all the words out before she paused again. Some of her words were slurred.

In *memory* testing, Cindy failed the tests of Free Recall from a Story, Uncued Delayed Memory, and Cued Delayed Memory.

In the *abstract thinking* section, Cindy struggled with Proverb Interpretation and gave up after one proverb. She said she felt too tired to continue after that.

Cindy took a deep breath and began to cry softly. "I should be telling you about my health problem, but I'm having a hard time saying what it is. I'm just so tired all the time and it seems to be worse during these hot days."

I leaned over in my chair and looked into her eyes, which regarded me with a jerky gaze. "That is all right, Cindy. I think I can guess what you want to tell me."

CHALLENGE
Your challenge is to carefully read the description and try to determine Cindy's underlying disorder.
SOLUTION

Cindy has **multiple sclerosis** (ICD-10 G35).

Multiple sclerosis is a progressive deterioration of nerve cells in the brain and spinal cord characterized by scanning speech, slurred speech, fatigue, heat sensitivity, depressed and labile mood, inappropriate affect, tremor, nystagmus, vision problems, muscle weakness, dizziness, lack of coordination, and paresthesias. When a patient with multiple sclerosis walks in your office and you see all these symptoms together, you will never forget them.

My first clue to Cindy's multiple sclerosis was her scanning speech (speech that occurs in rapid monotonic bursts separated by brief hesitation or silence) that is characteristic of multiple sclerosis. Also, "some of her words were slurred." When Cindy said that her fatigue was "worse during these hot days," she revealed heat sensitivity—the neurological problems of multiple sclerosis worsen when the weather is hot. Cindy mentioned depression, and depressed mood is common in multiple sclerosis. She also demonstrated labile mood by suddenly laughing and crying, and inappropriate affect by her over-cheerfulness during a sad story. I observed a coarse tremor in her right arm, and when I "looked into her eyes," I saw "jerky" movements of nystagmus, unconscious rhythmic movements of the eyes.

Some symptoms were equivocal. For example, stumbling over a table might be caused by vision problems, muscle weakness, dizziness, lack of coordination, or difficulty walking. Rubbing her left neck and face may have reflected sensory paresthesias like numbness and tingling.

Other Diagnostic Considerations

Cindy's deficits in *attention, language, memory,* and *abstract thinking* lead some clinicians to diagnose Mild Neurocognitive Disorder (DSM-5 331.83, ICD-10 G31.84). However, there is no evidence that these cognitive deficits are causing her to expend greater effort or use compensatory strategies in her daily activities. The physical symptoms and depression caused by multiple sclerosis are the source of Cindy's problems.

The presence of multiple, changing and seemingly unrelated physical symptoms in multiple sclerosis is often mistaken for Somatization Disorder, Factitious Disorder, or Malingering. However, Cindy did not have the multiple pain, gastrointestinal, sexual, and pseudoneurological symptoms necessary for Somatization Disorder. Cindy did not appear to be feigning physical or psychological symptoms to assume the rôle of a sick person, as in Factitious Disorder—in fact; she seemed to be trying to hide her physical condition. And there was no evidence that Cindy was seeking personal gain, which is essential for the diagnosis of Malingering.

Cindy's individual symptoms reflect dysfunction in several parts of the nervous system. Scanning speech, poor coordination (ataxia), intention tremor, and dizziness can arise from damage to the brain cerebellum. Nystagmus (eye movements) originate in the vestibular system, cerebellum, and brainstem. Tremors can result from damage to the brain neocortex, cerebellum, and brainstem. Heat sensitivity (also known as Uhthoff's syndrome) results from the effects of heat on damaged nerve cells at any place in the nervous system. The presence of simultaneous problems at many sites in the nervous system is typical of multiple sclerosis.

Bipolar Disorder, Schizophrenia with negative symptoms, Borderline Personality Disorder, and Schizotypal Personality Disorder often present with labile mood or inappropriate affect. Medications and drugs of abuse can cause slurred speech, fatigue, labile mood, tremor, nystagmus, dizziness, and lack of coordination. However, multiple sclerosis explains all of Cindy's symptoms.

Cognitive Testing

Cindy's Cognitive Examination demonstrated errors on tests that required sustained attention, including Vigilance, Free Recall from a Story, and both Uncued and Cued Delayed Memory. Without sustained attention, she is more likely to make errors on tests of *abstract thinking* or *sequential thinking*.

CLINICAL NOTES

Multiple sclerosis causes the loss of myelin insulation around nerve cells distributed throughout the central nervous system. Multiple sclerosis is present in 0.03% of the world's population. It is most common in white women and it is five times more prevalent in cooler climates than in the tropics. Symptoms come and go, depending on where the nervous system damage is located and the limited ability of the nervous system to repair itself. Prognosis is hard to predict, but multiple sclerosis can seriously impair patients' ability to function normally.

Depression and labile affect characterized by sudden laughing or crying, are often the first symptoms of multiple sclerosis, leading patients to seek help from psychiatrists, psychologists, social workers, and counselors. Moods of euphoria, sadness, anxiety, and anger can appear suddenly, fluctuate, and disappear. Symptoms resembling Manic Episodes have been reported late in the course of the disease. Cognitive testing often reveals poor *attention* and *abstract thinking*.

You will periodically find patients who have difficulty telling you their problems. Sometimes they begin by describing their problem as if it belonged to someone else. Sometimes they ramble vaguely through most of their evaluation and finally drop their bombshell a few minutes before the end of the session.

Cindy had many good reasons to hesitate before releasing her health information. Some patients wish to protect their family and friends from the painful knowledge of the gradual and potentially crippling deterioration that multiple sclerosis sometimes brings. Some multiple sclerosis patients fear gossip, discrimination, and pity if their secret gets out. Other patients try to deny the existence of their multiple sclerosis by refusing to face it or talk about it. Cindy demonstrated her wish to work on her problems by showing up at her appointment with me, and together, we helped address her problems.

I offered Cindy an SSRI antidepressant that has been shown to increase the release of brain-derived neurotrophic factor (BDNF), a substance the body produces to help heal and regrow cells in the brain. I encouraged her to begin weekly individual Interpersonal Therapy to address her depression and help her cope with her changing relationships. I referred her to a therapy group composed of other multiple sclerosis patients to learn coping skills. Together, these treatments were effective in helping Cindy come to grips with her illness and improve her level of function.

Cindy's case is not common, but people like Cindy frequently come to mental health clinicians for help. Do not be surprised if a patient like Cindy walks into your own office someday soon.

CASE 38
MISS ZELDA TUMBLES

Miss Zelda F was a 51-year-old, slightly overweight woman who came to my office on time for her appointment. Her brown hair was long and coiled around her head. Her blouse, skirt, and shoes reflected youthful styles that had been in the stores some ten years earlier. She entered my office, settled on my couch, and began to speak.

"I am coming to you, Doctor, because I can't go out of my house," she began.

"How did this happen, Zelda?" I inquired.

"Everything was fine in my life until I turned forty," Zelda replied. Suddenly, on my 40th birthday, I found that I could not leave my home."

"How were your emotions at that time?" I asked.

"I had some mild depression going back for years, but it hadn't changed any," Miss Zelda answered. "I had no anxiety, panic, or other strong emotions that I remember."

"Tell me more about why you cannot leave your home," I encouraged.

"I'm not sure what I was thinking before," Zelda explained, "but lately, I never go outside my house because I am embarrassed about my overweight condition. I don't want to run into any of my former boyfriends—that would be horrifying."

"I had so many former suitors who were willing to do anything to please me and win my affections," Zelda continued. "I was a fool to reject their advances when I was young because now they are gone from my life. Wherever they are, I am sure that my boyfriends still desire me. The possibility of reunion is out of the question because of the shame I feel from being overweight. Even if I looked and felt fine, it would be impossible to rejoin them because I am unable to leave my house."

"How do you spend your days?" I asked.

"I spend the majority of my time sleeping in bed to overcome my low energy and fatigue," Zelda answered.

In her Diagnostic Examination, Zelda said that she suffered from headache, neckache, lower back pain, joint pain, fatigue, urinary frequency, low sex interest, difficulty achieving orgasm, and poor concentration. Zelda said she suffered from poor-self esteem and employed overeating as a means to make her feel better. She complained of experiencing hopelessness and sadness nearly every day for the last five years, but she denied any strong feelings of anxiety, fear, irritability, anger, or guilt. She denied any history of a suicide attempt, suicidal thoughts, or any hospitalization for psychiatric reasons.

Zelda refused a Cognitive Examination with the comment that "such things don't apply to me."

I gave Zelda a diagnosis and treated her for one year using Behavioral Therapy in 50-minute weekly sessions. As a result of her therapeutic work, Zelda was finally able to run errands, keep appointments, and leave her home to walk down the block unassisted for about 10 minutes before she felt compelled to return to her residence.

A month in advance of Christmastime, I had informed Zelda that my office would be closed during the upcoming holiday and we would miss one session while I was out of town. This would be the first appointment we had missed since we had begun our therapy. I tried to prepare Zelda by discussing this brief separation during each of our sessions, but she always changed the subject. On our last appointment before the holiday, I reminded her again about our schedule change and told her, "So I guess we won't be seeing each other for a while." I then reassured her that if she had any problems, she could call a wise old doctor who was covering for me. She said nothing until the end of the session and then walked out the door without a word.

After I returned from my brief trip, I expected to see Zelda at her usual appointment time but she did not appear. When I checked with the office manager, he told me that Zelda had fainted within hours after last leaving my office—she was now on the inpatient neurology ward of a nearby hospital.

When I called the attending physician on the neurology ward, he told me that he had admitted Zelda on an emergency basis for bilateral paralysis of both legs and amnesia surrounding the event. He surmised that she had sustained a severe fall that had both damaged her spinal cord and produced amnesia. His neurological examination, a computerized tomography (CT) scan, and a magnetic resonance imaging (MRI) study of her spine had been normal, but he was considering the possibility of closed head injury or stroke.

I called on Zelda in her hospital bed and expressed my regret that she was in the hospital. I told her I was back in my office again and that I hoped to see her soon at her next appointment. Zelda was surprised to hear from me. She said, "The last thing I remember you saying to me was, 'We won't be seeing each other again,' and then you told me to call another doctor. I remember thinking that I would never see you anymore."

CHALLENGE

Miss Zelda has a complicated story. What diagnosis you would have given her when she first appeared in your office? Would you change her diagnosis or treatment now? If so, what changes would you make?

SOLUTION

Zelda is suffering from **Persistent Depressive Disorder** (DSM-5 300.4, ICD-10 F34.1) and **Conversion Disorder (Functional Neurological Symptom Disorder)** (DSM-5 300.11, ICD-10 F44.4):

On her first appointment, Zelda met the following criteria for **Persistent Depressive Disorder**:
A. **Depressed mood most of the day for more days than not, for at least two years**. Zelda complained of feeling "sadness nearly every day for the last five years."
B. **Present while depressed, of two (or more) of the following**:
  1. **Poor appetite or overeating**. (*Overeating*): Zelda said that she "employed overeating as a means to make her feel better."
  2. **Insomnia or hypersomnia**. (*Hypersomnia*): Zelda said she spent "the majority of my time sleeping in bed."
  3. **Low energy or fatigue**. Zelda suffered from "low energy and fatigue."
  4. **Low self-esteem**. "Zelda said she suffered from poor-self esteem."
  5. **Poor concentration or difficulty making decisions**. (*Poor concentration*): Although Zelda refused a Cognitive Examination, "she complained of poor concentration."
  6. **Feelings of hopelessness**. In her Diagnostic Examination, Zelda complained of "hopelessness."

When I discontinued our psychotherapy for a week, Zelda experienced a **Conversion Disorder**:
One or more symptoms of motor or sensory deficit. The neurologist "had admitted Zelda on an emergency basis for bilateral paralysis of both legs and amnesia," which he felt was caused by damage to her spinal cord, "closed head injury, or stroke."
The symptoms are incompatible with a neurological or medical condition. The neurologist's examination as well as the computerized tomography (CT) and magnetic resonance imaging (MRI) studies of her spine had been normal.
The symptoms cause clinically significant distress or impairment in school, work, home, or social function or warrant medical evaluation. (*Impairment*): Zelda could not have maintained a normal school, work, family, or social life while lying paralyzed. (*Warrants medical evaluation*): The attending neurologist felt that Zelda's problem warranted medical evaluation because he admitted her to the hospital on an emergency basis.
The symptoms are not better explained by another medical or mental disorder. There were no additional medical or mental disorders that accounted for Zelda's paralysis.

Other Diagnostic Considerations

Most clinicians seize on the diagnosis of Agoraphobia because Zelda stayed in her house. However, individuals with Agoraphobia are trying to avoid possible panic symptoms when they avoid places or situations where escape might be difficult, a Panic Attack might be embarrassing, or where help might be unavailable (such as standing in a crowd; waiting in a line; stopping on a bridge; or traveling in a bus, train, subway, automobile, or airplane). In contrast, Zelda said "I never go outside my house because I am embarrassed about my overweight condition" and "I don't want to run into any of my former boyfriends."

Because Miss Zelda reported depressive emotions, many clinicians think of Major Depressive Disorder. However, Zelda did not meet the criteria for unipolar Major Depressive Disorder, because her depressed mood was not a change from previous functioning—instead it was constant and chronic over the past five years. Zelda did not meet criteria for a Manic Episode because she did not exhibit an elevated, expansive, or irritable mood.

Zelda did not have symptoms of Panic Attacks (such as pounding heart, choking, dizziness or lightheadedness, excessive sweating, chest pain, feelings of unreality or detachment, trembling, nausea, stomachache, fear of losing control, shortness of breath, numbing or tingling sensations, chills or hot flushes, or fear of dying) that peaked over minutes. She did not have Generalized Anxiety Disorder because she did not complain of uncontrollable worries about events or activities occurring most days for at least six months. Neither did she complain of muscle tension, irritability, feeling keyed-up or edgy, restless sleep, or her mind going blank.

Patient's with Conversion Disorder are often considered for diagnoses of Factitious Disorder or Malingering. However, there was no indication that Zelda's condition was intentionally produced or feigned to adopt an invalid rôle, as in Factitious Disorder. There was no evidence that Zelda was seeking personal gain, which is essential for the diagnosis of Malingering.

Although Zelda had many physical complaints (including headache, neckache, lower back pain, constipation, joint pain, urinary frequency, low libido, difficulty achieving orgasm, and poor concentration), she did not have the excessive thoughts about the seriousness of her symptoms, excessive anxiety about her health, or excessive time and energy devoted to her physical problems necessary for the diagnosis of Somatic Symptom Disorder.

Zelda shows several characteristics of Narcissistic Personality Disorder, including an inflated sense of self-importance and a preoccupation with fantasies of power, attractiveness, and ideal love. She expected admiration from her former suitors and some might find her comportment arrogant or snobbish. When she has stabilized, she should be evaluated for Narcissistic Personality Disorder (see *Mental Status Examination for Personality Disorders,* Chapter 8).

CLINICAL NOTES

When I interrupted her psychotherapy and left town for a week, Zelda felt abandoned—many patients have this reaction when their therapist goes on vacation. However, Zelda had few social contacts in her life and my impending absence must have been sorely felt. In her mind, she heard me say "we won't be seeing each other again" and telling her "to call another doctor." She had turned a week-long absence into permanent abandonment. At that point, Zelda fainted and developed paralysis and amnesia. A few days after I called on Zelda in the hospital, her paralytic symptoms abated, her cognition cleared, and she appeared in my office for her next regular appointment

The list of medical and neurological differential diagnoses for conversion disorder is long, so the neurologist's workup served to ensure that no medical etiologies had been overlooked. All studies that were performed in the hospital came back with normal results. There was never any direct evidence that a serious fall had taken place and no physical injury was ever demonstrated.

Previously called Conversion Reaction or Hysterical Neurosis, accounts of "hysterical" numbness and paralysis abound in the earliest neuropsychiatric literature. However, Conversion Disorder now appears to be rare, occurring in about 0.02 % of the population.

One way of thinking about conversion symptoms is that they allow partial expression of a forbidden desire without the need to confront one's own impulses. In the context of psychotherapy, conversion symptoms can send a message about the therapeutic relationship that the patient cannot tolerate expressing directly. When threatened with perceived abandonment, Zelda's conversion symptoms sent a message to me that she was helpless and damaged and needed me to care for her. Although many conversion reactions have been described during Psychoanalytic Psychotherapy, Miss Zelda's conversion symptoms developed while she was receiving Behavioral Therapy.

After leaving the hospital, Zelda returned to her regular therapy schedule. Although I could have continued Behavioral Therapy, I elected to change her to Psychodynamic Psychotherapy because of the wealth of literature and experience treating conversion disorder, dysthymia, and personality disorders (neuroses) with this type of psychotherapy. She did well with this change and continues to improve.

CASE 39
TONY HAS A PERFECT PLAN

The sun was setting bright orange on a chilly Friday in December, early in my practice, when 29-year-old Tony P. walked into my office as a new patient. He was the last patient of the day and he was 30 minutes late, so our appointment time was limited.

Tony's face was bright and his manner was both dramatic and enthusiastic. Before I could speak, he launched into his story.

"OK, Wes. Here's my situation. I am the most successful person you'll ever meet—I am a studio executive—but I'm just not satisfied. I spend all my time working to get what I have but I feel like I'm capable of something truly wonderful. The stress makes me feel real edgy—it's hard for me to sit still. Also, my coworkers are all annoying. For weeks, the stress has made me lose my temper and it keeps me from sleeping. I am doing fine without much sleep, however. I just can't stand this stress.

"Also, my family and I fight all the time. My wife has put on some weight and my kids are not great students. I'm pissed off when my friends come over—I'm sure they are all thinking, 'How did a successful guy like Tony get stuck with this dumpy wife and these second-rate kids?' I deserve much better."

Tony denied experiencing muscle tension, fatigue, poor concentration, his mind going blank, palpitations, pounding heart, rapid heart rate, sweating, tremor, shortness of breath, choking, chest pain, nausea, stomachache, dizziness, fainting, numbness, derealization, or depersonalization, hypervigilance, exaggerated startle response, feeling dazed, amnesia, or fears of losing control, dying, or going crazy. He said he had never experienced a traumatic event.

On his Cognitive Examination, Tony did well on tests of *attention* and *language*. However, he was very talkative and his Quality of Speech was somewhat loud and rapid.

In the *memory* section, Tony could only repeat four out of seven digits on the Digit Span test. In the Cued Delayed Memory test, he could not remember any words without contextual hints.

In the *abstract thinking* section, Tony failed Proverb Interpretation. When asked to interpret the proverb, "Don't cry over spilt milk," he said, "There's no time like the present." When asked to interpret the proverb, "Rome wasn't built in a day," he replied, "When in Rome, do as the Romans do."

In the *sequential thinking* section, Tony failed Serial Sevens and the Arithmetic Story Problem.

At that point, I looked at the clock and found that our appointment time was up. I said, "Our session has come to an end, Tony, and I am not finished with your evaluation. I'd like you to come back on Monday so we can finish. In the meantime, I'll give you some evaluation material you can fill out yourself at home." I handed Tony a copy of the Diagnostic Questionnaire (Appendix II) and the Cognitive Questionnaire (Appendix IV), as well as some additional tests of *abstract* and *sequential thinking* to finish at home (Appendices VI and VII).

"That's fine with me," Tony replied, "but I don't want to go home without any treatment. I have anxiety and I want you to give me an SSRI antidepressant. I looked it up on the Internet, and I am positive that this brand of antidepressant would be just right for me."

"Sorry, Tony," I said. "It doesn't work like that. I have to match your medicine to your diagnosis and physiological profile. Also, we have to balance any potential benefits from an antidepressant with the possible risks that can come from taking it." At this point, I took a few minutes explaining the risks and benefits of the antidepressant he was suggesting, as well as other treatment alternatives.

"If you will not give this antidepressant to me, I will just get it from the Internet," Tony rejoined. "But I will make you a deal. Just give me three capsules of this antidepressant, just enough to get me through tonight and the weekend, and I'll be back in your office first thing Monday morning. Then, if I do not feel totally great, I will do whatever you suggest and work together with you to your satisfaction. I promise. I mean, what could go wrong in three days, right?"

I barely knew Tony and I felt I did not have enough evidence to make a definite diagnosis. However, he did have complaints of anxiety, edginess, and worried thoughts, so I assumed that he might have some anxiety disorder and I knew anxiety disorders can be treated with antidepressants.

Unfortunately, at this early stage of my career, I took the bait and gave Tony a prescription for three antidepressant capsules. Like Tony, I could not imagine what could go wrong in three days. I knew from my residency training that antidepressants did not even start working for three weeks. Tony left my office that evening feeling satisfied and I went home assuring myself that I had made another person's life a little brighter.

However, Tony did not come back in three days or even in three weeks. It was a full month before I saw Tony again.

CHALLENGE

What could have gone wrong with Tony's perfect plan? What would you have done differently?

SOLUTION

Tony has **Bipolar I Disorder, Most Recent Episode Manic, Severe** (DSM-5 296.43, ICD-10 F31.13).

On Monday, I reviewed Tony's clinical notes and I found that he met these criteria for a **Manic Episode**:

A. The following have been present most of the day nearly every day:

Increased goal-directed activity or energy. Tony was activated and energetic in my office and he said, "I spend all my time working."

Plus at least one of these:
  a. **Elevated mood.**
  b. **Expansive mood.** "Tony's face was bright and his manner was both dramatic and enthusiastic."
  c. **Irritable mood.** Tony gives examples of his irritability, saying that "for weeks, the stress has made me lose my temper," "my coworkers are all annoying," and "my family and I fight all the time."

These symptoms last at least one week or any duration if hospitalization is necessary.

B. At least three of the following symptoms (four if the mood is only irritable):

1. **Inflated self-esteem or grandiosity.**): (*Self-esteem*): "I am the most successful guy you'll ever meet." (*Grandiosity*): "I feel like I'm capable of something truly wonderful."
2. **A decreased need for sleep (needs <3 hours).** Tony said that his situation "keeps me from sleeping," yet he felt that "I am doing fine without much sleep."
3. **Talking more than usual or interrupting others (pressured speech).** (*More talkative*): Tony "was very talkative." (*Pressured*): He launched into his monologue without giving me a chance to speak.
4. **Rapid or racing thoughts.** Tony's Quality of Speech was "rapid."
5. **Distractibility.** Tony did not complain of distractibility but he failed Digit Span, Cued Delayed Memory, Serial Sevens, and the Arithmetic Story Problem on his Cognitive Examination, tests that are vulnerable to distractibility.
6. **Increased goal-directed activity or psychomotor agitation.** (*Goal-directed activity*): "I spend all my time working." (*Psychomotor agitation*): Tony said he felt "real edgy—it's hard for me to sit still."
7. **Excessive involvement in activities that have a high potential for painful consequences (costly or risky impulsive actions).**

These bipolar symptoms should have warned me not to give Tony an antidepressant.

A month later, Tony told me what had happened after his first appointment. After taking three antidepressant capsules, Tony felt on top of the world. He stayed up all Sunday night thinking and talking with himself. On Monday morning, Tony went to work and submitted his resignation. When the president and CEO asked why he quit, Tony screamed at them, "You have been holding me back and keeping me from my greatness!"

Tony drove his commuter car to the bank, withdrew all his savings, and closed his account. When he arrived back home, Tony took all the bottles from his liquor cabinet and loaded them into his family's expensive luxury convertible. Ignoring the objections of his wife and children, Tony drove away and turned north toward Washington. Along the way, he bought cases of beer and picked up hitchhikers alongside the road.

Tony drove day and night with the top down, drinking beer and singing with his new friends, only stopping to replenish his liquor supply. When he was too exhausted to drive, he stopped and rented suite in five-star hotels. There he sent out for more liquor and partied drunkenly all night with the hitchhikers and whomever else he could find in the hotel. In the morning, without sleep but still wide-awake, he and his friends hit the road again.

The next thing that Tony remembered was waking up on a cot in a Canadian jail cell two weeks later. His brother was sitting nearby, and when Tony could converse, his brother explained that the police had found him wandering down a snowy road in a daze, without any wallet, money, credit cards, or shoes. The police had found his name on an old credit receipt in his pocket and called his brother to get him. No one ever found the car.

After he began his exodus, Tony met these additional criteria for a **Manic Episode**:

A. The following have been present most of the day nearly every day:

Increased goal-directed activity or energy. Tony stayed up driving and partying 24 hours a day.

Plus at least one of these:

a. **Elevated mood.** "Tony felt on top of the world."
   b. **Expansive mood.**
   c. **Irritable mood.** Tony screamed at his company's president and CEO.

These symptoms last at least one week or any duration if hospitalization is necessary.

B. At least three of the following symptoms (four if the mood is only irritable):

1. **Inflated self-esteem or grandiosity.** . (*Grandiosity*): "Tony told his supervisors, "You have been holding me back and keeping me from my greatness!"
2. **A decreased need for sleep (needs <3 hours).** "Tony drove day and night" until "he was too exhausted to drive," when he stopped and "partied drunkenly all night." He left "in the morning, without sleep but still wide-awake."
3. **Talking more than usual or interrupting others (pressured speech).**
4. **Rapid or racing thoughts.**
5. **Distractibility.**
6. **Increased goal-directed activity or psychomotor agitation.** (*Increase in goal-directed activity*): "Tony drove day and night" and partied all night without sleeping.
7. **Excessive involvement in activities that have a high potential for painful consequences (costly or risky impulsive actions).** Examples include: running away from the responsibilities of work and family, driving with the top down in December, picking up hitchhikers, driving while drinking, driving with "cases of beer" in the car, and partying drunkenly with hitchhikers and other strangers in hotels. Ultimately, he woke up in jail, missing his expensive car, credit cards, money, and shoes.

Other Diagnostic Considerations

My initial impression was that Tony might have an anxiety disorder, but he did not. Tony experienced Generalized Anxiety Disorder symptoms of irritability, restlessness, feeling keyed-up, and edginess, but he did not complain of six month's duration of uncontrollable anxiety and worried thoughts about performance at work or similar activities. He denied Generalized Anxiety Disorder symptoms of muscle tension, fatigue, poor concentration, or his mind going blank. Tony did not have Panic Disorder, because he denied symptoms of palpitations, pounding heart, rapid heart rate, sweating, tremor, shortness of breath, choking, chest pain, nausea, stomachache, dizziness, fainting, numbness, derealization, or depersonalization that developed abruptly and reached a peak within minutes.

Tony did not suffer from Acute or Posttraumatic Stress Disorder because he denied trauma, hypervigilance, exaggerated startle response, poor concentration, feeling dazed, derealization, depersonalization, or amnesia.

There was no evidence of social avoidance suggesting Social Anxiety Disorder.

Cognitive Testing

I should have known that something was wrong with Tony during his first appointment—there was no reason why a successful executive should have such an abnormal Cognitive Examination, failing important tests of *memory*, *abstract thinking*, and *sequential thinking*.

CLINICAL NOTES

I gave Tony proper treatment for his Bipolar I Disorder (lithium salts or an anticonvulsant) and he gradually recovered. After his Bipolar Disorder was stable, Tony tried to put his life back together. However, by that time, his employers wanted nothing to do with him, his family had left him, his money was gone, and his house had been taken by creditors. As is often the case, a single Manic Episode had cost him everything that had given his life meaning.

Some experts suggest that over one-half of all individuals with Bipolar Disorder are misdiagnosed on their first presentation. These misdiagnosed patients may mistakenly receive antidepressants, which trigger Manic Episodes in 1-5% of bipolar patients. Antidepressants can also worsen bipolar mania and depression, trigger psychosis, and possibly worsen the course of Bipolar Disorder for life. Given the recent evidence that antidepressants do not help bipolar depression, it seems like an inappropriate risk to prescribe antidepressants to patients with known Bipolar Disorder.

Past bipolar symptoms, a family history of Bipolar Disorder, atypical depressive symptoms, or life tables showing cyclic mood changes may raise our index of suspicion that Bipolar Disorder is present. Nevertheless, a good mental status examination with complete, unhurried Diagnostic and Cognitive Examinations is the best way of catching Bipolar Disorder and ensuring that bipolar patients receive the correct treatment.

CASE 40
LOUISE'S PARTY SURPRISE

Louise was a slim, dark-eyed, 29-year-old architect. She entered my office, sat down, and began speaking.

"Three weeks ago, I had a great job, a great lifestyle, and an ideal relationship with the greatest guy in the world. Now I can't go to work and I can't talk to my friends or my family. I've never felt like this before," Louise said, and burst into tears.

"I just can't understand what happened," Louise continued. "Luis and I had been living together for two years and everything was going perfectly. Although we were waiting to announce our engagement, I always referred to him as my fiancé, and I was always talking to him about when we would be married, what kind of house we would have, and when we should have children. Over the last few months, I had been making wedding plans and I was going to announce our wedding at a big graduation party I threw for him and all my friends and family.

"You see, from the first day I met Luis, we were together every minute. We knew we were soul mates. He was trying to decide if he wanted to leave school or finish his last year and become an architect like me. We made a deal that he would move into my apartment to save money and I would support him through his last year of school. Then, when he graduated, we would get married and he would support me so that I could have our children. It took longer than he thought to finish school—he had to go an extra semester to pick up some classes he needed and then he spent another six months doing make-up work and taking examinations. Luis was so busy finishing school the last two months that he was in the library all day and didn't even come home until early morning. I kept myself busy thinking about our wedding and planning his big graduation party, inviting everyone I knew to celebrate the next stage of our lives. Finally, he handed in all his work, took his last test, and he was finished with school.

"The idea was that we would all wait at the party until he came home from his last test and then we'd all celebrate together. Well, the night of the party came and everyone showed up and began having a great time but Luis never even showed up for his own party. I was incredibly on edge, making excuses to everyone, and I expected him to walk in at any minute, but he never came. The party broke up at about 11:00 P.M. and it was the longest evening of my life. I managed to keep myself together until everyone was gone. Then I broke down and I cried for hours. I never even mentioned the subject of our wedding at the party. I would have looked so foolish to talk about marrying someone who never even showed up for the party that I threw him.

"Finally, Luis came home drunk at 3:00 A.M. He wouldn't talk to me but he just put his clothes into a big suitcase and walked out on me. He never came back and I haven't seen him since that night. I got a call from a woman who came over and took away his other belongings. She was horrible. She was a bleached blonde and she looked like an anorexic teenager just out of high school. I asked her about Luis and she said he had moved into her apartment.

"Since that time three weeks ago, I haven't been myself. Nothing makes me happy and I don't enjoy anything about my life, anymore. I can't eat and I've lost 10 pounds. Usually I wake up feeling the worst at 4:00 A.M., two hours before my alarm, and I can't get back to sleep. I'm too tired to go to work and I can't seem to keep focused. Everybody says it's like I'm moving in slow motion. My head is filled with angry thoughts about that horrible girl that won't go away. I just can't see how she could steal him away from me at the last minute, just as our life together was really starting. I feel guilty all the time and I wonder what I did to drive him to her. At first, I thought of how I could hurt her but lately I've been turning my anger against myself. You've got to help me make this stop!"

Louise denied any prior history of mental or emotional problems.

On her Cognitive Examination, Louise was alert and she did well on all tests of *attention, language, abstract thinking,* and *sequential thinking.*

However, on *memory* tests, Louise could only repeat four of seven numbers on a test of Digit Span. She could not recall more than two of the past Four Presidents, and she could only recall a few words in a test of Free Recall from a Story. Louise could not remember anything after three minutes on a test of Cued Delayed Memory.

CHALLENGE

Louise can't figure out how her life has gone awry—can you help her? What is wrong with Louise?

SOLUTION

Louise is experiencing unipolar **Major Depressive Disorder, Single Episode with Melancholic Features, Moderate** (DSM-5 296.22, ICD-10 F32.1):

At least five of the following symptoms nearly every day for at least two weeks:
1. **A sad, depressed mood.**
2. **A loss of interest or pleasure in most activities (anhedonia).** Louise said, "Since that time three weeks ago, I haven't been myself. Nothing makes me happy and I don't enjoy anything about my life, anymore."
3. **A significant change in appetite or weight (e.g., a change of more than 5% of body weight per month).** Louise said, "I can't eat and I've lost 10 pounds." Unless Louise weighs more than 200 pounds, this is more than 5% of her body weight.
4. **Insomnia or hypersomnia.** (*Insomnia*): Louise awakened two hours early and said, "I can't get back to sleep."
5. **Psychomotor depression or agitation.** (*Psychomotor depression*): Louise told us that "everybody says it's like I'm moving in slow motion."
6. **Fatigue or low energy.** Louise said, "I'm too tired to go to work."
7. **Thoughts of guilt or worthlessness.** (*Guilt*): Louise complained that "I feel guilty all the time and I wonder what I did to drive him to her." (*Worthlessness*): Louise said, "My life is ruined!"
8. **Difficulty concentrating or making decisions.** Louise said, "I can't seem to keep focused." Louise also failed several tests of *memory* on her Cognitive Examination.
9. **Recurrent thoughts of death, suicide, or a suicidal attempt or plan.**

The symptoms cause a significant impairment in school, work, home, or social life; and they must include either depressed mood or anhedonia. Louise said, "I can't go to work and I can't talk to my friends or my family."

Louise also met the criteria for **Melancholic Features**, thought by many to characterize *unipolar* major depression:

A. **Either of the following, occurring during the most severe period of the current episode**:
  1. **Loss of pleasure in all or almost all activities (anhedonia).** Louise said, "I don't enjoy anything about my life, anymore."
  2. **Lack of reactivity to usually pleasurable stimuli** Louise told us that "nothing makes me happy."

B. **Three or more of the following**:
  1. **Distinct quality of depressed mood characterized by despondent, morose, despair, or empty mood.** Louise was despondent.
  2. **Depression regularly worse in the morning.** Louise said, "I wake up feeling the worst at 4:00 A.M."
  3. **Early morning awakening at least two hours before the usual time of awakening.** Louise said that she awakened "two hours before my alarm."
  4. **Marked psychomotor depression or agitation.** (*Psychomotor depression*): Louise commented that "everybody says it's like I'm moving in slow motion."
  5. **Significant anorexia or weight loss.** Louise said, "I can't eat and I've lost 10 pounds."
  6. **Excessive or inappropriate guilt.** "I feel guilty all the time and I wonder what I did to drive him to her."

Other Diagnostic Considerations

Because of the extreme distress caused by Louise's breakup and her current functional impairment, you might consider a diagnosis of Adjustment Disorder with Depressed Mood. This diagnosis is sometimes referred as "exogenous depression" or "situational depression." However, DSM-5 states that an Adjustment Disorder cannot be diagnosed if the patient meets the criteria for Major Depressive Disorder.

Because breaking up with her boyfriend is an identifiable stressor that occurred less than a month before, you might consider a diagnosis of Acute Stress Disorder. However, relationship breakup is not an event that involves actual or threatened death, serious injury, or a physical threat to oneself or others, so Acute Stress Disorder cannot be diagnosed.

Was Louise suffering from psychotic delusions? Delusions are a belief in conditions that are not supported by fact or are not evident to other people. Louise believed that Luis was "the greatest guy in the world," without any facts to support that contention. She felt that she and Luis were "soul mates" who had "an ideal relationship" where "everything was going perfectly," although events proved this to be false. Louise also erroneously considered Luis her fiancé and imagined that he was planning for their wedding, their married life, their future home, and their children. Somehow, she believed that she and Luis were together every minute, although "the last two months, he was in the library all day and didn't even come home until early morning."

Nevertheless, despite these unfounded and incorrect beliefs, Louise was not having psychotic delusions. Her beliefs were influenced by common cultural mores and fantasies and facilitated by her impaired focus and cognition.

She was being purposely misled by her boyfriend whose tactics were more effective because Louise's thinking was impaired by her depression.

Cognitive Testing

Louise failed several tests of *memory* function. Impaired memory is often seen in unipolar Major Depressive Disorder.

CLINICAL NOTES

I treated Louise with an antidepressant and weekly Interpersonal Psychotherapy. Gradually, it became clear that her Major Depressive Disorder had been present longer and had grown worse than she had thought. Her depressive episode probably started before she ever met Luis. In addition to starting that ill-fated relationship, Louise remembered making other decisions that showed uncharacteristically poor judgment during that time. She had unaccountably let some of her professional society memberships lapse. Louise also remembered her supervisor pointing out an increasing number of mistakes in her usually impeccable work, including two serious errors in the last six months. As her cognition cleared and she began to reorganize the details of her life, Louise realized that the last two years had been filled with misconceptions and distortions. For example, she realized that Luis had shown no excitement about their upcoming marriage or her plans to have children. She realized that they had not gone out in the last two months and that she had spent very little time with him, lately. As her depression receded, Louise realized she had been living in a fantasy world.

The extent of this fantasy world was revealed when we found out more about Luis' recent activities. In reality, Luis had dropped out of school a week after he moved in with Louise. In addition to free room and board, the "college fees" and "expense money" Louise gave him were spent in bars and over poker games with his friends. Luis had never intended to repay Louise for supporting him, and as he approached the day of his "graduation," Luis had found a new woman to pay his way. His younger, thinner, new girlfriend had been surprised to learn that Louise existed. The new girlfriend believed that Luis had been dating her faithfully and exclusively over the previous two months. "How could he possibly have been going to get married?" she later asked. "From the first day I met Luis, we were together every minute. We knew we were soul mates."

Thankfully, after pharmacological and psychotherapeutic treatment, Louise was able to put herself back together and move on to the next stage of her life.

CASE 41
ANITA IS NOT THE WOMAN I MARRIED

Anita was a 49-year-old woman who came to my office at the behest of her husband, Christopher. He asked that I see him alone in my office before I interviewed his wife.

Christopher was a warm, quiet, 59-year-old man. He had been married to Anita for ten years and it was the first marriage for both. They had no children.

"Anita is not the woman I married," Christopher began.

"Can you explain that to me, Christopher?" I asked.

"Anita and I have always been quiet, retiring people. She has always been a gentle, caring woman. We met completely by accident at church. We don't have many friends because we spend almost all our time together. We are both librarians and we both share a passion for books. For ten years, we had the same routine. On the weeknights, we would have a light dinner and spend the rest of the time reading. Once a month, we would take a drive down the coast, stopping somewhere and eating sandwiches that Anita had prepared. Once a year, we would travel to Mexico, where we would lie in the sun and read for two weeks. Then we would both go back to our library jobs and take up our lives where we left off.

"However, over the last six months, Anita has become a different person," Christopher continued. "It started right after a trip she made to Louisville, Kentucky, to attend a librarians' conference. When she arrived home, Anita had a terrible headache and she went to bed for several days. Shortly thereafter, Anita began to act strangely. She never before had a temper but we began to have arguments. Her attention span was shortened and she was more impatient and irritated at things, especially anything involving me. The library director called me after Anita said some cruel things to him at work one day. He said that Anita's attendance had fallen and she had been missing from the library much of the week. I did not know what to tell him.

"Anita became too impatient to read in the evening and said it gave her a headache. She began staying up late at night and sleeping late in the morning. For the first time, Anita began to drink. First it was a beer every night and then hard liquor. I saw her smoking outside on our porch for the first time in my life. For some reason, she became very demanding in bed, although for most of our marriage, we had mainly just read in bed together until we fell asleep.

"One day Anita did not come home until after twelve o'clock in the morning, which would have been unheard of before. I stayed up and when she finally came in, she was drunk and she would not say where she had been. Now Anita goes out frequently by herself at night. I do not know where she goes because she has never asked me to go with her.

"Anita did not want to come today, doctor, but I insisted. Please help me get my wife back."

I told Christopher that I would do what I could and I brought Anita into my office to see me alone. Contrary to her retiring description, Anita's hair was cut short and dyed bright red to match the thin, cotton dress she was wearing. Her perfume was strong and her voice was loud. Instead of sitting calmly, she strode around my office, examining the furnishings and commenting on what she liked and disliked. Finally, she sat down.

"I don't know what my dumb husband has been telling you or why he wants to waste your time. He says I've changed but I can't tell any damned difference. I think he's gone cuckoo."

"Christopher mentioned that you had been drinking, lately," I said.

"Yeah and what of it? I don't drink any more than anybody else I see. In fact, I'm a cheap drunk. One drink and I'm out like a light. If I'm at a bar and there's no music or anything going on, I start nodding off."

"Tell me about your job, Anita."

"Deadly boring books and everybody who works there's a stuffed shirt. Jeez, those stiffs could bore you to death at 20 paces. It's a mausoleum. I'll be glad to get away from that bunch of cadavers. I'm gonna take an early retirement. I'd like to travel."

"Where would you like to go, Anita?"

"Someplace nice," she said, "that I used to read about. Maybe the Rivera. I certainly want to go where there are some real casinos. I've just begun gambling online—I'm winning like crazy and I'm having the time of my life. This could be a new career for me."

"I understand that you used to go to Mexico."

"Yeah. I don't know what I saw in that place. Now I hate the idea. The whole time I did nothing but sit on my ass. I want to be around some people who know how to have fun."

"Do you have any complaints right now, Anita?"

"Yes, my memory has clearly gotten worse, lately. I wish you could do something about that."

I told Anita that I would do what I could. I also asked her to arrange to have any past medical records sent to my office.

On her Cognitive Examination, Anita did well on all tests of *attention*, *language*, and *abstract thinking*. However, her responses were slow and she sometimes appeared drowsy. She did not exhibit a very large vocabulary and her sentence structure and word usage were rough and unlike her husband's.

In *memory* testing, Anita had no difficulty naming 16 items from the category of her choice, which were types of mixed drinks. She failed a test of Uncued Delayed Memory.

In the *abstract thinking* section, Anita struggled with Proverb Interpretation but her responses were appropriate. For example, for "Don't cry over spilt milk," she said, "Oh, wait. Yeah. If something has happened to you, don't feel so bad. Don't let it keep you from having a good life." For "Rome wasn't built in a day, she said, "Ahh. OK. Big projects are hard and they take a lot of time. Have you ever been to Rome?"

Anita also failed the *abstract thinking* test of Set Analysis—she could not comprehend that Truth and Justice were overlapping sets (not all that is true is just, and not all that is just is true) and she could not understand that poverty and misery were overlapping sets (you can be poor but not miserable, and you can be miserable but not poor). Anita could not understand that daises were a subset of flowers (that all daises are flowers, but not all flowers are daises)—she simply said, "Daises *are* flowers. What's the big deal?"

In *sequential thinking* tests, Anita failed Serial Sevens subtraction from 100 (although she had previously performed well on Simple Arithmetic). She puzzled a few moments over the Arithmetic Story Problem and then gave an absurd answer that she apparently made up on the spot. Anita required six tries to repeat the Luria Sequential Movements and she failed all three examples of Rhythm Reproduction. Although Anita had copied the Greek Cross figure well, when given the Luria Figure Drawing Test (see Appendix VII) containing many repeating loops, lines, and letters, she was slow and made many incorrect additions and omissions in her drawings.

Several days after Anita's evaluation, I received medical records from a hospital in Louisville, Kentucky, indicating that she had been seen in the Emergency Room six months before after a motor vehicle accident. When I questioned her, Anita remembered nothing of the event.

CHALLENGE

Your challenge is to diagnose Anita's condition and suggest a treatment. If you are puzzled, try comparing her symptoms to other patients you have evaluated in the past.

SOLUTION

Anita is experiencing **Personality Changes Due to Head Trauma** (DSM-5 301.1, ICD-10 F07.0) resulting from the **sequelae of a motor vehicle accident** (ICD-10 Y85.0) with probable **intracranial injury** (ICD-10 S06.9).

Anita met the following criteria for **Personality Changes Due to a Another Medical Condition**:
A. **A persistent personality change from the individual's previous characteristic personality.** Christopher told us that, "over the last six months, Anita has become a different person." She has been recently impatient, irritable, and cruel; missing work, staying up late, smoking, drinking, and gambling. Anita's personality changes caused her significant impairment in her original job, family, and social life.
B. **There is evidence from history, examination, studies, or laboratory findings that the change is a physiological consequence of a general medical condition.** Anita's Emergency Room record described a motor vehicle accident. This was followed by severe headaches and amnesia for the event.

When coding disorders Due to a Another Medical Condition, specify the exact cause: Head Trauma.

Other Diagnostic Considerations

Anita's deficits in *memory*, and *sequential thinking* lead some clinicians to diagnose Mild Neurocognitive Disorder (DSM-5 331.83, ICD-10 G31.84). However, there is no evidence that these cognitive deficits are causing her to expend greater effort or use compensatory strategies in her daily activities. Like her personality changes, they are just aspects of Anita's new identity.

You may consider a late-onset or organic bipolar Manic Episode because of Anita's irritable mood and inflated self-esteem (such as the belief that she could easily make a career as an online gambler). However, Anita's sleep duration was normal, her speech was not pressured, her thoughts were slow or normal speed, and she showed less rather than more goal-directed work activity. Anita was engaged in pleasurable activities like drinking, smoking, and carousing that might eventually have negative consequences, but they were neither excessive nor did they violate laws or cultural norms.

Cognitive Testing

In the *sequential thinking* section of her Cognitive Examination, Anita failed tests of Serial Sevens, the Arithmetic Story Problem, Luria Sequential Movements, Rhythm Reproduction, and the Luria Figure Drawing Test. Her examination was also notable for mental and physical slowing and a sense of drowsiness. Mental and physical slowing, impaired Level of Consciousness, and poor *sequential thinking* are all associated with injury to the frontal area of the brain,

CLINICAL NOTES

Anita's Louisville medical records revealed that she had signed herself out of the hospital against medical advice (AMA) in time for her return airplane trip. By the time I examined her, Anita had amnesia from the time of the accident until the time she returned home. A computerized tomography (CT) scan of Anita's head had been done in Louisville but the film had been lost. I ordered a repeat scan and scheduled a neurologist's consultation but by that time there was no pathology to be seen.

In sudden deceleration caused by motor vehicle accidents, the brain is most vulnerable at the points where it is closest to the skull, particularly in the prefrontal cortex and temporal horns. This location also agrees with the results of Anita's Cognitive Examination.

I have seen other patients with closed head brain injury who exhibited similar personality changes with increased irritability, roughness of speech and behavior, impulsivity, disinhibition, and heightened sexual interest. They most frequently complained of headache and memory problems that were not evident on testing (probably resulting from slowed cognition and lowered level of arousal). When I interviewed their family members, the biggest change they noticed was an increase in impatience, irritability, and anger episodes.

I explained the probable source of the problem to both Christopher and Anita. Christopher listened intently and wrote down the names of several books I recommended on the topic.

Anita, on the other hand, was somewhat flippant during the discussion. She said, "I do not see any changes in me, and if there are any, I think that they're all for the good. I think it is you people that have brain injury," she said. "The only thing happening with me is that I've opened my eyes to what I've been missing in life."

I began seeing Christopher and Anita in couples' therapy. Christopher also saw me in individual sessions but Anita did not want individual therapy. I treated Anita with a low dose of the anticonvulsant carbamazepine (Tegretol), which she took agreeably in the hope that it would improve her memory. On carbamazepine, Anita became less angry, stayed at her job, and reduced her drinking. I scheduled her for further cognitive testing but she did not go to the appointment.

After two months, Christopher came to his couples' appointment without his wife. She had retired from her job, stopped her medicine, left Christopher, and moved to Las Vegas. The couple was divorced by the end of the year. A year later, Anita wrote me a postcard from Europe, telling me that she was having a great time and that she was feeling fine.

When I first examined Anita, she was failing in her job and marriage, qualifying her for a clinical diagnosis. However, her new personality was not abnormal. When Anita changed her lifestyle to fit her new personality, she was happy with the change. She was successful in her new lifestyle as a retiree, a night owl, a bar-hopper, a sexual woman, and a (so far) successful gambler. Anita's desire to retire from her job, have fun, and travel to the Riviera is probably more normal in our culture than the desire to live a quiet life as a librarian. Her increased irritability and anger, decreased patience, blunt and nonempathic comments, and generally slack attitude are within normal limits in the population. As long as Anita is successful at her new work (retirement), social, and family activities, she does not qualify for a psychiatric diagnosis.

When I offered my condolences on his loss, Christopher simply repeated his first words to me: "Anita is not the woman I married."

CASE 42
I'LL BE YOUR EASIEST PATIENT

Diane was a 30-year-old woman who came to my office for her first appointment. She indicated that she had just moved to town and needed a new doctor. She said that her prior doctor of many years had recently died and his out-of-state office had lost her medical records.

Diane spoke softly, saying, "Doctor, I am *very* anxious. I have both Generalized Anxiety and Panic Disorder. Really. Sometimes I am anxious and worried, restless, edgy, fatigued, tense, and irritable. It's hard for me to sleep or concentrate. Other times I get a pounding heart, sweating, shaking, choking and it's hard to breathe. I also feel chest pain, dizziness, and I feel nauseous. I don't have any other health problems. Really."

Diane appeared somewhat agitated—her hands shook and she was perspiring, which I attributed to her anxiety. She sometimes mumbled while speaking. Diane's eyes were watery, as if she had recently been crying, and both her eyes darted rhythmically around the room as we spoke. Although she smiled frequently, Diane also appeared very sad at several times during her interview. Then her mood brightened and she became cheerful and chummy toward the end of her appointment.

Diane had come quite late for her first appointment, limiting our evaluation time. To save time, I had asked Diane to complete a Diagnostic Questionnaire (Appendix II) while she was in the waiting room. When I scanned that form, I saw that she had checked every symptom under the Panic Disorder and Generalized Anxiety Disorder categories and left almost all the other answers blank. Diane had endorsed insomnia with less than five hours of sleep nightly, checked symptoms of nausea, and denied any suicidal or violent thoughts or intentions. She also denied any symptoms of psychosis.

I had also given Diane a Cognitive Questionnaire (Appendix IV) to fill out in the waiting room.

Diane did well in tests of *attention* and *language*.

However, in tests of *memory*, Diane failed tests of Digit Span, recall of Four Presidents, Free Recall from a Story, and Cued Delayed Memory for six words after three minutes.

In tests of *abstract thinking,* Diane failed a test of Judgment by saying, "If I smelled smoke in a theater, I'd immediately run out before I got caught in a mob and burned to death. Really." She also failed a test of Insight by saying, "If you lie, you have to be really careful, or else the cops will throw you in jail." Diane's Greek Cross drawing was well-proportioned but her lines were shaky.

In *sequential thinking* tests, she failed a test of Serial Sevens subtraction (although she could perform Simple Arithmetic).

I found that Diane had an elevated pulse of 105 beats per minute (normal pulse=60-100 bpm).

"I'll be an ideal patient, doctor," Diane crooned. "I'm both brilliant and beautiful—I'm just glad I finally found a brilliant, talented doctor who can understand me. I will also be your easiest patient. I just sit around the house all day by myself—I'll never get in trouble. I already know what I need in order to be OK. Really."

Diane requested alprazolam (Xanax) for her anxiety. She said, "It's been effective for years without raising the dose but if I take any less, then I feel bad. I'm running out of alprazolam, so I need more right away."

Given the addictive nature of most sedatives, I was reassured when Diane asked for a very moderate dose of alprazolam. It hardly seemed enough to get her in trouble. I was also encouraged that she had taken such a moderate dose for a long time without the need for dose escalation. I wrote a prescription for alprazolam and gave her a 10-day supply (20 tablets). We agreed that she would return in a week to finish her assessment and reevaluate her treatment. As Diane left my office, she stumbled, had trouble opening the door, and she appeared somewhat unsteady on her feet.

CHALLENGE

Diane says that she is the perfect patient, but without past medical records, our fund of information is limited. Your challenge is to analyze the information presented so far and come up the most probable diagnoses.

SOLUTION

Diane is experiencing **Alprazolam (Xanax) Intoxication** (DSM-5 292.89, ICD-10 F13.229), **Alprazolam Withdrawal** (DSM-5 292.0, ICD-10 F13.239), and **Severe Alprazolam Use Disorder** (DSM-5 304.10, ICD-10 F13.20).

Diane's diagnosis was clarified by later events. One day after her appointment, Diane called and left a message requesting another prescription for alprazolam. She said that all the tablets from her first prescription had inexplicably fallen down the kitchen drain. This time, she said she would need enough medication for six weeks because she had to make a sudden, unexpected trip to the East Coast. For that reason, she could not come to her second appointment.

My telephone rang again before I could return Diane's call. The second caller was a pharmacist colleague who reported that he had received an alprazolam prescription for Diane written by another physician immediately after filling mine. Later that day, I received another telephone call from an internist. He informed me that he had provided Diane with increasing doses of benzodiazepines for the last year and he had just been informed that four other internists were providing Diane with alprazolam during the same period. The caller sounded angry and betrayed.

At that point, I reviewed my notes and I found that Diane exhibited the following symptoms of **Sedative, Hypnotic, or Anxiolytic Intoxication**:
A. **Recent ingestion of a sedative, hypnotic, or anxiolytic drug**. Diane told me that she was taking alprazolam, a sedative medication frequently prescribed for anxiety.
B. **Clinically significant maladaptive behavioral or psychological changes (inappropriate sexual or aggressive behavior, mood lability, impaired judgment, impaired social or occupational functioning) that developed during, or shortly after sedative ingestion**. (*Mood lability*): Diane initially smiled, then looked sad, and then brightened during her interview. (*Impaired judgment*): Trying to get medications illegally from five physicians at the same time shows poor judgment because pharmacy records are often reviewed. (*Impaired function*): Diane's examination and cognitive testing showed that her physical and cognitive function were impaired by her intoxication.
C. **One (or more) of the following signs, developing during, or shortly after, sedative use**:
   1. **Slurred speech**. What I initially interpreted as mumbling was really slurred speech.
   2. **Incoordination**. As Diane left my office, she "had trouble opening the door."
   3. **Unsteady gait**. As Diane left my office, she stumbled and "appeared somewhat unsteady on her feet."
   2. **Nystagmus** (repetitive, rhythmic vertical or horizontal movements of the eyes). "Both her eyes darted rhythmically around the room as we spoke."
   3. **Impairment in attention or memory**. Diane failed tests of *memory* and Serial Sevens subtraction (a memory intensive task).
   6. **Stupor or coma.**

In my office, Diane was already showing symptoms of **Sedative, Hypnotic, or Anxiolytic Withdrawal**:
A. **Cessation of or reduction in sedative, hypnotic, or anxiolytic use that has been heavy and prolonged**. Diane said, "I'm running out of alprazolam, so I need more right away."
B. **At least two of the following develop within several hours to a few days after cessation or reduction**:
   1. **Autonomic hyperactivity** (sweating or pulse rate greater than 100 beats per minute). Diane was perspiring, her eyes were watery, and her pulse was elevated at 105 bpm. These symptoms result from increased adrenaline/noradrenaline activity that is part of the withdrawal process.
   2. **Tremor**. Diane's hands shook and her drawing of the Greek Cross was shaky.
   3. **Insomnia**. Diane claimed that she slept less than five hours per night.
   4. **Nausea or vomiting**. Diane endorsed nausea on her Diagnostic Questionnaire.
   5. **Transient visual, tactile, or auditory hallucinations or illusions**.
   6. **Psychomotor agitation**. Diane appeared agitated during her interview.
   7. **Anxiety**. Diane claimed to have a marked problem with anxiety.
   8. **Grand mal seizures.**

Overall, Diane met the criteria for **Sedative, Hypnotic, or Anxiolytic Use Disorder**:
At least two of the following occurring within a 12-month period:
   1. **The patient takes a substance in larger amounts for a longer period than intended.** If we combined the prescriptions from all her doctors, Diane was using a much higher dose of alprazolam than her prescribing doctors had intended.
   2. **The patient tries or wants to reduce substance use.** Diane told us that when she took any less than her usual dose, "I feel bad."

3. **The patient spends considerable time obtaining, using, and recovering from the substance effects.** Diane apparently spent lots of time going to doctors and filling prescriptions in order to secure her alprazolam.
4. **The patient feels strong urges or cravings to use the substance.** Diane said, "I'm running out of alprazolam, so I need more right away."
5. **Substance use causes impairment in school, work, family, or social function.** Diane was not working and she stayed at home.
6. **Use continues despite social problems attributable to the substance.** Diane was running into trouble with pharmacists and physicians.
7. **School, work, home, or social activities are curtailed because of the substance.** Instead of going to school, working, or socializing, Diana said she just sat around the house all day by herself.
8. **Use continues despite physical danger attributable to the substance.**
9. **Use continues despite physical or psychological problems attributable to the substance.**
10. **Tolerance—increased amounts are needed and/or the effects of the substance decrease.** Diane was now seeking alprazolam from many physicians at the same time. Although Diane claimed her alprazolam had "been effective for years without raising the dose," the internist who called me said that Diane had needed increasing doses of the medication.
11. **Withdrawal—characteristic withdrawal symptoms and/or substances are taken to avoid withdrawal.** (Withdrawal): See above.

The disorder is characterized as Severe when 6 or more symptoms are present.

In coding substance-related disorders, record the name of the specific substance used rather than the name of the class. Thus her diagnoses were Alprazolam Intoxication, Alprazolam Withdrawal, and Alprazolam Dependence.

Other Diagnostic Considerations

Although Diane had symptoms of Panic Attack (pounding heart, sweating, shaking, shortness of breath, choking, chest pain, and nausea), Generalized Anxiety Disorder (poor concentration, fatigue, restless sleep, restlessness, edginess, and irritability), and Posttraumatic Stress Disorder (sleep problems, restlessness, and irritability), all these symptoms were caused by alprazolam intoxication and withdrawal. She should be reevaluated after she is free from symptoms of alprazolam to see if she has any other diagnosis.

Cognitive Testing

Diane failed tests of *memory, abstract thinking,* and *sequential thinking.* These are all explained by the effects of intoxication and withdrawal on multiple brain areas.

CLINICAL NOTES

I called Diane and told her that she would need to return to my office to complete her evaluation before I could prescribe more alprazolam. I gently mentioned the call from the pharmacist and she flew into a rage. After delivering a few, choice anatomical instructions, she hung up the telephone and I never heard from her again.

Clues to Diane's true diagnosis began with her carefully crafted story. She limited the amount of data that I could collect by coming to her appointment late. Once there, Diane kept me from accessing her history by fabricating a story about a deceased, out-of-state physician whose office had lost her records. She tried to sell herself as an ideal patient—easy, satisfied, and low-maintenance. When asked about her symptoms, Diane repeated the criteria for Generalized Anxiety Disorder and Panic Disorder verbatim. Once she had obtained her first prescription from me, she claimed that she had lost the medicine, needed extra medicine for a trip, and sabotaged her future follow-up. She knew just what to say because she had been through the routine of getting benzodiazepines many times.

Benzodiazepine dependence is a general medical concern, as well as a mental health problem. Prescription drug addiction is unhealthy for the addict and places an unnecessary load on the overall health system. Sedative intoxication is associated with increased motor vehicle accidents and falls as well as fatal medical conditions like aspiration pneumonia. Mixing benzodiazepines with alcohol or other sedatives can result in serious respiratory depression and sudden withdrawal can cause seizures.

Unfortunately, I never had an opportunity to help Diane with her substance problem. After I confronted her on the telephone, I never heard from her again. Without treatment, I suspect Diane is still milking physicians for more sedatives to continue her dependence. As a colleague commented, Diane's case is not rare, yet drug-seeking patients fool well-meaning, intelligent clinicians every day. Awareness of the problem is the first step in helping these patients.

CASE 43
ALICE FACTORY SMELLS FEATHERS

A 24-year-old woman named Alice Factory stepped into my office one morning for her first appointment. "I have the most awful smell in my head and it's ruining my life," she said.

Alice explained that for the last three months she had been experiencing an odd triad of problems—headaches, vision problems, and an acrid odor that never went away.

"I went to my internist first, then to a neurologist for the headache, and then to an optician for the vision. They all agreed that I should see you for the smell," Alice said brightly. I wondered if my colleagues were having a joke at my expense.

"Why don't you tell me about the headache and the vision problems, first," I suggested.

"Why not?" she replied. "My headache is dull and throbbing right between my eyes. Every week it gets a little worse. It gets worse when I cough or strain on the toilet or move my head suddenly. Sometimes it hurts so badly that I get a nosebleed. The weirdest thing is that my breasts have been getting swollen and tender—I don't know if that's related. The neurologist said everything was fine."

I reached over and gently pressed on the area between her eyebrows with my thumb. "Ow!" Alice barked. "What are you trying to do, anyway?"

"Sorry," I said. "Now tell me about the vision problems."

"OK. It's like I suddenly need glasses," Alice said. "The optician gave me new glasses but they didn't help."

"All right. Now tell me about the smell."

"Finally. For the last three months, I've been having this smell in my head," Alice continued. "It doesn't matter what is going on outside—in fact, I can't smell anything else and my food tastes like sand. The smell is like burning feathers. My girlfriend said that in Gothic times a smell of burning feathers signified that a death was going to happen."

"Actually, I think it was the smell of extinguished candles that presaged death," I replied, "but never mind. Did the other doctors give you anything that helped?"

"Naw, not really. The neurologist gave me some pain medicine but it didn't help at all. My internist said my examination was normal. He gave me a strong steroid nasal spray, anyway. That didn't help the smell but it made my headache get better. Go figure."

Alice denied any other past history of hospitalization, physical, mental, or emotional disease. Her father was in good health and her mother had died in middle age after a long bout with breast cancer. Alice denied taking medications, consuming alcohol, or abusing drugs.

In her Diagnostic Examination, Alice looked tired and she said that she was not sleeping well because of the pain. Alice complained of worsening fatigue that she attributed to her inability to sleep. She was not hungry and she was losing weight, which she attributed to the smell in her head. Alice denied any physical symptoms of pounding or racing heart, excessive sweating, trembling, shaking, chills, hot flushes, shortness of breath, choking, chest pain, nausea, stomachache, dizziness, lightheadedness, tingling, muscle tension, restlessness, edginess, feeling keyed-up, poor concentration, mind going blank, a sense of detachment, fears of losing control or fears of dying.

Alice admitted to being irritated at her worsening problem, but she denied sadness, hopelessness, anxiety, panic, loneliness, or emptiness. She said that she enjoyed her daily activities as much as she ever had and she kept up an active social life despite her current problems. There was no evidence of expansive or elevated mood, physical agitation, obsessive activities, or risk-taking behavior. Alice said she had never heard voices or seen visions. She denied obsessions, compulsions, or thoughts or intentions of injury to herself or others.

I gave Alice a copy of the Cognitive Questionnaire (Appendix IV), the Nonverbal Tests of Abstract and Sequential Thinking (Appendix VI), and the Luria Figure Drawing Test of *sequential thinking* (Appendix VII) to fill out in the waiting room before our appointment. On the Cognitive Questionnaire, she characterized herself as alert but distracted. Otherwise, she did well on all tests of *attention*, *language*, and *memory*.

CHALLENGE

What is wrong with Alice and why does she smell burning feathers? Is she psychotic? Does her illusory odor tie in with her other problems? What would you recommend that she do next?

SOLUTION

Alice has **cancer** in the form of a **frontal sinus neoplasm** (ICD-10 C31.2) and **Psychotic Disorder Due to a Frontal Sinus Neoplasm, with Hallucinations** (DSM-5 293.82, ICD-10 F06.0). When the tumor presses upon the olfactory nerve, it causes her to smell burning feathers. This was confirmed by an emergency consultation with a neurosurgeon.

Alice met the following criteria for **Psychotic Disorder Due to a Another Medical Condition**:
A. **Prominent hallucinations or delusions**. Alice was smelling burning feathers.
B. **There is evidence from the history, physical examination, or laboratory findings that the disturbance is the direct physiological consequence of a general medical condition**. An emergency consultation with a neurosurgeon confirmed the presence of frontal sinus cancer.
C. **The disturbance is not better accounted for by another mental disorder**. There was no evidence of another mental disorder (see below).
D. **The disturbance does not occur exclusively during the course of a Delirium**. Andi did not have a Delirium.

When coding Psychotic Disorders Due to a Another Medical Condition, always list the specific name of the condition: Psychotic Disorder Due to a Frontal Sinus Neoplasm.

Other Diagnostic Considerations

Alice's internist and neurologist must have thought that Alice was experiencing hallucinations from a psychotic mental disorder when they referred her to me. They probably did not realize that olfactory hallucinations are rare in psychotic mental disorders. However, olfactory hallucinations are not as rare in neurology and neurosurgery practice, where they are sometimes called "uncinate fits."

The olfactory nerves lie underneath the orbital frontal cortex, above the top of the nasal cavity, near the frontal sinuses. From there they project to the olfactory tubercle, the temporal lobes, and the amygdala. Olfactory hallucinations can result from pressure on the nerves and olfactory bulbs; or injury, stroke, or seizures of the other mentioned areas. Olfactory hallucinations are also seen with migraines and Parkinson's disease.

Many clinicians think first of Schizophrenia when they see patients with hallucinations, but a diagnosis of Schizophrenia requires the additional presence of delusions, disorganized speech, disorganized behavior, or negative symptoms (flat affect, minimal speech, or inactivity). Alice did not demonstrate any of those, so she cannot be given the diagnosis of Schizophrenia. Schizophreniform Disorder, Brief Psychotic Disorder, and Schizoaffective Disorder require the same criteria, so they cannot be diagnosed, either. Schizotypal Personality Disorder can present with sensory illusions, but it begins early and continues steadily throughout the lifespan. There was no evidence of a substance intoxication, withdrawal, or medication responsible for Alice's hallucinations.

Borderline Personality Disorder may present with brief psychotic symptoms. However, personality disorders do not arise rapidly over the course of three months.

Hallucinations, delusions, and formal thought disorder can be seen in psychotic unipolar Major Depressive Disorder but Alice denied depressed mood or anhedonia (that is, loss of enjoyment or interest in daily activities), one of which is necessary for a diagnosis of a Major Depressive Episode.

Hallucinations, delusions, and formal thought disorder can also be seen in Bipolar I Disorder but Alice showed no expansive or elevated mood, physical agitation, obsessive activities, or risk-taking behavior characteristic of Bipolar Disorder.

Patients with Generalized Anxiety Disorder complain of irritability, fatigue, and impaired sleep, but Alice denied the excessive anxiety and uncontrollable worried thoughts about activities such as work or school performance continuing for at least six months that are needed for a Generalized Anxiety Disorder diagnosis.

CLINICAL NOTES

Alice Factory began providing clues to the nature and location of her problem as soon as she walked into my office. The duration of Alice's condition was three months and it was getting worse—this is a sudden and rapid course for a neuropsychiatric disorder but not for a rapidly growing cancer.

Alice's headache felt deep inside her head and sometimes caused bleeding that discharged through her sinuses and nasal passages—bleeding is often a sign of a mass lesion such as a tumor pressing on surrounding tissues. Her headache was throbbing and her pain worsened on coughing, straining, moving her head suddenly, or pressure on her skull—just as you would expect of a large mass pressing on blood vessels and sinus cavities.

Alice also complained of a recent change in vision. This could easily have been caused by a tumor mass pressing on the soft tissue around the eye sockets.

Breast cancer ran in Alice's family and she noticed swelling and tenderness in her breasts. Breast cancer often metastasizes to the brain and may produce hormones like estrogen that can cause the breasts to swell. Fatigue and weight loss are common symptoms in patients with metastatic carcinoma. However, these turned out to be false clues, as she did not have breast cancer and her tumor was not metastasized from the breast.

In addition to smelling burning feathers that were not there, Alice noted that she could not smell odors in her environment, and that her food had no taste, a typical finding for loss of smell, or anosmia. Loss of smell is frequently caused by smoke inhalation but it can also be a sign of dysfunction in the olfactory areas of the nervous system.

I keep an "olfactory test kit" in my office, composed of a bottle of imitation coconut extract and a bottle of imitation maple flavor that can be procured easily from any market. These are both dissolved in alcohol, which is detected by the so-called common chemical pathway that is separate from the olfactory system. If patients sniff one of these extracts and report smelling only alcohol, their sense of smell is suspect. Alice was unable to name the smell of either test aroma but she correctly named the scent of alcohol on a swab. (Note that some books suggest testing smell with a tube of lip balm. However, these products contain volatile ingredients like menthol, camphor, and phenol that stimulate the common chemical sense and they should not be used to test olfaction.)

Based on the evidence for an organic etiology, I sent Alice for an emergency appointment with an Ear, Nose, and Throat (ENT) surgeon with a note that said, "Please rule out possible mass lesion." The surgeon called me from his office to say that Alice had been scheduled for exploratory surgery that day. When the pathology results returned, they indicated that Alice suffered from a rare frontal sinus adenoma. After it was surgically removed, Alice recovered fully, without headaches, visual problems, or funny smells.

We are often the courts of last resort for our patients, who come to us after other clinicians have failed to help them. In addition to our own mental health specialization, we must keep a weather eye open for problems that our colleagues have missed. If we miss a serious and treatable illness, our poor patients will get scant comfort from the knowledge that "it really wasn't my job."

CASE 44
MARY GETS A BITE

"My problem is not in my head," Mary said. "I'm only coming here because my regular doctor said you could help reduce the stress I'm going through. He said to give you this letter."

Mary handed me a sealed business envelope bearing a physician's return address.

"Three months ago, I moved into a new condominium," Mary began. "The first day I moved in, I saw an insect crawling on the wall. Then I saw tiny insects floating in the beams of sunlight coming in through the windows. Since then, whenever I go to sleep, these tiny insects come out, getting in all my stuff and causing the worst bites. I feel them crawling on my skin and they have a terrible smell. I looked up parasites on the Internet and there are tiny chewing lice and bugs that hide all day in your bed and come out at night to feed on you.

"After I got all these bites, I had the place fumigated, checked the screens, and ran tests for asbestos and fiberglass, but nothing helped. I thought about insects from other people's pets but this building has strict rules against keeping any animals."

Mary was wearing a sleeveless top under a billowy jacket that covered her neck, arms, and legs. When she took off her jacket, I noted deep, weeping sores and excoriations on her neck, shoulders, and lower arms. However, I could not see any inflamed macules or papules that resembled the focal bites of insects.

"Tell me more about these insect bites," I said. "Could they possibly be due to any other causes?"

"No! They are definitely insects, like I told you! The dermatologist said that I caused them by scratching, but they don't itch and I never scratch them, anymore." Mary absent-mindedly scratched a lesion on her calf until it bled.

Despite her problem, Mary was able to perform her job and maintain a stable social life. She denied any former medical illness, mental illness, or hospitalization. Mary was taking no medications and she denied using any alcohol or drugs of abuse. She said that she had not changed her soap or hair products, nor had she been in contact with any household chemicals.

Mary's vital signs were normal, with a pulse of 70 beats per minute and a blood pressure of 118/78 millimeters of mercury.

In her Diagnostic Examination, Mary said that her sleep, appetite, and energy level were "Fine." She denied symptoms of poor concentration, mind going blank, fatigue, muscle tension, restless sleep, restlessness, edginess, or feeling keyed-up. Mary maintained that her attention, memory, task organization, and ability to relax were all normal. She endorsed occasional irritability and sadness, but denied feelings of hopelessness, anxiety, panic, loneliness, or emptiness. Mary said that she continued to enjoy the activities of her busy life.

I gave Alice a copy of the Cognitive Questionnaire (Appendix IV). She did well on all tests of *attention, language, memory, abstract thinking,* and *sequential thinking*.

Finally, I opened the envelope and took out a sheet of physician's stationary containing a brief handwritten note. It merely said, "There are no insect bites. Mental illness! Can you help her?"

CHALLENGE

You may have seen cases like this one. Give this condition a name, suggest a treatment, and consider which conditions you must rule out before making the diagnosis. Then go on to the solution.

SOLUTION

Mary suffered from **Delusional Disorder**, **Somatic Type**, (DSM-5 297.1, ICD-10 F22.0).

Delusions have been present for at least one month. Mary's condition began "three months ago," when she moved into a new condominium.

Schizophrenia Criterion A, with hallucinations, delusions and/or disorganized speech, has never been met. Any hallucinations are minimal and are related to the delusional theme. Mary said she felt the insects "crawling on my skin" and detected "a terrible smell"—these are related to her delusions of insect infestation.

Apart from the impact of the delusion, functioning is not impaired and behavior is not odd or bizarre. (*Functioning*): "Despite her problem, Mary was able to perform her job and maintain a stable social life." (*Odd or bizarre*): There was no evidence of odd or bizarre behavior in Mary's history or examination. Arthropod bites and stings are a commonplace, real-life problem—they are not strange or fantastic.

Manic or Major Depressive Episodes have been absent or brief compared with the delusional periods. Mary endorsed only "occasional irritability and sadness."

Delusional Disorders include Erotomanic, Grandiose, Jealous, Persecutory, Somatic, Mixed, or Unspecified Types.

Other Diagnostic Considerations

Many clinicians consider giving Mary Excoriation (Skin-Picking) Disorder (DSM-5 698.4, ICD-10 L98.1) but this diagnosis is ruled out if the picking is better explained by Delusional Disorder.

Delusional Disorder is a diagnosis of exclusion after ruling out the effects of substances or other medical causes. Dermatitis can be caused by contact with irritants such as acids, alkalis, solvents, detergents, asbestos, and fiberglass. Soaps, hair dyes, household chemicals, or allergic reactions to pharmaceutical drugs can cause allergic dermatitis. However, Mary said that she had done "tests for asbestos and fiberglass," had "not changed her soap or hair products," had not "been in contact with any household chemicals," and was "taking no medications."

Intoxication by stimulants like methamphetamine and cocaine is associated with scratching and picking at the skin. Delusions of insects are also common in withdrawal from alcohol, methamphetamine, and cocaine. However, Mary "denied using any alcohol or drugs of abuse," her vital signs were normal, there was no evidence of Substance Use Disorder in her Diagnostic Examination, and she had a normal Cognitive Examination.

Bedbugs (*Cimex lectularius*) are 5 mm (0.2 inch) nocturnal insects that feed on blood but do not transmit pathogens. Usually there is no reaction to bites, but sometimes rapidly-resolving, itchy maculopapular lesions are seen and rarely allergic reactions are reported. Mexican bedbugs (*Reduviidae*) feed on sleepers at night—they are vectors for Chagas disease but they rarely cause widespread dermatitis. Human lice (*Anoplura*) may carry typhus, which causes a rash that starts start on the torso and is accompanied by fever, red conjunctivae, tinnitus, and avoidance of light. Fleas and mosquitoes can cause itchy lesions, but Mary had checked her screens and fumigated without relieving the problem. Generalized pruritis or itching can result from hepatic cirrhosis and Hodgkin's disease, but Mary denied that her lesions itched.

Mary complained of occasional irritability, but she lacked the symptoms of sleep problems, restlessness, feeling keyed-up, edginess, muscle tension, easy fatigability, poor concentration, or mind going blank needed for a diagnosis of Generalized Anxiety Disorder.

CLINICAL NOTES

Neither the dermatologist's examination nor my own examination of Mary's skin revealed anything that looked like an insect bite. The dermatologist said that Mary "caused them by scratching," and this is the only etiology I could observe. Needless scratching and picking at one's skin can cause skin damage called *psychogenic excoriation*. Weeping or crusted lesions are usually found on the body areas most accessible to scratching, such as the face, neck, shoulders, lower arms, and calves. The condition occurs in about 2% of dermatology patients and women predominate.

The delusional belief that invisible insects are attacking you is called *formication* (after the ant genus *Formica*). Internists prefer the label *delusional parasitism* and entomologists include the phenomenon in *entomophobia* (fear of insects). A Professor of Entomology at Purdue University showed me jars of bath water and bottles of invisible arthropod specimens he had received from sufferers throughout his career.

As with most delusions, trying to talk the patient out of their odd notions is not productive. Psychogenic excoriation and formication have been treated with behavioral therapy, antidepressants, and antipsychotics such as pimozide (Orap), a medication with a long half-life (55-110 hours) that binds to serotonin and dopamine receptors.

I treated Mary for her problem and its resulting stress with pharmacotherapy and stress-reduction exercises (see Chapter 8), while keeping watch for the emergence of an underlying mental disorder that was heralded by her focal delusion. She never recanted her beliefs but as her treatment progressed and her sores healed, I heard less about the insects. One year later, the sequelae of Mary's lesions were gone and the episode was largely forgotten. If pressed on the subject, Mary still made feeble assertions that she had been the victim of an infestation, but she was at a loss to explain the details of her ordeal.

CASE 45
BOBBIE THE TERROR

Bobbie was an 8-year-old boy who came to my office with his worried mother, Francine. "We're very confused about Bobbie's diagnosis," said the mother. "A year ago, our family doctor thought his **Anxiety Disorder** was caused by high thyroid, but his thyroid tests were normal. Then he gave Bobbie a benzodiazepine sedative for his anxiety, but it didn't work and it made Bobbie more impulsive."

"What happened next?" I asked.

"We took Bobbie to a child psychologist after that. She also thought Bobbie was anxious because he had **Attention-Deficit/Hyperactivity Disorder**. She gave him play therapy and called a doctor who gave him a stimulant medication but it only made him angrier.

"Then we took Bobbie to a psychiatrist who was a psychopharmacologist," Francine said. "He thought Bobbie had an anxiety disorder called **Obsessive-Compulsive Disorder**. He gave Bobbie several antidepressants but they didn't help and they made Bobbie more hyperactive and he couldn't sleep.

"The last doctor we took Bobbie to see was a neurologist who said that Bobbie's anxiety was caused by something called **Autism Spectrum Disorder**, partly because Bobbie has no friends. Other children don't like Bobbie. The neurologist put Bobbie on an antipsychotic, which he is still taking."

"So what do you think of that treatment?" I queried.

"I'm worried about giving a powerful antipsychotic to my little boy. I mean, they give them to people with Schizophrenia. But it's the only thing that has helped him at all. It calms him a little but it doesn't do anything for the rest of his problems."

"When did this whole situation start?" I asked.

Francine replied, "As a five-year-old, Bobbie was really cheerful and entertaining, but in the last two years he has become a terror. He gets wild and violent whenever we don't do what he says. He takes over an hour to get ready in the morning. Every time I help him put on one set of clothes he starts screaming, 'No good! No good! You can't make me wear that!' Then I try other clothes and he does the same thing."

"Is there anything else?" I asked Francine.

"His room is a terrible mess, with papers all over the place, but whenever anybody tries to move them, he flies into a rage and screams, 'You can't touch my things! I will not let you!' So we just have to leave his things in a mess."

"Is there anything else you are concerned about that you have not told me?" I queried.

"I'm terribly worried about Bobbie's sleeping and eating," Francine answered. "He's so active that he stays up all night and he's so picky that he will only eat certain foods. He's awfully thin for his age."

I watched the behavior of both mother and son in my office. The mother sat quietly, seemed relatively deferential, and even let Bobbie hit her when he raged. Bobbie, on the other hand, moved around on my couch restlessly. He had a bag of toys and occasionally he picked one out, only to throw it down a few seconds later. Bobbie directed much of his energy toward his mother, yelling at her and trying to hit her. Periodically, he lunged at his mother's neckline, trying to pull one of her breasts out of her dress.

Most notable was Bobbie's language. He showed great proficiency with language—in fact, he kept up a constant monologue that was so rapid that it was difficult to interrupt. Most of the time he shouted and screamed loudly. His speech was also very perseverative.

At one point, Bobbie gave me an angry look and threw himself on the floor, kicking his legs in the air and shouting, "I don't want to be here! You can't make me stay here! I want a soda! I'll only talk to the doctor if you get me a soda. I want a soda and I have to have it *now*!"

Bobby kept screaming "You can't make me! You can't make me! I won't stop until you get me a soda!" nonstop for almost ten minutes, punctuating his discourse with punches to his mother's midsection. Finally, his mother reached in her bag and took out a bottle of soda. She opened it up and gave the bottle to him but he only threw it on the floor.

Immediately Bobbie began shouting again. "Get me a pony! Now! You *have* to get me a pony! Right now! Right now!" Bobbie screamed. "I want a pony right now and I won't do anything until you get me one!"

His mother said that this behavior was commonplace for her son. He would demand something repeatedly, and if he were given what he requested, he would immediately lose interest and scream for something else. She said that Bobbie would request objects that were unreasonable or impossible to obtain and obsess about them for weeks at a time. At first, she and her husband worked hard to fulfill these requests, but as soon as Bobbie received the object he demanded, it was summarily thrown away and forgotten.

In my office, Bobbie was quite hyperactive. During our interview, he ran around, sat in every chair, bounced on the couch like a trampoline, and tried to sit upside down with his feet in the air. He seldom looked at my face when he was talking, but his facial expressions, gestures, posture, interpersonal distances, and orientation were normal for his age. Random sights and sounds in the office easily captured Bobbie's attention. His affect was restricted and his mood was angry. There was no evidence of formal thought disorder or response to internal stimuli.

It was impossible to administer even minimal cognitive testing to Bobbie. However, it was clear from his speech and behavior that he was distractible, tangential, and perseverative. His speech was loud, rapid, continuous, and abundant but I saw no evidence of aphasia, aprosody, anomia, or word-finding problems. His thought content was solely about himself (egocentric)—other people were only mentioned in the context of what they could do for him.

CHALLENGE

See if you can figure out what is wrong with Bobbie. Which of the different diagnoses he has received is the right one? Or is it something altogether different?

SOLUTION

This is a fairly common presentation for **Bipolar I Disorder, Most Recent Episode Manic, Moderate** (DSM-5 296.42, ICD-10 F31.12), in a young child.

The diagnostic criteria for Bipolar Disorder are the same for children as for adults. Once you consider that Bobbie may be manic, the diagnosis is quite obvious. Bobbie met the following criteria for a **Manic Episode**:

A. The following have been present most of the day nearly every day:
Increased goal-directed activity or energy. Bobbie was activated, agitated, and he stayed "up all night."
Plus at least one of these:
  a. Elevated mood.
  b. Expansive mood.
  c. Irritable mood. The only emotion Bobbie displayed during his appointment was anger and it had been persistent. We heard that "in the last two years he has become a terror" and "he gets wild and violent"—he raged, shouted, and screamed angrily, punched and hit his mother, and threw a tantrum on the floor of my office.

These symptoms last at least one week or any duration if hospitalization is necessary.

B. At least three of the following symptoms (four if the mood is only irritable):
  1. **Inflated self-esteem or grandiosity.** (*Grandiosity*): Bobbie acted as if he were all-powerful by ordering adults around, demanding unreasonable items, asserting that adults could not touch his belongings or defy his demands, and expecting to be rewarded after behaving inappropriately.
  2. **A decreased need for sleep (needs <3 hours).** Francine said, "He's so active that he stays up all night."
  3. **Talking more than usual or interrupting others (pressured speech).** (*Talkative*): Bobbie's speech was "continuous and abundant." (*Pressured*): He kept up a monologue that "was difficult to interrupt."
  4. **Rapid or racing thoughts.** "His speech was "loud, rapid," and "so rapid it was difficult to interrupt." Rapid speech often reveals flight of ideas.
  5. **Distractibility.** "Bobbie's attention was easily captured by random sights and sounds in the office." "He was distractible, tangential."
  6. **Increased goal-directed activity or psychomotor agitation.** (*Goal-directed activity*): Bobbie was obsessively persistent in his demands for soda and a pony, overfocussed on his dressing and belongings, and he would persist in his demands "for weeks at a time." (*Sexual*): "He lunged at his mother's neckline, trying to pull one of her breasts out of her dress." (*Psychomotor agitation*): "Bobbie was quite hyperactive." He "ran around, sat in every chair, bounced on the couch like a trampoline, and tried to sit upside down with his feet in the air."
  7. **Excessive involvement in activities that have a high potential for painful consequences (costly or risky impulsive actions).** This is hard to evaluate in an eight-year-old, but Bobbie was certainly over-involved in inappropriate misbehavior that had a high potential for painful consequences like rejection and punishment.

Taking a long time to get ready, poor appetite, picky eating, unreasonable demands, perseverative speech and action, and an egocentric outlook are all nondiagnostic features that are common in childhood Bipolar Disorder. Most notably, Bobbie's interpersonal strategy was maladaptive and very ineffective. If he had just politely asked his mother for what he wanted, he would have been much more likely to get it, without wasting so much energy on screaming, hitting, and demanding. Most children know how to do this.

Other Diagnostic Considerations

What of Bobbie's prior diagnoses? Bobbie's doctors had focused on a few symptoms rather than looking for a pattern uniting many symptoms. The clue to making the correct diagnosis was the recognition that Bobbie's prevalent emotion was not anxiety—it was anger. I have seen numerous child patients who fumed, screamed, raged, threw objects, and threw tantrums in my office, after which their caretakers said, "See how anxious he is?"

Several prior clinicians had seen Bobbie's agitation and assumed it was caused by anxiety. However, psychomotor activation, not anxiety or worried thoughts, accounted for Bobbie's agitation.

The diagnosis of Obsessive-Compulsive Disorder was probably based on the presence of recurrent and persistent thoughts and impulses plus repetitive, perseverative behaviors. However, Bobbie's repetitive thoughts did not meet the criteria for obsessions because Bobbie did not recognize that his thoughts and impulses were excessive and unreasonable and he showed no attempts to ignore, suppress, or neutralize them. Although Bobbie's behavior was inflexible, his behaviors were not compulsions—there was no evidence of nonfunctional routines, rules, or rituals to prevent a dreaded event or situation. These distinctions are important because persistent, recursive thoughts and recurrent, perseverative behaviors are common in many clinical patients as well in normal individuals under stress.

Overall, Bobbie fulfilled none of the official diagnostic criteria for any anxiety disorders, including Separation Anxiety Disorder, Panic Disorder, Agoraphobia, Specific Phobia, Generalized Anxiety Disorder, Social Anxiety Disorder, Acute Stress Disorder, Posttraumatic Stress Disorder, Obsessive-Compulsive Disorder, or Substance-Induced Anxiety Disorder. Anxiolytic medications did not help but only made him more impulsive. Antidepressants made him more hyperactive.

Bobbie's diagnosis of Attention-Deficit/Hyperactivity Disorder was based on his failure in schoolwork, listening, following instructions, organizing tasks and activities, and performing tasks requiring sustained mental effort and memory. All these problems can be caused by distractibility and distractibility is one of the key criteria for Bipolar Disorder. However, Attention-Deficit/Hyperactivity Disorder cannot be diagnosed if the symptoms occur exclusively during or are accounted for by a mood disorder such as Bipolar Disorder.

Bobbie's diagnosis of Autism Spectrum Disorder was probably influenced by his failure to meet others' gaze and his lack of friends. In my evaluation, Bobbie did not meet the diagnostic criteria for Autism Spectrum Disorder. Although Bobbie "seldom looked at my face when he was talking," his nonverbal interpersonal communication, including "his facial expressions, gestures, posture, interpersonal distances and orientation were normal for his age." Although Bobbie had few peer relationships, a diagnosis of Autism Spectrum Disorder is not necessary to explain why a child who rages, screams, tantrums, bullies, orders, hits, and kicks does not make friends.

Unlike Autism, where individuals do not spontaneously share their emotions or interests, Bobbie was aggressive in communicating his angry emotions. He clearly communicated his interest in avoiding doctor's appointments, choosing his clothing, arranging his belongings, getting his preferred food, and acquiring sodas and ponies.

Peer relationships suffer whenever a child has any severe mental or physical disorder—they are not proof of Autism Spectrum Disorder. Although there was no evidence that Bobbie engaged other children in social play or games, he certainly involved his mother and me in intense interpersonal interactions during his session. Bobbie's behavior revolved around his angry, grandiose interactions with others—his outbursts served as a substrate for interpersonal control and Bobbie discarded them as soon as they were no longer effective.

Cognitive Testing

Bobbie demonstrated loud, rapid, pressured speech, distractibility, and tangentiality. Pressured speech and distractibility are diagnostic criteria for bipolar Mania. Tangential speech, with many digressions from the point, is another sign of distractible thoughts. I have often found perseveration while testing patients with active Bipolar Disorder.

CLINICAL NOTES

Bobbie's bipolar diagnosis was confirmed during the course of his three-year follow-up and his response to mood-stabilizing treatment.

The atypical antipsychotic Bobbie received was licensed as a treatment for Bipolar Disorder—which is why it somewhat helped his bipolar symptoms. I started Bobbie on a first-line mood stabilizer (lithium salts or an anticonvulsant) and tapered the dose up to therapeutic levels. Then I tapered and withdrew the unneeded antipsychotic. Over the course of treatment, Bobbie's condition improved dramatically. He gradually developed the ability to calm himself, first for minutes at a time, and later for hours at a time. His tantrums decreased from hourly events to a frequency of one or two per week.

With a clear diagnosis and effective treatment plan, Bobbie's mother and father were able to resume their rôles as caring parents and spend less time supervising and containing Bobbie's emotions and behaviors. They spent more time with their other children and began meeting weekly as a couple for dinner and a movie. They induced the school to pay for a tutor three times a week so that Bobbie could make progress in school studies. Gradually, Bobbie was able to resume life as a regular kid.

Emil Kraepelin believed that many bipolar patients had their first Manic Episode before 10 years of age and current research shows that over half of all adults with Bipolar Disorder had an onset of symptoms before 19 years of age. There has been recent speculation that most mood disorders of early childhood are Bipolar Disorder. Nevertheless, children who exhibit hypomanic or manic symptoms are frequently misdiagnosed.

CASE 46
JULIE'S NOCTURNAL ADVENTURE

I arrived at my office at 7:00 A.M. and found Julie waiting outside my door for her first appointment. "I've come to try to rectify a terrible problem that occurred at work," she said, after she had come inside and taken a seat.

"I'm 39 years old and I'm the managing partner at a large firm where I have worked for several years. I am known in my company for my calm demeanor and fair judgment. I take the time to get to know all the members of my staff personally, from the office manager down to data entry personnel. I'm highly respected by all my employees and I assure you that they are wonderful, competent people who would never let me down.

"Yesterday was just an ordinary day. I finished work late, as usual. Then I went home to my apartment, ate dinner, and went to bed at my usual time of 11:00 P.M. I awoke at my usual time of 6:00 A.M., to find that I was fully dressed in my work clothes, sprawled in an armchair in my living room. All the lights in my apartment were on and when I went into my kitchen to fix breakfast, I found a dirty teacup and part of a sandwich on my kitchen table. My clothes were all wrinkled—while I was changing them, I looked in the mirror and I saw a huge, purple bruise on my thigh.

"When I finally got to work, half of my ten staff was missing. The rest of them were really quiet all morning, like they were avoiding me. Finally, I called my office manager into my office and asked what was going on. He said that I had called him at home at 3:00 A.M. As soon as he answered his telephone, I began screaming at him, accusing him of poor performance, lateness, and a bad attitude. I cursed at him and used unprofessional language, including ethnic and gender-related slurs. Then I told him that he was terminated and that I never wanted to see him in the office again.

"When he arrived at work, he talked to the other staff members and called the ones who didn't come in for work—they had all received a call like his, where I screamed at them and terminated them. When I heard what I had done, I ran home and made the first available appointment with you." Julie began to sob deeply.

"I don't remember any of that. As far as I can tell, I must have awakened in the middle of the night, put on my work clothes, and called up and fired all my staff. I must have been completely awake, because I apparently made a cup of tea and a sandwich. I must have fallen down during the night because I have that bruise. Then I apparently fell back asleep in the living room with all my clothes on."

Julie denied any prior psychiatric hospitalization or outpatient treatment. She reported a past history of mild insomnia about a year ago. She said she had a bout of mild depressive symptoms about six months ago but it had subsided without treatment. Last week, when Julie had her yearly checkup, she casually mentioned to her primary physician that her insomnia had started again. He urged her to take some samples of a sleeping medication and she had her first dose the night of the incident.

In her Diagnostic Examination, Julie denied physical symptoms of Panic Disorder and Generalized Anxiety Disorder. Julie said she had no problems with hyperactivity, or impulsivity, but she had been somewhat distractible recently. Julie said she had been in a particularly good mood lately and she denied emotions of sadness, hopelessness, anxiety, panic, irritability, loneliness, or emptiness. She said that she enjoyed her life and her job, and denied any obsessions, compulsions, hallucinations, delusions, suicidal thoughts, or violent intentions.

Julie performed well on all the tests of *attention, language, memory, abstract thinking,* and *sequential thinking* on her Cognitive Examination. Her Quality of Speech was loud and rapid.

Personality testing with the Personality Inventory Scale (see *Mental Status Examination for Personality Disorders*, Chapter 8), showed no evidence of personality disorders.

CHALLENGE

Julie's experience seems like a psychotic break but her usual level of function is high. What caused this episode and what is her diagnosis? What treatment do you recommend?

SOLUTION

Julie experienced **Zolpidem (Ambien) Intoxication** (DSM-5 292.89, ICD-10 F13.929).

She met the following criteria for **Sedative, Hypnotic, or Anxiolytic Intoxication**:
A. **Recent use of a sedative, hypnotic, or anxiolytic**. Her doctor "urged her to take some samples of a sleeping medication and she had her first dose the night of the incident."
B. **Clinically significant maladaptive behavioral or psychological changes (inappropriate sexual or aggressive behavior, mood lability, impaired judgment, impaired social or occupational functioning) that developed**

during, or shortly after, ingestion of a sedative, hypnotic, or anxiolytic. (*Inappropriate sexual or aggressive behavior*): Julie screamed, accused, cursed, fired, and insulted her staff, using inappropriate "ethnic and gender-related slurs." (*Mood lability*): Although Julie told us she that is noted for her "calm demeanor and she denied emotions of sadness, hopelessness, anxiety, panic, irritability, loneliness, or emptiness; she clearly flew into a rage in the middle of the night, showing mood lability. (*Impaired judgment*): Although Julie said she is known for her "fair judgment," it showed poor judgment indeed to scream and curse at her staff and summarily fire them. (*Impaired functioning*): Firing her staff demonstrated significant occupational impairment on the part of the managing partner of a large firm.

C. **One (or more) of the following signs, developing during or shortly after sedative, hypnotic, or anxiolytic use**:
  1. **Slurred speech**.
  2. **Incoordination**. Julie saw a "huge, purple bruise" on her thigh and she hypothesized that she "must have fallen down during the night." If so, this would demonstrate poor coordination.
  3. **Unsteady gait**.
  2. **Nystagmus** (repetitive, rhythmic vertical or horizontal movements of the eyes).
  3. **Impairment in attention or memory**. (*Impaired memory*): Julie said, "I don't remember any of that." She had amnesia for the entire event.
  6. **Stupor or coma**.

In coding substance-related disorders, the clinician should record the name of the specific substance used rather than the name of the class. Thus, Julie received the diagnosis of Zolpidem (Ambien) Intoxication.

Other Diagnostic Considerations

Non-Rapid Eye Movement Sleep Arousal Disorder, Sleepwalking Type (DSM-5 307.46, ICD-10 F51.3), is another condition where individuals rise from sleep, followed by amnesia for the experience in the morning. However, sleepwalking is most prominent in children, and sleepwalkers are typically unresponsive to communication and have the appearance of being asleep. Julie communicated so well with others that they thought she was awake. Her behavior was purposeful, not the purposeless wandering of sleepwalking.

Hypno*pompic* hallucinations occur in the semiconscious state just before normal waking. Hypna*gogic* hallucinations occur in the semiconscious state just before sleep onset. However, Julie's problem occurred in the middle of the night after the ingestion of a hypnotic medication.

CLINICAL NOTES

I have personal knowledge of over a dozen such incidents characterized by midcycle waking, unpredictable behavior, mood changes, and consequent amnesia for the event after patients took brief-acting, rapid-onset hypnotic medications. There have been case reports in the literature and anecdotal reports about patients who woke from sleep, dressed, held conversations, prepared food, ate voluminous meals, drove recklessly at high speeds, and committed violent acts with no memory for the events in the morning.

Usually intoxication is not observed with hypnotics because their effects take place while the patient is sleeping. It has long been known that benzodiazepines can cause activation and amnesia for the period following ingestion—even after just one dose. This is probably caused by rapid withdrawal effects that are greatest after taking short-acting sedatives and their relatives. Short-acting sedatives include propofol (Deprivan: half-life=45 minutes), zolpidem (Ambien: half-life=2 hours), midazolam (Versed: half-life=2 hours), and triazolam (Halcion: half-life=3 hours). By comparison, the half-life of alprazolam (Xanax) is 11 hours, lorazepam (Ativan) is 14 hours, clonazepam (Klonopin) is 23 hours, and diazepam (Valium) is 43 hours.

One short-acting hypnotic label lists aggression, amnesia, bizarre behavior, extroversion, and hallucinations as possible side effects. The warning suggests that the emergence of such symptoms "may be the consequence of an unrecognized psychiatric or physical disorder." However, Julie denied physical problems of anxiety or attention. There was no evidence of sadness, anhedonia, irritability, expansive mood, mood elevation, or hallucinations in her Diagnostic Examination, and Julie was not impaired in her work or social life prior to her intoxicated episode.

I counseled Julie that her nocturnal behavior was the result of a drug reaction that was beyond her control. I advised her to avoid sedatives, hypnotics, and anxiolytics in the future to avoid a possible repeat episode. Julie and I met in several psychotherapeutic sessions while she resolved problems at work and recovered from the shame and discomfort caused by her nighttime episode. Then she was able to return to her former life activities.

CASE 47
FREDDI HANGS OUT AT THE FAIR

It was a bright, crisp September morning when Freddi and Ralph walked into my office. I had treated Freddi for Bereavement after her mother died several years before and I already had her evaluation and chart on my desk.

Ralph sat on the edge of his chair, anxious to speak, while his wife Freddi leaned back in the cushions of the couch, as far away from me as she could get.

"My wife Freddi didn't want to come today, but I convinced her that she couldn't avoid this thing anymore. She has such terrible anxiety and doesn't like to go out of the house or do anything. It's been going on this way for a year."

"When did this anxiety start, Freddi?" I asked.

"I don't really want to talk about this but I guess I have to," she said plaintively. "It was my birthday and Ralph took me to the State Fair. He likes to go on the carnival rides but I'm afraid of them, so I will only go on the one that has little boxes and bright red umbrellas and goes around like a little Ferris wheel. Well, I was on the ride and when we got to the top where I close my eyes, the car tilted and I fell right out."

"My goodness," I exclaimed. "How did you survive?"

"Well, I didn't fall all the way out. Before I went crashing down to the ground, my hand got caught in the door and I was left hanging from the base of the car by my wedding ring."

"I was sure glad we were married, then," Ralph added dully.

"The Fair people didn't know what to do. They stopped the ride with us at the top and they let me hang there for over an hour before they figured out what to do. I was terrified. Eventually, they just let the ride go around slowly and pulled me out when I got close to the ground. Actually, I was completely unhurt physically but I haven't felt right since. I don't even like to think about it."

"That sounds like a terrible experience!" I said. "What happened afterwards?"

"I didn't want to go to work or even leave the house for over a month. I just sat around home doing crosswords, knitting, and other things I like."

"How else has this experience affected you?" I asked.

"Well, I'm never going on another carnival ride as long as I live," said Freddi emphatically. "I get nervous just seeing commercials for the State Fair on television."

"Things haven't been quite the same for us in our marriage in the last year, either," said Ralph. "Freddi used to be such a warm person, but it seems that she has cooled off to me. Things aren't quite the same in the bedroom, either, if you know what I mean." I saw Freddi's face redden.

On her Diagnostic Examination, Freddi said it took her 30-60 minutes to fall asleep each night. "If I hear any kind of noise at night, I jump right out of bed to see what it is," she said. "Sometimes I dream about hanging there and Ralph says I wake up screaming.

"I'm just a wreck," Freddi said. "If I hear a loud noise, I jump out of my skin. I start sweating, trembling, and my heart starts pounding."

Freddi denied feelings of choking, dizziness, chest pain, nausea, shortness of breath, paresthesias, or fear of losing control or dying. She endorsed strong anxiety and uncontrollable worries but she denied fatigue, muscle tension, edginess, poor focus, or inadequate attention. She endorsed emotions of sadness, hopelessness, and irritability, but said, "They never last very long." Freddi denied thoughts of suicide or violence toward others.

Freddi did well on all tests of *attention, language, memory, abstract thinking,* and *sequential thinking.*

CHALLENGE

What is causing Freddi's anxiety? What would you do to help correct it?

SOLUTION

Freddi is suffering from **Posttraumatic Stress Disorder** (DSM-5 309.81, ICD-10 F43.10):

Exposure to actual or threatened death, serious injury, or sexual violation to self or others. Hanging from the bottom of a car high in the air, anchored only by your wedding ring for over an hour is certainly an event that involved the threat of injury and death.

One or more of the following:
   1. Recurrent, involuntary, and intrusive memories of the trauma. "I don't even like to think about it," Freddi told me.

2. Recurrent distressing dreams of the trauma. Freddi said, "Sometimes I dream about hanging there." "Ralph says I wake up screaming."
   3. Flashbacks of the trauma.
   4. Distressed by reminders of the trauma. Freddi said, "I get nervous just seeing commercials for the State Fair on television."
   5. Physiological reactions to reminders of the trauma.
One or more of the following:
   6. Efforts to avoid feelings and thoughts about the trauma. "My wife Freddi didn't want to come today," said her husband. Freddi confided, "I do not really want to talk about this but I guess I have to."
   7. Efforts to avoid external reminders of the trauma. "I'm never going on another carnival ride as long as I live," Freddi asserted.
Two or more of the following:
   8. Inability to remember an important aspect of the trauma.
   9. Negative cognitions about oneself, others, or the world.
   10. Unrealistically blaming self or others for the trauma.
   11. Persistent negative emotions (e.g., fear, anger, or shame)
   12. Diminished interest or participation in important activities. Freddi said, "I didn't want to go to work or even leave the house for over a month."
   13. Feelings of detachment or estrangement from others. "Freddi used to be such a warm person but it seems that she has cooled off to me," her husband said.
   14. Persistent inability to experience positive emotions (e.g., happiness, love, satisfaction). "Things aren't quite the same in the bedroom," said Freddi's husband.
Two or more of the following:
   15. Irritable behavior and angry outbursts (e.g., verbal or physical aggression to people or objects).
   16. Reckless behavior.
   17. Hypervigilance. "If I hear any kind of noise at night, I jump right out of bed to see what it is," said Freddi.
   18. Exaggerated startle response. "If I hear a loud noise, I jump out of my skin."
   19. Poor concentration.
   20. Sleep problems. Freddi told me that "it took her 30-60 minutes to fall asleep each night."
The disturbance lasts more than one month. Freddi had her symptoms for "a year."
The disturbance causes clinically significant distress or impairment in school, work, home, or social function.
   Freddi's symptoms caused problems in her work, family, and social life.

Other Diagnostic Considerations

The physical symptoms of impaired sleep, anger, poor concentration, hypervigilance, or startle response are the most objective markers of Posttraumatic Stress Disorder. However, to make the diagnosis of Posttraumatic Stress Disorder, you must establish that these arousal symptoms were not present before the trauma. In Freddi's case, I had her previous evaluation with a Diagnostic Examination, Cognitive Examination, and personality testing that confirmed that she had not been experiencing arousal problems before this incident.

Freddi endorsed pounding heart, sweating, and tremor that suggest Panic Disorder, but these symptoms did not peak over minutes and she did not have the other symptoms necessary for a Panic Disorder diagnosis.

Freddi admitted to anxiety, uncontrollable worries, and restless sleep that suggest Generalized Anxiety Disorder but she denied any of the other physical criteria needed to make the diagnosis.

Freddi cannot be given a diagnosis of unipolar Major Depressive Disorder because her feelings of sadness "never last very long" and she told us that she does "crosswords, knitting, and other things I like," indicating that she is not anhedonic.

Similarly, Freddi does not qualify for a diagnosis of Bipolar Disorder because we see no evidence of periods of activity, elevated or expansive mood, and her irritable emotions "never last very long." Furthermore, these incorrect diagnoses do not explain all of Freddi's symptoms like Posttraumatic Stress Disorder does.

CLINICAL NOTES

After hanging from the top of a carnival ride for an hour, Freddi experienced Posttraumatic Stress Disorder. Although most of the cases of Posttraumatic Stress Disorder you will hear about are predicated on warfare experiences or childhood abuse, PTSD can be triggered by many other stressful life experiences.

I treated Freddi with Behavioral Therapy, where we agreed on assignments that placed her incrementally closer to reminders of her experience until she gradually became desensitized to them. We also did Interpersonal Therapy, where we reviewed her associations and motivations during important social interactions, to help make her feel more comfortable in her work, family, and social relationships. Six months later, Freddi had put most of her experience behind her and was going on with her life.

CASE 48
HARRY HAS A HANG-UP

The sun had just broken through cloudy skies when Harry walked into my office. He was a tall, slender young man in an attractive, close-fitting grey coat and stylish grey shoes with white patches over the toes. He looked all around my office before curling up on the leather sofa.

"I'm been having trouble at work for years," Harry began. "I'm uncomfortable going to meetings in our conference room—it's just too crowded for me. I travel in my job and I have trouble riding in crowded airplanes and difficulty riding the subway when I go to Chicago and New York. I even have difficulty eating in the crowded little restaurants that my wife and her friends like to frequent."

"What is the most troubling part of these situations for you, Harry?" I asked.

Most frequently, I worry that I will have to get up suddenly to urinate and I won't be able to make it to the bathroom in time. Sometimes at business or personal dinners, I worry that I will get sick and I won't be able to get to the bathroom in time. These things have never happened in my life, but I worry about them when I feel closed in.

"I also worry that I'll start blushing if I say something stupid—when I blush, I turn a deep, beet-red color. I wear shirts and jackets that don't show dampness, but I still worry that business clients or my wife's friends will see that I'm perspiring. I worry that I will be holding a drink and my hands will start to shake or I will choke on my food and look absurd. Sometimes I worry that I will get dizzy and fall over someone. These fears are all excessive and unreasonable worries, but I can't shake them, and they're interfering with my work and social life. They only occur when I'm in these situations and afterwards they go away."

On his Diagnostic Examination, Harry denied sleep, appetite, or energy problems. He said he had no difficulties with chest pain, racing heart, tremor, chills, hot flushes, shortness of breath, choking, stomachache, nausea, poor concentration, mind going blank, restlessness, edginess, tingling, a sense of detachment, or fears of losing control or dying. He denied emotions of euphoria, sadness, or irritability. He denied worried thoughts occurring most days, or thoughts of hopelessness, guilt, worthlessness, suicide or violence.

On his Cognitive Examination, Harry did well on all tests of *attention, language, memory, abstract thinking,* and *sequential thinking.*

CHALLENGE

Does Harry have a mental illness? If so, what is it and what will you do to help him?

SOLUTION

Harry has **Social Anxiety Disorder** (DSM-5 300.23, ICD-10 F40.10):

Excessive fear and avoidance of social situations where patients might be humiliated, embarrassed, or rejected because of their anxiety symptoms. Harry is afraid of being in crowded "conference rooms," "airplanes," "subways," and "restaurants" that are filled with strangers who may be scrutinizing him. Harry says that he fears he will have "to get up suddenly to urinate" or vomit and not being able to reach the bathroom in time. He worries about saying "something stupid," blushing, "perspiring," shaking, choking, feeling "dizzy," or falling.

This fear typically lasts for six months or more. Harry has been having trouble "for years,"

These symptoms cause clinically significant distress or impairment in work, family, or social function. These symptoms make Harry "uncomfortable" and cause him to "worry." It is difficult for him to travel to work, attend meetings, or go to dinners for work or with friends.

Other Diagnostic Considerations

It is natural to think of Panic Disorder when hearing of Harry's worries about vomiting, blushing, perspiring, shaking, choking, and dizziness. However, although Harry worries about these symptoms, he rarely or never experiences them. His disorder is about fears of having panic symptoms.

Clinicians usually consider Generalized Anxiety Disorder when a patient presents with anxiety. However, Harry worries only when he is in anxiety-provoking social situations—he does not have excessive anxiety and uncontrollable worried thoughts about activities such as work or school performance that have been present most days for six months. Moreover, Harry denies poor concentration, mind going blank, fatigue, muscle tension, restless sleep, restlessness, edginess, or irritability.

Whenever you consider Social Anxiety Disorder, you should also rule out Avoidant Personality Disorder (DSM-5 301.82, ICD-10 F60.6). Patients with both conditions avoid interpersonal contact at work or school for fear of criticism, disapproval, or rejection. Both feel reticent around strangers or in new social environments and both may feel inept or unappealing. However, patients with Avoidant Personality Disorder fear internal feelings of shame and inadequacy, whereas Social Anxiety Disordered patients fear physical panic or panic-like symptoms. Also, the symptoms of Avoidant Personality Disorder begin early in life and persist throughout the lifetime in many situations, while Social Anxiety Symptoms are limited to specific social environments.

CLINICAL NOTES

We are used to associating Social Anxiety Disorder with difficulties in public speaking, addressing authority figures, initiating or maintaining conversations, or dating. Harry's case gives us the opportunity to see a common presentation of Social Anxiety Disorder where the emphasis is on panic and panic-like symptoms in close social situations.

Fear of urinary urgency is common in Social Anxiety Disorder. Urinary urgency, palpitations, pounding heart, rapid heart rate, excessive sweating, tremor, shortness of breath, choking, chest pain, nausea, stomachache, dizziness, lightheadedness, fainting, numbness, tingling, derealization, depersonalization, and fears of losing control, dying, or going crazy are all driven by stress neurotransmitters (like adrenaline and noradrenaline) and stress hormones (like cortisol). These are all part of the body's stress reaction.

The prevalence of Social Anxiety Disorder varies between studies but ranges between 0.5-7%. The mean onset is around 12 years-of-age, and onset after 25 years is rare. Social Anxiety Disorder occurs more frequently in women than men. Clinically it must be distinguished from normal shyness and Avoidant Personality Disorder. Experimental work has associated social anxiety with brain areas such as the amygdala and caudate nucleus, and with neurochemicals such as dopamine, serotonin, and prolactin. It can be treated with Behavioral Therapy, Cognitive Therapy, and Interpersonal Psychotherapy; and with serotonergic antidepressants and the MAO Inhibitor phenelzine (Nardil). Sedatives, beta-blockers (such as propranolol/Inderal), and alpha-agonists (such as clonidine/Catapres) can decrease physical symptoms.

Harry and I agreed on a five-month course of a serotonergic antidepressant which significantly relieved his discomfort. During this time, we treated his Social Anxiety Disorder symptoms with Behavioral Therapy, gradually increasing his exposure to crowded and confined conditions while monitoring his expectations of physical stress. We discussed the expectations he had formed through his past experiences with strangers and authority figures. When he needed to travel for business, I gave him a mild sedative to take with him in crowded, confined environments like airplanes and subways. He faithfully carried these pills in his pocket for years, but he never felt the need to take any.

CHAPTER 7
THE MENTAL STATUS EXAMINATION IN LEGAL AND FORENSIC SETTINGS

In forensic psychiatry, clinicians are called upon to evaluate patients with a variety of behavioral, social, and mental problems. Forensic clinicians have a responsibility to the law and they may be asked to offer opinions to defenders, prosecutors, and the court.

CASE 49
RICHARD RUNS IN FEAR

I opened the door and ushered Richard and his wife Celine into my office for their first appointment. Richard handed me his completed Diagnostic and Cognitive Questionnaires while his wife settled back into my couch. He was dressed in a shiny blue, pinstriped polyester suit, blue tie, and shiny black straw hat, whereas his wife was wearing a long, dark, maroon dress and patent leather shoes. They looked like they had just come from church. Celine spoke first.

"My husband Richard had a terrible experience at his work and he has not been the same, since. My brother is a personal injury attorney and he said we should come here to see if you think he has a diagnosis." Celine's voice sounded slightly nervous.

"What diagnosis do you or your brother think that Richard might have?" I asked.

"We would prefer not to say and let you form your own conclusions," Celine replied. "Go ahead, Richard, tell the doctor what happened to you."

"I am a bonded night watchman at the Lincoln Shopping Mall," Richard said, slowly. "Really what I do is to watch the parking structure all night. It is five floors of parking. I have a little bicycle and I ride up and down the parking ramp from the ground floor to the top fifth level and around each level all night long, keeping an eye on things. No one is supposed to be in there while the shops are closed, but sometimes young people sneak up there in their cars to make out or bums come in with a bottle of wine to find a place to sleep. My job is to politely insist that they leave because, really, they are trespassing on shopping center property."

"Do not forget to explain to the doctor about the truck parked on the roof," Celine reminded.

"Yes," said Richard. "The shopping center allows vans and small trucks to park in the parking structure overnight if they are delivering clothes or other merchandise to the stores in the morning. However, big vans and trucks have to stay on the ground level because the ramp that goes between levels is too steep and narrow for commercial vehicles to use. I was told that a big van got stuck on the narrow ramp going up to the second level years ago and since then no commercial vehicles are allowed past the first floor. The ramp was only built for cars but even some big cars have trouble going on the ramp, it's so narrow.

"Three weeks ago, at 3:00 A.M., the parking structure seemed deserted. I was riding my bicycle up the ramp to the top fifth level. I always ride up to the top level and work my way down to the other four levels because it's easier to coast down than pedal up that steep, narrow ramp. On the top level, I saw a big truck parked—I don't know how it fit up the ramp. I rode over, woke up the trucker, and said his rig was too big to park there. Then I turned into the ramp to coast down to the fourth level.

"Suddenly I heard a really loud noise behind me and this big truck was trying to go down the ramp really fast. There wasn't any place for me to go and I yelled and waved my hands but he didn't see me and he kept on coming down the ramp fast. There's no room to turn off on that narrow ramp and I had to peddle my bicycle as fast as I could down that steep ramp. I was scared that the trucker was mad because I told him to move and that he was trying to run over me and kill me. I was going too fast to turn onto another level and this giant truck chased me all the way down four floors. I could smell the diesel in my nose, he was so close. When I got down to the ground level, he chased me across the parking lot and right out the door until I skidded my bicycle and fell over into the bushes. When I picked myself up, I was shaking and I couldn't continue working—I had to go home from work early."

"That sounds terrible," I said. "So, what happened after that?"

"Richard was not the same when he came home," continued Celine. "He did not seem to know who he was or even that he was at home with me. He kept wandering around the house in a daze. Usually my husband is very warm and polite but that night he was cold and emotionless. At first, he could not remember what had happened to him and it was hard to get him to talk about it."

"I don't want to think about that night ever again but my thoughts keep coming back to it," Richard added. "The next day, my thoughts were so painful whenever I rode down the ramp again that I had to take off work for a while. I only started feeling normal a couple of days ago."

Richard had been to his primary care doctor before coming to me and his physical examination was normal. He had never carried a psychiatric diagnosis and he denied using any drugs or medications.

On his Diagnostic Questionnaire, Richard noted difficulty sleeping, feelings of restlessness, and emotions of irritability. He said that these were not present before his incident.

On the Cognitive Questionnaire, Richard did well in tests of *attention*, but he put the wrong date on his forms and overlooked several questions, indicating that his concentration was poor.

Richard did well in all tests of *language*.

In *memory* testing, Richard could only remember four numbers in a Digit Span test of working memory, and he failed the Free Recall from a Story test of short-term memory.

Richard did well in all *abstract thinking* tasks, although he overlooked tests of Set Analysis and Insight, as mentioned above.

In tests of *sequential thinking*, Richard failed the Arithmetic Story Problem.

CHALLENGE

Richard has experienced an ordeal. What diagnosis, if any, would you suggest for the attorney? If Richard and Celine want treatment, what would you suggest?

SOLUTION

Richard is experiencing **Acute Stress Disorder** (DSM-5 308.3, ICD-10 F43.0).

Exposure to actual or threatened death, serious injury, or sexual violation to self or others. Being chased down a steep narrow ramp, fearing that he would be run over by a big truck any second, is an event that involved potentially serious injury and death.

Nine or more of the following:
1. **Recurrent, involuntary, and intrusive memories of the trauma.** "My thoughts keep coming back to it," Richard told us.
2. **Recurrent distressing dreams of the trauma.**
3. **Flashbacks of the trauma.**
4. **Distress and/or physiological reactions to reminders of the trauma.** Richard noted that he experienced painful thoughts "whenever I rode down the ramp" after the incident.
5. **Persistent inability to experience positive emotions (e.g., happiness, love, satisfaction).** After the event, Richard's wife Celine said that he was "cold and emotionless."
6. **Depersonalization (feeling detached from oneself) or derealization (feeling detached from one's environment).** (*Depersonalization*): Celine said that "he did not seem to know who he was." (*Derealization*): Celine said that Richard "kept wandering around the house in a daze." His wife also said that Richard did not seem to know "that he was at home with me."
7. **Inability to remember an important aspect of the trauma.** "At first, he could not remember what had happened to him."
8. **Efforts to avoid feelings and thoughts about the trauma.** "I don't want to think about that night ever again," said Richard.
9. **Efforts to avoid external reminders of the trauma.** "My thoughts were so painful whenever I rode down the ramp again that I had to take off work for a while."
10. **Sleep problems.** On his Diagnostic Questionnaire, Richard noted "difficulty sleeping."
11. **Irritable behavior and angry outbursts (e.g., verbal or physical aggression to people or objects).** On his Diagnostic Questionnaire, Richard noted "irritability."
12. **Hypervigilance.**
13. **Poor concentration.** Richard's performance on his Cognitive Questionnaire indicated that "his concentration was poor." Richard wrote the wrong date and omitted two tests. He failed tests of Digit Span, Free Recall from a Story, and the Arithmetic Story Problem, tests that are sensitive to distractibility and concentration problems.
14. **Exaggerated startle response.**

Other Diagnostic Considerations

Acute Stress Disorder may not be diagnosed if the symptoms are the result of a substance or a another medical condition, but Richard denied using any drugs and he had just had a normal physical examination. Acute Stress Disorder cannot be diagnosed in the presence of Brief Psychotic Disorder, but there was no evidence of psychosis.

Acute Stress Disorder also may not be diagnosed in the presence of another preexisting psychiatric disorder. This criterion is critical because many mental conditions can mimic the symptoms of Acute Stress Disorder or amplify the intensity of normal life experiences to the point that they seem very stressful. However, Richard denied any previous psychiatric condition and his reaction to being chased by a giant truck seemed reasonable.

Cognitive Testing

Richard demonstrated *attention* errors when he put the wrong date on his forms and overlooked several questions. He failed tests of Digit Span, Free Recall from a Story, and the Arithmetic Story Problem, tests that are sensitive to distractibility and concentration problems. Thus, Richard's poor *attention* could account for his other errors downstream. Richard should be retested when he has returned to baseline.

CLINICAL NOTES

To diagnose Acute Stress Disorder, it must cause significant impairment in school, work, family, or social life, or prevent the patient from tasks like telling family members about the traumatic experience. Richard was clear that his symptoms had caused work impairment when he said that "I had to go home from work early" and "I had to take off work for a while." At home, Richard was initially cold, emotionless, would not talk to his wife, and appeared not to notice that she was in the room with him, indicating transitory impairment in family function.

To meet criteria for Acute Stress Disorder, the symptoms must last between three days and four weeks. Richard said that the incident happened "three weeks ago" and that he "started feeling normal a couple of days ago." Thus, the duration of the incident was about 19 days, a little less than three weeks, and this is consistent with the Acute Stress Disorder diagnosis.

Unfortunately for the bank accounts of Richard, Celine, and their attorney; Richard's Acute Stress Disorder appeared to be resolving at the time of his evaluation and he concurred that he had been "feeling normal" for "a couple of days." There appeared to be no lasting conditions that would support a claim for disability.

I reassured the couple that Richard's symptoms were probably self-limiting and were unlikely to progress to a case of Posttraumatic Stress Disorder. I offered Couple's Therapy if Richard and Celine thought they needed to work through any details of the experience that were still troublesome for their relationship and I offered to speak to Richard's employer if he needed a few more days off work to recover. I also invited the couple to return if any of Richard's symptoms resurfaced in the future.

Richard and Celine thanked me politely and left my office. I never saw or heard from them again.

CASE 50
DON'S CURIOUS CRIME

A judge of the juvenile court called me one day to perform a mental status examination on Don D, a 17-year-old Hispanic boy accused of shoplifting.

Don had been arrested for shoplifting before and he faced serious consequences if he was convicted again. At the public defender's request, the court asked me to render an opinion on whether the boy had been acting on his own free will or if his actions were beyond control by reason of insanity. If he was insane, the court wanted me to tell them whether Don was too insane to be tried. On the telephone, the public defender said that Don seemed "funny," but he had no mental health, medical, or hospital records.

According to the police report, the crime had been committed around 1:00 P.M. in a small, crowded neighborhood convenience store. Don was well known to the store manager and all the regular customers because he came to the market frequently. On the afternoon of his arrest, Don was observed putting an ice cream bar into the front of his tee shirt and pulling the shirt up over his head. Subsequently, Don ran through the crowded market, past the manager at the cash register, and out the door. Several customers ran outside, tackled Don, and held him until the police arrived. Subsequently, the ice cream bar was found melting in the bushes outside the store.

Don came to my office for his examination. He was a tall, slightly overweight adolescent dressed in a shabby tee shirt and jeans. Don said that he lived alone with his invalid mother in a small apartment located in the center of the city near the convenience store. He had no siblings and his father had left the family when Don was small. The mother could not work and she received state disability. He had no social relationships outside of work except for his invalid mother. Don had failing grades in grade school. He left high school after one year and found a job loading trucks in a printing warehouse, a job that he still held at the time of the shoplifting incident.

"I'm a psychiatrist, Don," I began. "The court asked me to evaluate your mental health and tell the judge and other legal representatives my opinion. I cannot be your doctor and I cannot keep anything you say to me confidential. I don't know if my report will help or harm your case and you do not have to answer any questions you don't want to. Do you consent to be evaluated?"

"Sure, that's OK," Don replied.

When I asked him about the crime, Don was in agreement with the police report but he seemed at a loss to explain his behavior.

"I don't know why I acted that way in the store. I went to the store to buy an ice cream. When I found the ice cream, I found out that I couldn't buy the ice cream because I didn't bring any money. I didn't have any money so I just grabbed the ice cream and ran. I wrapped it up in the tee shirt and held the shirt over my head but I guess somebody recognized me, anyway."

"Can you give me a reason why you tried to steal from the store instead of handling the situation some other way?" I asked.

"I guess I just like ice cream," was his reply.

On his Cognitive Examination of *attention,* Don did well on all tests.

In tests of *language,* Don's Quality of Speech was slow and halting and he did poorly on Object Naming.

In tests of *memory,* Don could only repeat back three of seven numbers I read to him on a test of Digit Span (working memory). On other tests of memory, Don could not name any of the prior Four Presidents and he could only recall two items on tests of Free Recall from a Story, Uncued Delayed Memory, and Cued Delayed Memory. Don's Category Recall was good for current animation and comedy shows on television.

In *abstract thinking* tests, Don failed Proverb Interpretation. When asked to interpret the proverb, "Don't cry over spilt milk," Don said, "I never spill milk anymore. I used to when I was a kid, but my mom told me milk costs too much money to waste. So I never spill milk anymore." When asked to interpret, "Rome wasn't built in a day," Don was puzzled. "I go to the Roman Catholic church on Sunday. Is that what you mean?" he asked.

Also in *abstract thinking,* Don failed the Greek Cross test because his drawing was poorly proportioned. In a test of Judgment, when Don was asked what to do if he were in a movie and smelled smoke, he said, "I don't go to movies. Movies are expensive and television is free." In a test of Insight, when asked why it was good to tell the truth, Don said, "I never lie anymore. I used to lie when I was a kid, but my mom told me it was bad. So I never lie anymore."

In *sequential thinking* tasks, Don could only follow two steps in a Four-Step Sequential Command. He was only able to subtract 7 from 100 once on the Serial Sevens test. He failed the Arithmetic Story Problem, but at my request, he correctly explained how to make change from a dollar. He failed the Luria Sequential Movements and Rhythm Reproduction tasks.

The court needed certain information to determine if Don could be put on trial. Don accurately described the charges against him and he correctly explained the purpose and mechanics of the trial process. I was unsure of the correct diagnosis until I performed an additional test—then I was able to complete my report and make my recommendations to the court.

CHALLENGE

Your challenge is to consider the evidence and render your opinion. Think about Don's general comportment, cognitive testing, and the additional test that helped clarify my conclusions. After you have formulated your solution, decide what professional advice you will give to the judge about trying this case.

SOLUTION

Don has mild **Intellectual Disability** (DSM-5 319, ICD-10 F70).

The additional test I administered was a standardized intelligence test. Together with his poor school achievement, social limitations, and poor performance on his Cognitive Examination, Don met the following criteria:

A. **Intellectual deficits in *memory* and learning, *abstract thinking*, reasoning and planning, confirmed by both clinical assessment and standardized intelligence testing.** (*Memory*): Don failed tests of Digit Span (working memory), Four Presidents, Free Recall from a Story, Uncued Delayed Memory, and Cued Delayed Memory. (*Abstract thinking*): Don tests of Proverb Interpretation, the Greek Cross drawing test, a test of Judgment, and a test of Insight. (*Reasoning and planning*): His hapless criminal behavior showed poor reasoning and planning.
B. **Failure to meet developmental and sociocultural standards for personal independence and social responsibility in one or more activities of daily life, such as communication, social participation, and independent living across school, work, home, and social environments.** (*Communication*): Don's speech was "slow and halting" and "he did poorly on the *language* test of Object Naming." (*Social participation*): "He had no social relationships outside of work except for his invalid mother." (*Self-care*): "Don was overweight and "dressed in a shabby tee shirt and jeans."
C. **The deficits begin in childhood.** Don's problems first surfaced when he earned failing grades and left high school.

Other Diagnostic Considerations

Sometimes disorders such as Bipolar Disorder, Schizophrenia, Substance-related Disorders, physical brain injury, or illness can make a patient appear to have a low native intelligence. However, these effects are usually transient or cyclic. There was no evidence that Don had any other psychiatric disorders and his poor school performance suggested that his cognition had been impaired since childhood.

Cognitive Testing

Don failed cognitive tests of *language*, *memory*, *abstract thinking*, and *sequential thinking*, although his *attention* was good. He failed many tests of *abstract thinking*, and he had difficulty remembering more than two items at a time. Don's speech was very linear in style, with frequent repetitions. All these are consistent with mild Intellectual Disability.

CLINICAL NOTES

Don's crime is puzzling for its extremely poor planning and execution. Robbing a convenience store in the middle of the day amid many familiar witnesses suggests poor competence in the art of crime. Furthermore, using your tee shirt to hide your face will not fool people who know you well, and running from the scene with your shirt in a twist is not an example of a clever "get away." The fact that Don had previously been apprehended for shoplifting in the same store marks Don as a poor criminal indeed. The key to understanding Don's actions is to understand that he had mental limitations, limited simultaneous memory capacity, and had received no remediation or social services support for his disability.

Intellectual deficits become a mental disorder when they cause problems in school, work, family life, and social life; or when they affect communication, self-care, use of community resources, self-direction, leisure, health, or safety. Don's usual, predictable, low-confrontation, low-stress lifestyle usually kept his intellectual deficits from causing problems in his life. He did what was expected of him at work, watched television and took care of his mother at home, and went to a nearby church on Sundays. However, Don's limitations were unmasked in new and stressful situations. In Don's case, he responded impulsively to his appetite for an ice cream bar, then panicked and demonstrated poor judgment in his attempt to escape.

Under other circumstances, we might have expected Don's deficit to be picked up early in life and addressed with special services including school and social programs. However, in an environment of social isolation and poverty, Don had not received any special help for his condition and he had managed as well as he could on his own.

My report to the judge stressed the functional limitations imposed by intellectual deficits and the fact that Don had never received any professional help because his condition had never been recognized. The situation was explained to the shop owner, who agreed to drop the charges, and Don was scheduled for a Social Services evaluation to determine his eligibility for public services and support.

Intellectual Disability has been estimated to occur in about 1% of the population, although estimates vary widely. It is estimated that 4-10% of prison inmates are mentally retarded. Diagnosis requires a childhood intelligence quotient of 70 or less, plus impairments in adaptive living. It is an error to base a diagnosis on IQ test results alone, because functional impairment is necessary to demonstrate that a disorder is present. When their life becomes stable; with appropriate work, social, and family performance; individuals will still have a low intelligence quotient, but they will no longer have a mental disorder.

CASE 51
JACK SEES RED

As I sat in the tiny holding cell that was my office, I smelled a strong aroma of old cigarette smoke. When I looked out into the corridor, I realized that the smell came from Jack, who was standing alone outside the door—the guard who was supposed to accompany him was nowhere to be seen. Consequently, I left the door open when he walked in and I arranged the little metal table that served as my desk so that either Jack or I could make a fast break for the door without getting in each other's way.

Jack was a small, wiry, rail-thin man with dark, unkempt black hair and a thin face covered with several days of black stubble. It was cold in the prison at night, although you could not tell the hour because no windows could be seen, and Jack was shivering in his short-sleeved orange prison shirt. Jack hunched in his metal chair looking uneasy.

Jack's police report said that police officers had been called to the cheap Norwegian Wood apartment house by Jack's neighbor, after hearing Jack screaming inside his one-room apartment. When the police arrived, they heard his screaming and broke the door open. Inside the messy, smelly room, they found Jack sitting in the corner, crying. They brought him in for causing a public disturbance.

The only other record I had was a quarter-screen note from the computerized records of a free public clinic, written five weeks ago. It did not give a reason for Jack's visit to the clinic at that time. The note alluded to "Many previous hospitalizations in the past," but it mentioned no specifics. The diagnosis was "Psychotic," and the note indicated that Jack had been given a prescription refill for his usual antipsychotic.

"Hello, Jack," I began. "I am a psychiatrist. Your judge asked me to visit you and evaluate you to see if any mental or emotional problems were going on. Do you understand that?"

"Yes," replied Jack, passively.

"And is it OK with you if I evaluate you and make a report for your judge and others to read?" I continued. "I cannot promise that it will help or hurt your case but it may help your judge better understand what is happening with you. I cannot be your doctor and I cannot keep your comments confidential but you don't have to answer any of my questions if you don't want to."

"Yes," replied Jack. "That's OK."

"I read the police report and they said they found you in your apartment, sitting in the corner crying. Do you remember what was going on?"

"Yes, doctor. I remember what was going on because I was afraid. That's why I was sitting in the corner crying. Because I was afraid," Jack explained.

"You were crying because you were afraid," I returned. "Can you tell me why you were afraid?"

"Yes, doctor. I was in the corner crying and afraid because of the walls," Jack replied.

"I see. You were crying and afraid because of the walls," I echoed. "Can you tell me why you were afraid of the walls?"

"Yes, doctor. I was crying and afraid because the walls were bleeding," Jack said.

"You were afraid because the walls were bleeding. How were the walls bleeding?" I asked. "Help me understand what you were experiencing."

"I was in the corner crying and afraid because I saw red blood pouring out of the walls. It poured out of the walls like a hose. And while the red blood poured out of the walls like a hose, I heard the walls screaming." Jack looked miserable.

"I see. While you watched red blood come out of the walls, you heard the walls screaming. Do you remember what the walls were screaming?" I inquired.

"Yes, doctor," Jack continued. "The walls were screaming that the world was coming to an end and everybody was going to die. And I was afraid of the world coming to an end and everybody dying and I tried to stop them from screaming. But I couldn't think of any way to stop the walls from screaming that everybody was going to die. So I just sat there crying." Jack looked desperate.

"I see. Had you been drinking or smoking or taking any drugs that week?" I asked.

"I thought of that, too, doctor," Jack said. "I thought that if I had been taking any drugs, then they could have made the walls scream at me. But I hadn't been taking anything that week, so that couldn't have made the walls scream at me."

"Uh-huh," I rejoined.

174

Jack suddenly grinned weakly. "Except for my cigarettes. I had been smoking my cigarettes. I always have to have my cigarettes. And my coffee."

"I can understand that," I replied. "And do you watch television?"

"Yes, doctor. I have a television in my room and I watch it all night when I can't sleep. I smoke my cigarettes and drink my coffee and I watch my television all night every night."

"Do you remember any television shows you had been watching that week?" I asked. "Were there any television shows that stick in your memory?"

Jack creased his forehead in thought and then looked up. "There's only one show I can remember. I remember that show because it scared me. It was about how a volcano went off underground and red hot stuff came out of the ground and burned everybody up. They said how everything was burned up and everybody died."

"It's sort of a coincidence that you should watch a show about everybody dying and then the walls started screaming that everybody was going to die, don't you think?" I asked.

Jack looked up again, puzzled. "Do you think the *walls* were watching the television and they heard it too?" he ventured cautiously.

"No, I wasn't thinking that the walls were watching television," I said, "but *you* were watching television and maybe that show helped put the thought of everybody dying in your head."

This time Jack didn't look up at me. "Yeah, I guess," he said, unconvinced.

"Have the walls ever bled or screamed before, Jack? Or anything similar to that?"

"Yes, doctor," Jack said. He did not sound puzzled any more. "In the last three weeks they sometimes bled a little. But it was not very much and I just would look the other way. Oh, also, I remember last year they did the same thing. Blood poured out and the walls screamed that everybody was going to die. That time they sent me to the State Hospital for a month. They said it was because I wasn't taking my medicine. But I was."

"How was it being in the State Hospital for a month?" I queried.

"Oh it was OK, I guess. They always had coffee." Jack smiled wanly again, showing a block of rotten, yellow-stained teeth. "And nobody was screaming at me."

"Is that what you want me to do, Jack? Do you want me to send you to the State Hospital this time?" I asked.

"No, you better not send me to the State Hospital this time," Jack said slowly. "My social worker and my conservator told me to stay out of the State Hospital. They say I'm lucky to have an apartment that I can afford, and they told me not to leave it or I might lose it. Sometimes I think I'd like to lose it, though."

Although Jack seemed tired, he stuck with the assessment and answered many of my Diagnostic Interview questions. Jack said he did not sleep or eat very much in prison. His chain smoking and constant coffee drinking might have had something to do with that. He denied physical symptoms of Panic Disorder or Generalized Anxiety Disorder and said he was experiencing no problems with attention, memory, listening to others, or organizing his activities. He did admit to restlessness and difficulty sitting in one place, but this also may have been due to nicotine and caffeine.

Jack said he did not know whether he felt hopeless, anxious, irritable, angry, or empty. He said that he felt afraid about what might happen if he went back to his apartment. Jack denied feelings of depression or a decreased interest in his usual activities. He said he was a loner but he did not go out of his way to avoid people. Jack showed no evidence of expansive or elevated mood.

Jack denied any history of suicidal attempts or any current thoughts of killing himself or doing harm to anyone else. He denied experiencing hallucinations in any sensory modality. I saw no evidence of formal thought disorder. When I asked him whether he really believed that walls could bleed and scream, now, he told me that he wasn't sure. "I know I saw it and heard it then, but here in the prison I don't think about it," he explained.

Jack worked heroically on his shortened Cognitive Interview, but he was fatigued and somewhat slow. In *attention* tests, he was Oriented to person, place, and time, but he did not know the date or the day of the week. His Basic Verbal Comprehension was normal.

In *language* tests, Jack's Quality of Speech was perseverative. His voice was monotonic and hoarse, probably as a result of his chain smoking. He did well on tests of Verbal Registration and Immediate Repetition, and Object and Part Naming.

In *memory* testing, Jack repeated only three of seven numbers in the Digit Span task. He could not recall any presidents. In a test of Category Recall, I asked him to tell me every type of clothing that there was as fast as he could. Jack looked down at his clothing and said, "Shoes, socks, pants, and shirt." After that, he just smiled, a little embarrassed. When I read Jack a short story and asked him to repeat it to me (Free Recall from a Story), he looked up with a blank look on his face. "I just don't remember it," he told me. In a test of Cued Delayed Memory, Jack could not remember any of the target words after three minutes, but he could pick two of them from a list I read to him.

In *abstract thinking* tests, Jack could not perform Simple Arithmetic. In the Proverb Interpretation task, his interpretation of the proverb, "Don't cry over spilt milk" was "Don't cry. It's only milk. It's not important." In response to the proverb "Rome wasn't built in a day," he replied, "It took a long time to build Rome." When I asked him to explain the difference between a daisy and a flower, he said, "They're the same thing. Daisies and flowers are the same."

In *sequential thinking* tests, Jack easily completed a Four-Step Sequential Command. He stumbled over Simple Arithmetic, so I did not give him the Serial Sevens test or the Arithmetic Story Problem. He easily reproduced the three Luria Sequential Movements on his first trial and he brightened when I told him he was correct. "That one was easy," he said.

Finally, I was able to say, "Thanks, Jack. You've done everything I wanted you to do, and you were very cooperative. Do you have anything you want to say before we finish?"

"I'm glad I talked to you," said Jack. "I finally figured out what to do if the walls ever start bleeding and screaming again. I got the idea when you were talking about that volcano movie I saw. I feel better now that I know what to do."

"Yes. And what would you do?" I inquired.

Jack shook his head and would not answer, but only gave me his funny wan smile again.

CHALLENGE

What is Jack's diagnosis? What would you write in your report to the judge and what treatment recommendations would you make? What did Jack mean when he said he now knew what to do about the recalcitrant walls? There is much to learn from this quiet interview.

SOLUTION

Jack has **Schizophrenia** (DSM-5 295.90, ICD-10 F20.9):

At least two of the following usually present during a one-month period (at least one must be 1, 2, or 3):
1. **Hallucinations.** (*Auditory*): Jack heard the walls screaming. (*Visual*): He saw red blood pouring out as if from "a hose."
2. **Delusions.** Jack believed that his screaming walls would cause everybody to die.
3. **Disorganized speech (with frequent stopping, derailment or incoherence).**
4. **Disorganized or catatonic behavior (immobility, stereotypies, posturing, mannerisms).**
5. **Negative symptoms—diminished expression of emotion (flat affect), diminished words or content in speech (alogia), or failure to engage or persist in activities (avolition).** Although Jack's interpersonal style was quiet and passive, and his voice was monotonic, he smiled and looked uneasy, desperate, puzzled, cautious, or embarrassed, depending on the social context. There was no evidence of flat affect or negative symptoms.

Continuous signs of the illness must persist for at least six months—during this time two symptoms may be milder or only negative symptoms may be present. Jack's symptoms have been present for years.

There has been significant impairment in self-care, school, work, family, or social function since the onset of the disturbance. Jack's symptoms impaired his ability to go to school, work, or have a normal family or social life. They also contributed to his interpersonal isolation, poor hygiene, and poor self-care.

Other Diagnostic Considerations

Some clinicians would consider a diagnosis of Bipolar I Disorder, which would be consistent with his crying, his failure to sleep, and his depressing story. However, Jack showed no evidence of abnormally and persistently elevated, expansive, or irritable mood necessary for a Manic Episode. His thought and speech content suggested Major Depressive Disorder, but Jack demonstrated neither sadness nor anhedonia—his main emotion was fear.

Cognitive Testing

Jack's Cognitive Examination was significant for *memory* problems across all the tests measuring working memory, distant memory, immediate recall, and delayed recall. He also did poorly on tests of *abstract thinking*—his Proverb Interpretations were concrete and he did not comprehend the notion of overlapping sets. His speech was very linear and content overlapped between successive sentences. I have seen these characteristics before in patients with Schizophrenia.

CLINICAL NOTES

Jack's repetitive, serial style of speech arose from his inability to hold multiple thoughts in working memory. Instead of holding several words/concepts in working memory at once, a mind with limited simultaneous memory capacity must break words and concepts into smaller bits that are processed sequentially—that is, ordered into repetitive sequences that are communicated one after the other. Limited working memory also impairs *abstract thinking*. Instead of comparing multiple concepts at the same time, analysis must be reduced to small steps that can be evaluated one at a time by *sequential thinking* processes. In this way, no more than three thoughts must be held in working memory at once—the past thought, the current thought, and the expectation of the next thought.

What triggered Jack's terrifying episode? He denied taking anything, so Jack may have stopped taking his antipsychotic medications. Refills are usually given in one-month or six-month intervals. His clinic prescription was dated five weeks previously so Jack may have run out of his medications. It is also notable that Jack did not specifically deny drinking alcohol. Alcohol can work against antipsychotic medications to increase psychotic symptoms.

Chain-smoking and constant coffee drinking are common among individuals with Schizophrenia, and Jack's habits may have had a significant influence on his overall mental health. Nicotine stimulates cholinergic receptors, whereas the caffeine and theophylline found in coffee stimulate noradrenergic alpha-1 receptors in the cerebral cortex and alpha-2 receptors in the striatal part of the brainstem. Both cause significant stimulation, and at high doses, both have been known to cause psychosis in otherwise normal individuals. Moreover, nicotine tends to lower the blood levels of antipsychotics, while overhydration and diuresis from excessive coffee intake can also dilute medications and lower their blood levels. Although his medication levels may have been adequate for his stays in the hospital; when Jack began staying up all night, his nicotine and caffeine intake increased in proportion to the number of extra hours he spent awake, smoking and drinking coffee. It is a vicious cycle—smoking and drinking coffee provide extra stimulation that suppresses sleep and causes patients to stay up later so they smoke more cigarettes and drink more coffee. The resultant sleep deprivation and impaired nutrition from the anorexic effect of stimulants cause further vulnerability to decompensation and psychosis.

In my report to the court, I said that Jack was quiet and no longer psychotic. However, I strongly emphasized that there was nothing in place to keep his psychotic event from recurring, as it had in the past. In fact, Jack was vulnerable to recurrent psychosis because of his excessive nicotine and caffeine intake and his belief that forces in his apartment posed a threat to the world. If his psychosis returned, he might pose a danger to himself or others.

I urged the court to send Jack to the State Mental Hospital again for his own safety. There he could be enrolled in an inpatient smoking cessation program. I also advised that Jack be moved out of his apartment into structured group living. This would remove the threat posed by his apartment delusions, surround him with other people in a relatively supportive atmosphere, and help him develop a more reasonable sleep-wake cycle so that he would no longer stay up smoking and drinking coffee all night. This setting would also help Jack maintain a regular medication schedule. I also requested increased Social Services support in his new living situation, to catch any relapses before they became too severe.

I encouraged Jack's doctors to reevaluate his treatment plan and consider a stronger pharmacotherapeutic strategy to prevent psychosis. If there was ongoing concern about missed medications, depot forms of medications could be considered.

I was glad to hear that Jack was released from prison and a meeting between his doctor, social worker, and conservator was scheduled to consider my recommendations. Unfortunately, Jack was not hospitalized and none of my other recommendations was followed. Jack's terrifying psychotic experience with the screaming and bleeding walls recurred after three months. This time, instead of cowering in the corner, Jack quietly set fire to his apartment and perished in the flames.

CASE 52
ME AND MY UNCLE

I was asked by the court to interview Thomas, who was being held on a murder charge after shooting his uncle in the face with a double-barreled shotgun at point-blank range. He had been arrested several times before for assault.

I arrived early at an outlying Men's Prison, situated far away from the city. The facility was a modern, well-kept building where the guards worked from inside a centrally located, glass-walled room that looked impregnable. I stood outside the glass in the common area, spoke to them through a microphone, and I was quickly passed through the waiting area to the locked wing where prisoners were housed.

Thomas was paged and arrived in the common area, out of sight of the guard station. Thomas was in his fifties, with gray-white hair and a sunburn that clashed with his orange uniform.

I introduced myself and began the interview. "Hello, Thomas. I'm a psychiatrist. I was asked to give my opinion of your mental health to the judge and others. I don't know if it will help or hurt your case. I cannot be your doctor and I cannot keep anything you tell me confidential. However, you don't have to answer any of my questions. Is that OK with you?"

"It's OK, doc," Thomas replied. "I guess I'm here because I lost my cool. But it's partly my uncle's own fault. And my brother's. They put me up to it." Thomas spoke with a glib, disarming charm.

"You see, Doc, I'm usually a very easy-going guy," Thomas explained. "I live in a nice little house with my brother and we usually get along fine. It was Saturday afternoon, my uncle had come over, and we were watching the ball game and drinking some beer. I get bored easily and I like to have the television on if nothing else is happening. It was a perfectly normal day."

"And what happened that caused you to come to prison?" I asked.

"It was my brother's and my uncle's bickering," Thomas said, tersely. "Whenever they are together, they always start yelling at each other. Well, they were at it again, so I told them to shut up. I told them three times and then I just moved into my bedroom to watch my little TV and get away from them. But they still wouldn't leave me alone. They came in my room with me and started arguing in there. I was lying on the bed and I told them again to shut up and they wouldn't."

"What happened then?" I asked.

"Well, they pissed me off no end, so I just reached under my bed and got the shotgun I keep there. I stuck it in my uncle's face and pulled both triggers. Then I finally got to watch my television in peace until the cops came," Thomas concluded.

"I gather that this bickering between your uncle and your brother was a common occurrence," I said. "What was it about this particular time that made you react the way you did?"

Thomas looked thoughtful. "I guess I just never had a gun close by when he was pissing me off before."

"So, do you regret what you did?" I asked.

"No, not really," Thomas said seriously, then smiled. "I finally got him to shut up, though"

Thomas denied any prior history of treatment for mental disorders or other medical problems. He said he was currently retired and living on social security benefits. When asked if he had been married, Thomas replied, "Yeah, I was married three times—two more if you count the girls I've lived with."

In his Diagnostic Examination, Thomas demonstrated little emotion in his voice, facial expressions, or gestures. He maintained that his sleep, weight, exercise, and nutrition were adequate and stable. Thomas denied heart problems, breathing problems, stomach problems, fatigue, muscle tension, restlessness, excessive sweating, trembling, chills, hot flushes, dizziness, poor concentration, a sense of detachment, fears of losing control, or fears of dying. Thomas admitted to being angry on the occasion of the murder, but he denied any prominent feelings of irritability, sadness, hopelessness, anxiety, panic, or fear. He said he led an active life and enjoyed his usual activities very much. He was comfortable around others and denied having euphoric or overly optimistic, expansive moods. He denied prior suicide attempts, obsessive thoughts, or impulsive behaviors. He denied any past or present hallucinations, delusions, or suicidal thoughts. He said that he never intended any harm to anybody unless they crossed him.

I gave Thomas the Cognitive Questionnaire to fill out (Appendix IV). He did well on all tests of *attention*, *language*, *memory*, and *sequential thinking*.

In the Proverb Interpretation test of *abstract thinking*, Thomas interpreted "Don't cry over spilt milk" by replying "Just get out of the kitchen before anyone sees you." Then he grinned and said, "Tell them the cat did it." For the proverb "Rome wasn't built in a day," Thomas chuckled and said, "They had to take time off to burn the Christians, right?" Thomas failed a test of Judgment by replying that he would "Run as far away as I could before all the doors got blocked" if he were caught in a burning theatre. He said that the reason it was good to tell the truth was "So you don't get caught on your income tax."

I also gave Thomas the Personality Inventory Scales to assess personality symptoms (from the book *Mental Status Examination for Personality Disorders*, Chapter 8).

CHALLENGE

What's going on with Thomas?

SOLUTION

Thomas has **Antisocial Personality Disorder** (DSM-5 301.7, ICD-10 F60.2) and **Psychopathic Personality**.

Thomas met the following criteria for **Antisocial Personality Disorder**:
There is a pervasive pattern of disregard for and violation of the rights of others occurring since age 15 years, as indicated by three (or more) of the following:
1. **Failure to conform to social norms with respect to lawful behaviors as indicated by repeatedly performing acts that are grounds for arrest**. Thomas "had been arrested several times before for assault."
2. **Deceitfulness, as indicated by repeated lying, use of aliases, or conning others for personal profit or pleasure**.
3. **Impulsivity or failure to plan ahead**. (*Impulsivity*): Thomas shot his uncle impulsively. He said that he had never shot his uncle before because "I guess I just never had a gun close by when he was pissing me off." (*Failure to plan*): Thomas fired without thought of future consequences, such as prison or execution.
4. **Irritability and aggressiveness, as indicated by repeated physical fights or assaults**. (*Irritability and aggressiveness*): "They pissed me off no end and so I just reached under my bed and got the shotgun I keep there." (*Assaults*): Thomas "had been arrested several times before for assault."
5. **Reckless disregard for the safety of self or others**. Murder in plain view of a witness shows disregard for Thomas' own safety, and of course, the safety of the uncle that he killed.
6. **Consistent irresponsibility as indicated by repeated failure to sustain consistent work behavior or honor financial obligations**.
7. **Lack of remorse, as indicated by being indifferent to or rationalizing having hurt, mistreated, or stolen from another**. (*Indifference*): Thomas never spoke of his uncle's death with remorse, and when he was asked if he felt regret, he answered, "No. Not really. I finally got him to shut up."

Antisocial Personality Disorder cannot be diagnosed unless the patient met the criteria for Conduct Disorder (DSM-5 312.8, ICD-10 F91.1) as a youth. Thomas met these criteria by endorsing more than three of the following items from the Conduct Disorder scale of the Personality Inventory Scales:

Conduct Disorder

As a child, I often played hooky or ditched school................................	T
As a child, I ran away from home twice or more....................................	T
As a teen, I damaged other people's things on purpose............................	T
As a teen, I caused people physical pain against their will	T
As a teen, I had sex with a partner who didn't want to.............................	T
As a teen, I often needed to be intimidating or threatening........................	T
As a teen, I often started physical fights with others................................	T

Because Conduct Disorder is a requirement for the diagnosis of Antisocial Personality Disorder, when a diagnosis of Antisocial Personality Disorder is made, the additional diagnosis of Conduct Disorder is documented but not recorded.

Thomas' crime went far beyond a mere "disregard for and violation of the rights of others." To spatter your relative's brains around the room while you continue to watch television is horrific. In this context, the construct of "psychopathy" is useful.

Thomas satisfies the following six of the criteria for **Psychopathic Personality** from the book *Mental Status Examination for Personality Disorders* (See Chapter 8):
1. **Glib and charming**. "Thomas spoke with a glib, disarming charm."
2. **Narcissistic and grandiose**. It is grandiose to expect your uncle and brother to obey your commands and it is especially grandiose to believe that you have the right to kill them if they do not do as you ask.
3. **Bored and stimulation-seeking**. Thomas said, "I get bored easily and I like to have the television on if nothing else is happening."
4. **Shallow affect**. In his Diagnostic Examination, "Thomas demonstrated little emotion in his voice, facial expressions, or gestures."
5. **Lacks empathy**. It shows callousness and lack of empathy for Thomas to think that murdering someone is an appropriate response when they talk too much.
6. **Leads a parasitic lifestyle** (despite ability to work, patient relies on family, relatives, friends, or disability status to obtain food, money, and shelter).
7. **Sexually promiscuous**.
8. **Frequent short-term marital relationships**. Thomas said that he had three marriages and two common law marriages.
9. **Poor self-control over emotion and behavior**. It shows poor self-control to murder a family member when "pissed off."
10. **Does not accept responsibility for own actions**. Thomas rationalized, "It's partly my uncle's own fault. And my brother's. They put me up to it."
11. **Commits many types of crimes**. In addition to charges of assault and murder, Thomas admitted to juvenile acts of vandalism and possible rape.
12. **Revocation of conditional release** (such as jumping bail or violating parole conditions).

Other Diagnostic Considerations

Experts have pointed out that the criteria of irritability, grandiosity, and impulsivity in Antisocial Personality Disorder overlap the DSM-5 diagnosis of Bipolar Disorder. Psychopathic criteria of glib speech, grandiosity, and promiscuous sexual behavior also overlap the diagnostic criteria for Bipolar Disorder. However, Thomas demonstrated only episodic irritability when his wishes were thwarted, not a distinct period of abnormally and persistently elevated, expansive, or irritable mood, as required for a Manic Episode, so he cannot be given a bipolar diagnosis.

CLINICAL NOTES

Hervey Cleckley first popularized the term "psychopath" in 1950, to characterize a particularly dangerous type of antisocial criminal. DSM-5 and ICD-10 subsume the terms "psychopathy" and "sociopathy" under the category of Antisocial Personality Disorder but they do not describe a separate psychopathic diagnosis. However, Thomas' story provides an example of an antisocial individual who eclipses the criteria for Antisocial Personality Disorder. In this case, the notion of Psychopathic Personality is useful for the clinician.

Cleckley's theories were characterized in Robert Hare's *Psychopathy Checklist PCL-R* (See Chapter 8). Hare's *Psychopathy Checklist* contains some criteria that duplicate the diagnosis of Antisocial Personality Disorder and additional items that characterize Psychopathic Personality. See *Mental Status Examination for Personality Disorders* (Chapter 8), for more details.

The diagnosis of Psychopathic Personality is particularly linked with sadistic and sexual violence. Individuals with Psychopathic Personality are more likely to repeat their crimes than individuals with Antisocial Personality Disorder alone. Neither treatment nor punishment has been found to curtail their objectionable behavior satisfactorily. Moreover, psychopaths can be dangerous to treat.

Popular literature emphasizes psychopaths' tendencies to view other people as objects, existing only for the psychopathic individuals' use and gratification. In Thomas' case, it seemed perfectly right to him that if his uncle should annoy him, then his uncle should be killed. He even seemed somewhat puzzled that he should be punished for what seemed like a reasonable act to him.

CHAPTER 8
RESOURCES

American Psychiatric Association, *Diagnostic and Statistical Manual of Mental Disorders, Fifth Edition (DSM-5)*. American Psychiatric Association, 2013.

Wes Burgess. *The Mental Status Examination for Personality Disorders. Volume 2 of the Mental Status Examination Series*. CreateSpace, 2013.

Wes Burgess. *Calm Your Mind: Exercises to Reduce Stress, Improve Focus, and Control Anxiety, Anger, and Depression*. CreateSpace, 2011.

Wes Burgess. *Transtorno Bipolar. Perguntas da Vida Real com Prespostas Atualizadas*. Editora Gaia, São Paulo, Brazil, 2010. (Portuguese)

Wes Burgess. *The Depression Answer Book*. Sourcebooks, 2009.

Wes Burgess. *The Bipolar Handbook for Children, Adolescents, and Families*. Avery/Penguin Press, 2008.

Wes Burgess. *Guia del Bipolar*. Ediciones Robinbook, Barcelona, Spain, 2007. (Spanish)

Wes Burgess. *The Bipolar Handbook*. Avery/Penguin Press, 2006.

Wes Burgess. Neurocognitive Impairment in Personality Disorders. *Psychiatry Research*, volume 42, pages 283-290, 1992.

Wes Burgess & V. P. Zarcone. Cognitive Impairment in Dramatic Personality Disorders. *American Journal of Psychiatry*, volume 149, page 136, 1992.

Wes Burgess. The Personality Inventory Scales: A self-rating clinical scale for the diagnosis of personality disorders. *Psychological Reports*, volume 69, pages 1235-1246, 1991.

Wes Burgess. A Standardized Quantified Mental Status Examination Discriminating Four Psychiatric Diagnoses. *Hospital and Community Psychiatry*, volume 43, pages 937-940, 1992. (Swedish translation: 1994).

Wes Burgess. The Relationship of Depression and Cognitive Impairment to Self-Injury. *Psychiatry Research*, volume 38, pages 77-87, 1991.

Wes Burgess. Neurocognition in Acute and Chronic Depression. *Biological Psychiatry*, volume 30, pages 305-309, 1991.

Wes Burgess. Cognitive Information Processing in Borderline Personality Disorder: A Neuropsychiatric Hypothesis. *Jefferson Journal of Psychiatry*, volume 8, pages 34-49, 1990.

Wes Burgess & D. Spoor. Seven Faces in a Crowd: Parallel or Serial Information Processing. *International Journal of Neuroscience*, volume 12, pages 93-98, 1981.

Hervey Cleckley. *The Mask of Sanity*. C.V. Mosby, 1950.

A. Colby & L. Kohlberg. *The Measurement of Moral Judgment*. Cambridge University Press, 1987.

Hans O. Doerr & Albert S. Carlin, Editors. *Forensic Neuropsychology*. The Guilford Press, 1991.

C. J. Golden. A Standardized Version of Luria's Neuropsychological Tests. In S. B. Filskov and T. J. Boll, Editors. *Handbook of Clinical Neuropsychology*. Wiley-Interscience, pages 608-642, 1992.

Donald Rex Gorham. *A Proverbs Test for Clinical and Experimental Use*. Southern Universities Press, 1956.

Igor Grant & Kenneth Adams. *Neuropsychological Assessment of Neuropsychiatric Disorders*. Oxford University Press, 1986.

R. K. Hahn, C. Reist, & L. J. Albers. *Psychiatry*. Current Clinical Strategies Publishers, Seventh Edition, 2005.

J. G. Hardman and L. E. Limbird, Editors. *Goodman and Gillman's The Pharmacological Basis of Therapeutics*. McGraw-Hill, 2001.

R. D. Hare. *The Hare Psychopathy Checklist- Revised.* Multi-Health Systems, Inc., 1991.

Muriel D. Lezak. *Neuropsychological Assessment.* Oxford University Press, 1983.

A. R. Luria. *Cognitive Development.* Harvard University Press, 1976.

A. R. Luria. *The Working Brain.* Basic Books, 1973.

A. R. Luria. *Higher Cortical Functions in Man.* Basic Books, 1962.

J. S. Maxmen & N. G. Ward. *Essential Psychopathology and its Treatment.* W.W. Norton, 1995.

Medline Plus provides diagnostic information. See: http://www.nlm.nih.gov/medlineplus/mentalhealthandbehavior.html

J. Morrison. *Diagnosis Made Easier: Principles and Techniques for Mental Health Clinicians*. The Guilford Press, 2006.

B. J. Sadock & V. A. Sadock. *Kaplan and Sadock's Comprehensive Textbook of Psychiatry.* Lippincott Williams & Wilkins, 2005.

R. L. Spitzer, M. B. First, M. Gibbon, & J. W. Williams, Editors. *Treatment Companion to the DSM-IV-TR Casebook.* American Psychiatric Publishing, 2004.

R. L. Spitzer, M. Gibbon, A. E. Skodol, & J. W. Williams. *DSM-IV-TR Casebook: A Learning Companion to the Diagnostic and Statistical Manual of Mental Disorders*. American Psychiatric Publishing, 2002.

Otfried Spreen & Esther Strauss. *A Compendium of Neuropsychological Tests.* Oxford University Press, 1991.

Richard Strub and F. William Black. *The Mental Status Examination in Neurology.* F. A. Davis, 2000.

E. C. Toy & D. L. Klamen. *Case Files in Psychiatry.* McGraw-Hill, 2006.

J. Vitkus. *McGraw Hill Casebook in Abnormal Psychology.* McGraw Hill, 2004.

World Health Organization. *International Statistical Classification of Diseases and Related Health Problems*. 10th Revision. The World Health Organization Press, 2011. See: http://apps.who.int/classifications/icd10/browse/2010/en#/F21

M. Zimmerman. *Interview Guide for Evaluating DSM-IV Psychiatric Disorders, and the Mental Status Examination.* Psych Products Press, 1994.

APPENDIX I
THE DIAGNOSTIC INTERVIEW

© Wes Burgess, M.D., Mental Status Examination

Reason for Visit

"Please tell me why we are seeing each other today." Write down patient's short statement verbatim:

_____

1. Activity Patterns

"Tell me about your average sleeping, eating, and exercise patterns over the last *7 days*."
"What time do you usually go to bed at night?" _____ o'clock

"About how long do you sleep each night?"	__ 5-9 hr	__ 0-4 hr	__ > 9 hr
"How long does it take you to fall asleep?"	__ 5-20 min	__ 30-60 min	__ > 1 hr
"How long are you awake during the night?"	__ 0-20 min	__ 30-60 min	__ > 1 hr
"How long do you lay awake in the morning?"	__ 0-20 min	__ 30-60 min	__ > 1 hr
"How long do you oversleep in the morning?"	__ 0-20 min	__ 30-60 min	__ > 1 hr
"How much weight did you lose this month?"	__ 0-5 lb	__ 5-10 lb	__ > 10 lb
"How much weight did you gain this month?"	__ 0-5 lb	__ 5-10 lb	__ > 10 lb
"How much do you usually exercise per day?"	__ 0-30 min	__ 1-2 hr	__ > 2 hr
"How was your nutrition in the last 30 days?"	__ Good	__ Fair	__ Poor
"When did you last go 24 hr without sleep?"	__ 1-3 wk ago	__ 1-12 mo ago	__ > 1 yr ago

2. Physical Anxiety (4)

"Which of these have you experienced in the last *2 weeks*?"

__ pounding or racing heart   __ excessive sweating   __ trembling or shaking   __ chills or hot flushes
__ shortness of breath   __ feeling of choking   __ chest pain or discomfort
__ nausea or stomachache   __ dizzy or lightheaded   __ tingling fingers or face
__ fear of losing control   __ fear of dying   __ feeling detached

"Did these ever peak together within a period of 10 minutes?" .... __ Yes __ No

3. General Anxiety (3)

"Which of these has been a problem for you in the last *2 weeks*?"

__ poor concentration OR your mind goes blank   __ easily fatigued   __ muscle tension   __ restless sleep
__ uncontrollable worries lasting at least 6 months   __ feeling restless, keyed-up, or edgy   __ irritability

4. Other Physical Symptoms

"Which of these has been a problem for you in the last *7 days*?"

__ headache   __ joint pain   __ frequent urination
__ neckache   __ abdominal pain   __ low sex interest
__ back pain   __ diarrhea   __ problems with orgasm

5. Focus Problems (6)

"Which of these problems have you experienced in the last *2 weeks*?"

__ attention to details OR careless mistakes   __ maintaining attention   __ listening to others
__ finishing projects   __ organizing tasks & activities   __ doing work or homework
__ losing things   __ too distractible   __ too forgetful

6. Activity Symptoms (6)

"Which of these problems have you experienced in the last *2 weeks*?"
__ fidgeting or squirming __ problems sitting in one place __ restless feelings or behavior
__ difficulty quieting down __ on the go or driven like a motor __ talking excessively
__ blurting out answers __ problems waiting your turn to speak or act __ interrupting others

7. Emotions

"Which of these feelings have you felt in the last *2 weeks?*"
__ on top of the world! __ sad __ hopeless __ anxious __ irritable __ angry __ lonely __ empty

"Which of these feelings have you felt nearly every day during the last *2 years?*"
__ on top of the world! __ sad __ hopeless __ anxious __ irritable __ angry __ lonely __ empty

8. Low Feelings (5)

"Which of these problems have you experienced in the last *2 weeks*?"
__ depressed most of the time __ a loss of interest or pleasure in most activities
__ change in appetite or weight __ sleeping too little or too much __ slowed down or restless
__ feeling fatigue or low energy __ feeling guilty or worthless
__ hard to concentrate or make decisions __ having recurrent thoughts of death

9. Atypical Low Feelings (3)

"Which of these have you experienced in the last *2 weeks*?"
__ good news is cheering __ hungry & gaining weight __ want to sleep too much
__ feel paralyzed and unmotivated __ sensitive to rejection

10. Emotional Activation (1)

"In the last 2 years, which of these problems have you had for *a week or more*?"
__ feeling quite irritable __ feeling quite expansive __ feeling super good

Behavioral Activation (3/4)

"Which did you have during this period of irritability, expansiveness, or feeling super good?"
__ feeling like you "could lick the world" __ needing less sleep
__ talking more than usual or interrupting others __ rapid or racing thoughts
__ easily distracted __ agitated OR overfocussed on activities __ impulsive actions

Other Activated Conditions

"In the last 2 years, which of these conditions have you had for *a week or more*?"
__ feeling tremendous energy __ not sleeping for days __ intense work/social life
__ spending too much money __ feeling lots more sociable __ more sexually aware
__ can't finish projects __ working >12 hr per day __ working all night
__ need constant distraction __ feeling overwhelmed __ can't cope
__ jumping out of your skin __ morning panic __ overactive thoughts
__ not feeling right in your body __ worrying about diseases __ taking sudden trips

11. Adult Experiences

"Which of these have you *ever* experienced as an adult (when not intoxicated)?"
__ a ringing in your ears — knowing others' thoughts __ a sense of leaving your body
__ having visions __ amnesia episodes __ hear noises OR voices others can't hear

12. Social Anxiety

"Are you often,"

__ excessively anxious in social situations?   __ afraid of being embarrassed in front of others?

If so, ask, "Do these feelings interfere with your life?"……............................ __ Yes __ No

13. Past Behaviors

"Which of these have you *ever* done on purpose as an adult?"

__ binge eating   __ using laxatives to diet   __ suicide attempt(s)

14. Thoughts and Behaviors

"Do bad thoughts keep coming into your head even when you don't want them?" __ Yes __ No

If Yes, say, "Give me an example:" _____

"Do you feel a pressure to perform excessive or senseless behaviors?"................ __ Yes __ No

If Yes, say, "Give me an example:" _____

15. Past Trauma

"Are you still recovering from a traumatic experience in the past?"...................... __ Yes __ No

If Yes, say, "Give me an example:" _____

"Do you try to avoid reminders of this traumatic experience?"............................. __ Yes __ No

If Yes, say, "Give me an example:" _____

16. Dangerous Thoughts

"Have you been thinking that your life is not worth living?"................................ __ Yes __ No

If Yes, say, "Give me an example:" _____

"Have you been having thoughts of hurting anyone else?".................................... __ Yes __ No

If Yes, say, "Give me an example:" _____

APPENDIX II
THE DIAGNOSTIC QUESTIONNAIRE

© Wes Burgess, M.D., Mental Status Examination

Please fill out this report to allow more time for personal attention to you. It covers all areas of physical condition, stress, attention, and emotions.

In a few words, why are you being seen today? _____

1. Activity Patterns

Tell me about your average sleeping, eating, and exercise patterns over the last *7 days*:
What time do you usually go to bed at night? _____ o'clock

About how long do you sleep each night?.....	__ 5-9 hr	__ 0-4 hr	__ > 9 hr
How long does it take you to fall asleep?......	__ 5-20 min	__ 30-60 min	__ > 1 hr
How long are you awake during the night?...	__ 0-20 min	__ 30-60 min	__ > 1 hr
How long do you lay awake in the morning?	__ 0-20 min	__ 30-60 min	__ > 1 hr
How long do you oversleep in the morning?.	__ 0-20 min	__ 30-60 min	__ > 1 hr
How much weight did you lose this month?.	__ 0-5 lb	__ 5-10 lb	__ > 10 lb
How much weight did you gain this month?.	__ 0-5 lb	__ 5-10 lb	__ > 10 lb
How much do you usually exercise per day?.	__ 0-30 min	__ 1-2 hr	__ > 2 hr
How was your nutrition in the last 30 days?..	__ Good	__ Fair	__ Poor
When did you last go 24 hr without sleep?....	__ 1-3 wk ago	__ 1-12 mo ago	__ > 1 yr ago

2. Physical Anxiety (4)

Which of these have you experienced in the last *2 weeks*?
- __ pounding or racing heart
- __ excessive sweating
- __ trembling or shaking
- __ chills or hot flushes
- __ shortness of breath
- __ feeling of choking
- __ chest pain or discomfort
- __ nausea or stomachache
- __ dizzy or lightheaded
- __ tingling fingers or face
- __ fear of losing control
- __ fear of dying
- __ feeling detached

"Did these ever peak together within a period of 10 minutes?"... __ Yes __ No

3. General Anxiety (3)

"Which of these has been a problem for you in the last *2 weeks*?"
- __ poor concentration OR your mind goes blank
- __ easily fatigued
- __ muscle tension
- __ restless sleep
- __ uncontrollable worries lasting at least 6 months
- __ feeling restless, keyed-up, or edgy
- __ irritability

4. Other Physical Symptoms

Which of these has been a problem for you in the last *7 days*?
- __ headache
- __ joint pain
- __ frequent urination
- __ neckache
- __ abdominal pain
- __ low sex interest
- __ back pain
- __ diarrhea
- __ problems with orgasm

5. Focus Problems (6)

Which of these problems have you experienced in the last *2 weeks*?
- __ attention to details OR careless mistakes
- __ maintaining attention
- __ listening to others
- __ finishing projects
- __ organizing tasks & activities
- __ doing work or homework
- __ losing things
- __ too distractible
- __ too forgetful

6. Activity Symptoms (6)

Which of these problems have you experienced in the last *2 weeks*?
__ fidgeting or squirming   __ problems sitting in one place   __ restless feelings or behavior
__ difficulty quieting down   __ on the go or driven like a motor   __ talking excessively
__ blurting out answers   __ problems waiting your turn to speak or act   __ interrupting others

7. Emotions

Check all the ways you have felt in the last *2 weeks*:
__ on top of the world!   __ sad   __ hopeless   __ anxious   __ irritable   __ angry   __ lonely   __ empty

Check all the ways you have felt nearly every day for the last *2 years*:
__ on top of the world!   __ sad   __ hopeless   __ anxious   __ irritable   __ angry   __ lonely   __ empty

8. Low Feelings (5)

Which of these have you experienced in the last *2 weeks*?
__ depressed most of the time   __ a loss of interest or pleasure in most activities
__ change in appetite or weight   __ sleeping too little or too much   __ slowed down or restless
__ feeling fatigue or low energy   __ feeling guilty or worthless
__ hard to concentrate or make decisions   __ having recurrent thoughts of death

9. Atypical Low Feelings (3)

Which of these have you experienced in the last *2 weeks*?
__ good news is cheering   __ hungry & gaining weight   __ want to sleep too much
__ feel paralyzed and unmotivated   __ sensitive to rejection

10. Emotional Activation (1)

In the last 2 years, which of these have you had for periods lasting *a week or more*?
__ feeling quite irritable   __ feeling quite expansive   __ feeling super good

Behavioral Activation (3/4)

In the last 2 years, which of these have you had for periods lasting *a week or more*?
__ feeling like you "could lick the world"   __ needing less sleep
__ talking more than usual or interrupting others   __ rapid or racing thoughts
__ easily distracted   __ agitated OR overfocussed on activities   __ impulsive actions

Other Activated Conditions

In the last 2 years, which of these conditions have you had for *a week or more*?
__ feeling tremendous energy   __ not sleeping for days   __ intense work/social life
__ spending too much money   __ feeling lots more sociable   __ more sexually aware
__ can't finish projects   __ working >12 hr per day   __ working all night
__ need constant distraction   __ feeling overwhelmed   __ can't cope
__ jumping out of your skin   __ morning panic   __ overactive thoughts
__ not feeling right in your body   __ worrying about diseases   __ taking sudden trips

11. Adult Experiences

Which of these have you *ever* experienced as an adult (when not intoxicated)?
__ a ringing in your ears   — knowing others' thoughts   __ a sense of leaving your body
__ having visions   __ amnesia episodes   __ hear noises OR voices others can't hear

12. Social Anxiety

Are you often excessively anxious in social situations?............................……....... __ Yes __ No

Are you often afraid of being embarrassed in front of others?............................…....... __ Yes __ No

If so, Do these feelings interfere with your life?...........…..........................…....... __ Yes __ No

13. Past Behaviors

Which of these have you *ever* done on purpose as an adult?

__ binge eating   __ using laxatives to diet   __ suicide attempt(s)

14. Thoughts and Behaviors

Do bad thoughts keep coming into your head even when you don't want them?.. __ Yes __ No

If Yes, give a brief example:_____

Do you feel a pressure to perform excessive or senseless behaviors?.................... __ Yes __ No

If Yes, give a brief example:_____

15. Past Trauma

Are you still recovering from a traumatic experience in the past?........................ __ Yes __ No

If Yes, give a brief example:_____

Do you try to avoid reminders of this traumatic experience?................................ __ Yes __ No

If Yes, give a brief example:_____

16. Dangerous Thoughts

Have you been thinking that your life is not worth living?..................................... __ Yes __ No

If Yes, give a brief example:_____

Have you been having thoughts of hurting anyone else?....................................... __ Yes __ No

If Yes, give a brief example:_____

APPENDIX III
THE COGNITIVE INTERVIEW

© Wes Burgess, M.D., Mental Status Examination

Tests of Attention

1. Level of Consciousness

Say, "How are you feeling right now?:" __Alert, __Distracted, __Sluggish, __Confused, __Fuzzy/Spacey/Out of It?"

Score: Alert=8, Distracted=6, Sluggish=4, Confused=2, Fuzzy/Spacey/Out of It=0. Score:___/8

2. Orientation

Say, "What's your name?"_____, "this place?"_____, "the date?"__-__-__, "the time?"__:__

The score is the total number of blanks filled in correctly plus 1 (Total+1)...................... Score:___/8

3. Basic Verbal Comprehension

Say, "Hold up your left hand." Do *not* hold up your own hand to demonstrate.

The score is 9 minus the number of tries needed to hold up either hand (9-Tries)............ Score:___/8

If the score of questions 1-3 is low, stop testing and evaluate for Delirium.

4. Vigilance

Say, "I'm going to read some numbers to you. Please raise your finger whenever

you hear a '**5**.'" Read the numbers at a rate of one per 2 seconds. Circle each **5** identified.

" 9 0 5 8 6 7 2 6 5 5 0 8 5 9 3 4 5 2 1 9 9 5 1 5 3 4 2 4 5 0 "

The score is the sum of correct answers.. Score:___/8

Tests of Language

5. Quality of Speech

Check the following speech qualities, if present:

__ Loud __ Rapid __ Tangential __ Pressured __ Derailed

__ Scanning __ Aprosodic __ Dysarthric __ Blocked

The score is 8 minus the number of checked items (8–Total)...….......….................. Score:___/8

6. Verbal Registration and Immediate Repetition

Say, "I'm going to say some words. I'd like you to say them back to me when I'm done."

"Ready?" Say, "a *Red Ball*, a *Blue Car*, and the *City of Chicago*."

Speak at about one word per second. If the patient does not repeat the words correctly

on the first trial, say, "Let's try again," and repeat the above.

The score is 9 minus the trials needed to repeat all words correctly (9-Trials).................. Score:___/8

Now say, "**Now see if you can remember these words when I ask you again, later.**"

7. Object and Part Naming

Say, "I'm going to touch some things and I want you to tell me their names."
Show a wristwatch. Touch watch and band with your fingertip and say, "What's this?"
If the patient answers "watch," check .... Correct __
Say, "This is my WATCH. What's the name of this part of the watch?" Touch the band.
If the patient says "band" or "bracelet," check.. Correct __
Say, "What's the name of this part of the watch?" Tap on the watch crystal.
If the patient says "crystal" or "face," check .... Correct __
Take out a pen, rub your fingertip along its length and say, "What's this?"
If the patient answers "pen" or "pencil," check .... Correct __
Say, "This is my PEN. What's the name of this part of the pen?" Touch the pen point.
If the patient answers "point or tip," check .... Correct __
Show your shoe, rub your fingertip along its length and say, "What's this?"
If the patient answers "shoe," check... Correct __
Say, "This is my SHOE. What's the name of this part of the shoe?" Touch the length of the sole.
If the patient answers "sole," check.. Correct __
Say, "What's the name of this part of the shoe?" Touch the heel of the shoe.
If the patient answers "heel," check.. Correct __
The score is the sum of correct answers... Score:___/8

Tests of Memory

8. Digit Span (Working Memory Capacity)

Say, "I'm going to say some numbers. Just say them back to me when I'm done. Ready?"
Then say the following numbers at one per second and write down the replies in order.

"3 2 6 0 9 1 0"   Reply: ___(3) ___(2) ___(6) ___(0) ___(9) ___(1) ___(0) ___ ___
"8 1 5 3 7 2 9"   Reply: ___(8) ___(1) ___(5) ___(3) ___(7) ___(2) ___(9) ___ ___
The score is the total number of correct answers divided by 2 plus 1 [(Total/2)+1].......... Score:___/8

9. Four Presidents (Distant Memory)

Say, "Name the last four presidents." _____ _____ _____ _____
Count the correct current or previous president and the three preceding him or her as one point each.
The score is the number of correct answers in any order, times 2 (Totalx2)..................... Score:___/8

10. Category Recall

Say, "Which do you like best, animals or clothes?" Use the category that patient picks.
"When I say GO, I want you to name as many (animals/clothes) as you can, as fast as you can."
"Ready? GO!" Let the patient continue for 30 sec.
Record the number of different names: _____ and the number of repeats:_____
The score is the sum of different names minus repeats / 2 [(Total-Repeats)/2]................. Score:___/8

11. Free Recall from a Story

Say, "I'm going to tell you a story. When I'm done, say everything back to me."
"OK? Ready?" Tell the following story, speaking slowly and clearly.
  "__*Thursday* was __*Jackie's* __*9th* __*birthday*. He __*woke* up, __*brushed* his teeth,
  __*dressed*, and __*walked* to __*Lincoln* __*School* on __*5th* Street. In __*Classroom*
  __*Seven*, he said __*'Good Morning'* to __Ms. *Thomas*, his __*teacher*. __She *said*
  __*'Happy Birthday'* and __*handed* him a __*baseball*."
When you have finished telling the story say, "Now repeat everything back to me."
Check every italicized word that the patient repeats correctly.
The score is the sum of correct answers, divided by 2 (Total/2)……................……. Score:___/8

23. Uncued Delayed Memory (transfer here from the end of examination)................ Score:___/8

24. Cued Delayed Memory (transfer here from the end of examination).................. Score:___/8

Tests of Abstract Thinking

12. Simple Arithmetic

Say, "I'm going to give you some arithmetic questions." Read each problem and record response:

"What's 4 plus 7?" ___ (11)   "What's 17 plus 5?" ___ (22)   "What's 48 divided by 4?" ___ (12)

"What's 23 minus 6?" ___ (17)   "What's 13 times 3? ___ (39)   "What's 6 times 9?" ___ (54)

The score is the sum of correct answers plus 2 (Total+2)... Score:___/8

13. Proverb Interpretation

Say, "Proverbs teach a lesson. I'll tell you a proverb and you tell me what it means to *you*."

Say, "Don't Cry Over Spilt Milk." (write response):_____

Scoring: assign points for the answer closest to the example (see Chapter 2).
Don't be upset over problems in the past/Don't let past mistakes bother you... 4 Points __
Little things don't matter/Don't worry about the past/What's done is done..... 2 Points __
Concrete Answers: It spilled, forget it/Clean it up and go on.......................... 0 Points __
Irrelevant Answers: Don't worry, be happy/You win some, you lose some.... 0 Points __

Then say, "I'm going to tell you another proverb. Tell me what it means to *you*."

Say, "Rome Wasn't Built in a Day." (write response):_____

Scoring: assign points for the answer closest to the example (see Chapter 2).
It takes time to achieve something great/Great things take time...................... 4 Points __
Don't do things too fast/Have patience/Great things need special attention..... 2 Points __
Concrete Answers: You can't do some things in a day/It takes too much time   0 Points __
Irrelevant Answers: In Rome, do as the Romans do/Haste makes waste......... 0 Points __

The score is the sum of all points... Score:___/8

14. Set Analysis

Say, "You know how some things are different?"
"I'm going to tell you two things and I want you to tell me how they are *different*."

If the patient just defines the words (like "justice means fairness") or restates them (like "truth means being true"), then say, "Yes, but what is the *difference* between them?"

Scoring: assign points for the answer closest to the example (see Chapter 2).

Say, "How are *truth* and *justice* different?" (write response):_____

Score: Something can be true but not just/Something can be just but not true............. 3 Points __

Say, "How are *poverty* and *misery* different?" (write response):_____

Score: You can be poor but not miserable/You can be miserable but not poor............ 3 Points __

Say, "How are a daisy and a flower different?" (write response):_____

Score: A daisy is a type of flower/All daisies are flowers, not all flowers are daisies.. 2 Points __

The score is the sum of all points... Score:___/8

15. The Greek Cross

Give the patient a sheet of paper containing the Greek Cross (below), and a pen.
Say, "Here is a picture. I want you to draw a copy of it anywhere on this page."
"Make your copy the same size and shape as the original."
Watch to make sure the patient does not fold the paper or trace the outline of the figure.

To score, measure each of the twelve lines in the patient's drawing with a ruler.
Score one error for each line that is ¼ inch longer or ¼ inch shorter than the original.
Also, score one error if the circle is drawn anywhere other than to the lower right of the copied Greek Cross, or if the circle is omitted.
The score is 8 minus the number of errors—the lowest score is 0. (8-Errors)...................... Score:___/8

16. Judgment

"Say, "Imagine you were watching a movie in a crowded theater and you discovered that the building had caught on fire. What would you do?"
Write down the entire response: _____

Scoring: assign points for the answer closest to the example (arranged by public responsibility).
Find someone in authority and tell her there is a fire, then leave quietly......... 8 Points __
Call 911 and then tell the people around me to file out quietly........................ 7 Points __
Call 911 OR the fire department and report the fire.. 6 Points __
Make a calm announcement that there is a fire so everyone can get out........... 3 Points __
Scream fire as loud as I can, then run out... 2 Points __
Run out real fast/Find the nearest door and save myself, etc............................ 0 Points __
The score is the number of points.. Score:___/8

17. Insight

Say, "It's important that people tell the truth. Why is it important to *you* to tell the truth?"

Write down the entire response: _____

Scoring: assign points for the answer closest to the example (arranged by type of values).
Global/Cultural: We all live together/For harmony/For civilization to work.... 8 Points __
Personal: For self-respect/Because I'm not a liar/To be a good person............. 7 Points __
Interpersonal: To earn respect/So I won't be called a liar/So others trust me.... 7 Points __
External Rules and Punishment: To stay out of trouble/You're supposed to.... 5 Points __
No answer, doesn't know, or answer is irrelevant... 0 Points __
The score is the number of points.. Score:___/8

Additional Abstract Information
Check if the patient shows:
Right vs. Left Confusion (Patient holds up the wrong hand in questions 3 or 18)....... __
Part vs. Whole Confusion (Patient names object instead of the part in Question 7).... __
Finger Agnosia (The patient holds up the wrong finger in Question 18).................... __

Tests of Sequential Thinking (Executive Function)

18. Four-Step Sequential Command

Say, "I'm going to tell you something and I want you to do it. Ready? OK."
Say, "Touch your left ear with the little finger of your right hand and smile."

Check: __ touch left ear __ using little finger __ using the right hand __ smiling
The score is the sum of correct responses times 2 (Totalx2)...………………............. Score:___/8

19. Serial Sevens (Arithmetic and Sequential Thinking)

Say, "What is 100 minus 7? Ninety-three, right? What is 93 minus 7? Keep taking 7 away."
Record each response. After an error, the next correct answer is 7 minus the prior answer.
100 – 7 = 93... ___86 ___79 ___72 ___65 ___58 ___51 ___44 ___37
The score is the sum of correct answers.………………................……..…...................... Score:___/8

20. Arithmetic Story Problem (Arithmetic and Sequential Thinking)

Say, "I'm going to tell you a story problem and I want you to figure the answer in your head."
"Ready?" "A man drove 275 miles in 5 hours. What was his speed in miles per hour?"
If the patient answers "55," check.. 8 Points __
If the patient gives any number between 50-60 other than 55, check................ 4 Points __
If the patient gives any other number that is not between 50-60, check............ 2 Points __
If the patient cannot answer, check.. 0 Points __
The score is the number of points...…………...……...……..…….…..….................. Score:___/8

21. Luria Sequential Movements

Sit across from patient. Make sure both of you are sitting with feet flat on the floor and your hands on your knees. Say, "I'm going to do something with my hands. I want you to watch and do the same thing when I'm done. Ready? OK." Make the following movements in this order, at a rate of about one movement every 2 seconds:

1) Make a fist with your right hand and place the heel of your hand on your right knee. Lift and relax your hand.

2) Spread your right hand out flat and place it palm down on your right knee. Lift and relax your hand.

3) Make a ring with your thumb and forefinger in the "OK" sign and place place the heel of your hand on your right knee so that the loop is horizontal. Lift and relax your hand.

Say, "Now you do it just like me." If the patient fails, say, "OK. Try it again." Then repeat the movements.

The score is the number of trials needed to copy all 3 correctly, minus 9 (9-Total)....... Score:___/8

22. Rhythm Reproduction

Sit across from patient. Make sure both of you are sitting with feet flat on the floor and your hands on your knees.
Say, "Do you like music? I'm going to tap out some rhythms on my knee. I want you to watch
and do the same thing when I'm done. Ready? OK."

Tap the following rhythms. For each "*", tap at a rate of one tap per second. This is the *short* tap.
For each "—", tap at a rate of one tap per 3 seconds. This is the *long* tap.
Record all the patient's taps using "*" for short taps, and "—" for long taps. Check if all taps in a sequence are correct.

Tap:
* * * — — — * * *   Response: __ __ __ __ __ __ __ __ __   Correct = 3 Points __

Tap:
— — * * * — — —   Response: __ __ __ __ __ __ __ __   Correct = 3 Points __

Tap:
— — * * — —   Response: __ __ __ __ __ __ __   Correct = 2 Points __

The score is the sum of all points. There is no partial credit……………..............…….. Score:___/8

Additional Sequential Information

Check if the patient shows:
___ Omission of movements or numbers   ___ Perseveration (extra movements or numbers)
___ Slowed response (>5 sec)   ___ Transposition (movements/numbers out of order)

Tests of Delayed Memory

(Transfer the scores for questions 23 and 24 to the memory section)

23. Uncued Delayed Memory

Say, "Tell me the three things I showed you today." Check if correct: __ Watch __ Pen __ Shoe

The score is the sum of all correct answers, times 2, plus 2 [(Totalx2)+2]......................…..... Score:___/8

24. Cued Delayed Verbal Memory

Say, "Do you remember the words I asked you to remember before? Tell me."

Check if correct: __ RED __ BALL __ BLUE __ CAR __ CITY __ CHICAGO

The score is the sum of all correct responses plus 2 (Total+2)……………............................… Score:___/8

When patients miss the Cued Delayed Memory task, the following questions assess whether the words ever reached longer-term memory.
They are not scored and they do not contribute to the total score.

Memory with Associated Cues

If patient missed any words on the first try,

Say, "One was RED, one was BLUE, one was a CITY. Tell me the other words."

Check all words correctly remembered with cues: __ BALL __ CAR __ CHICAGO

Memory from a List

If the patient still misses a word on the second try, present that word again in a list:

If BALL was missed, say, "Was it a red pen, a red ball, or a red table?"........... Correct __

If CAR was missed, say, "Was it a blue box, a blue flower, or a blue car?"...... Correct __

If CITY was missed, say," Was it Chicago, New York or San Francisco?"....... Correct __

TOTAL SCORE

The TOTAL SCORE is the sum of all points... TOTAL SCORE ____/192

AVERAGE SCORE

The AVERAGE SCORE is the TOTAL SCORE, divided by the number of tests given (24).

TOTAL SCORE / 24=..…............................. AVERAGE SCORE ____/8

15. The Greek Cross
Please copy the figure below anywhere on the page. Try to make your drawing as similar as possible to the original.

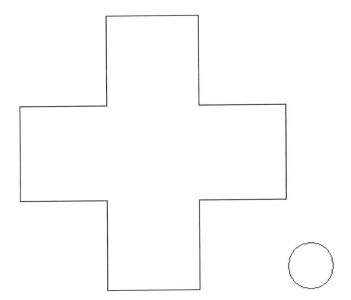

APPENDIX IV
THE COGNITIVE QUESTIONNAIRE

© Wes Burgess, M.D., Mental Status Examination

Please write a brief answer for each question. The questions cover numerous topics—some are easy and others are hard. Do these in your head and do not get help from anyone else. If you cannot answer a question, just write an X in the blank and go on.

1. Level of Consciousness
How are you feeling right now?: __Alert, __Distracted, __Sluggish, __Confused, __Fuzzy/Spacey/Out of It?"

2. Orientation
Fill in the blanks with the right answers. Don't look at a watch or clock and don't get help from anyone else:

Write your name:_____, the name of this place:_____, the date:___-___-___, the time:___:___

3. Verbal Registration and Immediate Repetition
Read the following words once:
Red Ball, Blue Car, City of Chicago.
Now, cover the words with your hand.

Without looking back, write all the words you remember here:

_____

Now see if you can remember these words in a few minutes.

4. Object Naming

Please name the three simple items pictured below: _____, _____, _____

5. Object Part Naming
Arrows point to parts of these three objects. Write the name of each part on the arrow pointing to it. Don't change your answers or ask for help.

6. Digit Span
Read the following numbers once:
3 2 6 0 9 1 0
Now cover the numbers with your hand.

Without looking back, write the numbers that you read here:
_____

7. Four Presidents
Write the names of the last 4 presidents: _____, _____, _____, _____

8. Free Recall from a Story
Read the following story once:

Thursday was Jackie's 9th birthday. He woke up,
brushed his teeth, dressed, and walked to Lincoln School
on 5th Street. In Classroom Seven, he said "Good Morning"
to Ms. Thomas, his teacher. She said "Happy Birthday"
and handed him a baseball.
Now cover the words with your hand.

Without looking back, write everything that you remember here:
_____
_____
_____
_____
_____

Do not change your answers.

9. Simple Arithmetic
This question involves some simple arithmetic. Read each problem and write the answer.
Do these problems in your head and do not change your answers after they are written:

4+7= ____   17+5= ____   48/4= ____   23-6= ____   13 x 3= ____   6 x 9= ____

10. Proverb Interpretation
Proverbs teach a lesson. What do these proverbs mean to *you*?:

Don't cry over spilt milk: _____

Rome wasn't built in a day: _____

11. Set Analysis

How are these 2 things *different* to *you*?: Truth + justice:_____

How are these 2 things *different* to *you*?: Poverty + misery:_____

How are these 2 things *different* to *you*?: A daisy + a flower:_____

10. The Greek Cross
Please copy the figure below anywhere on the page. Try to make your drawing as similar as possible to the original.

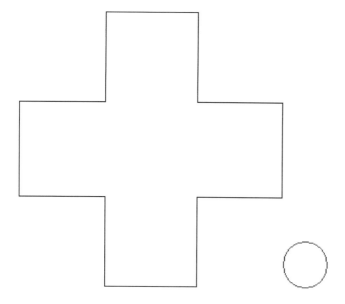

When you are finished, go on to the next page.

13. Judgment

Imagine you were watching a movie in a crowded theater and you discovered that the building had caught fire.

What would you do?:_____

14. Insight

It's important to tell the truth. Why is it important to *you* to tell the truth?"_____

15. Serial Sevens

Start at 100 and count backward by 7s, taking 7 away each time.
Do this in your head and do not change your answers after they are written:

_100_   _93_   _____   _____   _____   _____   _____   _____   _____

16. Arithmetic Story Problem

Read this story and write down the answer.
Do this in your head and do not change your answer after it is written:

A man drove 275 miles in 5 hours. What was his speed in miles per hour? _____

17. Uncued Delayed Verbal Memory

Do you remember those 3 pictures I asked you to name?
Write down the names of those objects below. Do not turn back to the previous pages:

_____   _____   _____

18. Cued Delayed Verbal Memory

Do you remember those words I had you write down and then asked you to remember?
Write down those words below. Do not turn back to the previous pages:

_____

APPENDIX V
THE COGNITIVE QUESTIONNAIRE SCORE SHEET
© *Wes Burgess, M.D., Mental Status Examination*

Tests of Attention

1. Level of Consciousness Check the patient's answer below.

Score: Alert=8, Distracted=6, Sluggish=4, Confused=2, Fuzzy/Spacey/Out of It=0. Score:___/8

2. Orientation

Check all correct answers- __Name __Place Date:___-___-___ Time:___:___

The score is the total number of blanks filled in correctly plus 1 (Total+1)...................... Score:___/8

Tests of Language

3. Verbal Registration and Immediate Repetition

Check all words remembered correctly: __RED, __BALL, __BLUE, __CAR, __CITY, __CHICAGO

The score is the sum of the correct answers, plus 2 (Total+2)..........……..................... Score:___/8

4. Object Naming Check each object named correctly: __Watch __Pen __Shoe

The score is the sum of the correct answers, times 2, plus 2 [(Totalx2)+2]...................... Score:___/8

5. Object Part Naming Check each object and part named correctly:

__band/bracelet __hand/face __buckle/clasp
__cap/top __clip __point/tip __heel __sole

The score is the sum of the correct answers..................................…………................. Score:___/8

Tests of Memory

6. Digit Span Record the answers: ___(3) ___(2) ___(6) ___(0) ___(9) ___(1) ___(0) ___

The score is the total number of correct answers plus 1 (Total+1)........................... Score:___/8

7. Four Presidents check the correct answers below. Any order is acceptable.

__Current or Prior President __Previous President __Previous President __Previous President

The score is the sum of correct answers, times 2 (Totalx2)…….….......................... Score:___/8

8. Free Recall from a Story Check the word(s) repeated correctly in any order:

__Thursday __Jackie's __9th __birthday __woke __brushed
__dressed __walked __Lincoln __School __5th __Classroom
__Seven __Good Morning __Thomas __teacher __said
__Happy Birthday __handed __baseball

The score is the sum of correct answers divided by 2 (Total/2)...…….................. Score:___/8

17. Uncued Delayed Memory (transfer score from the end of the examination)............. Score:___/8

18. Cued Delayed Memory (transfer score from the end of the examination)................ Score:___/8

Tests of Abstract Thinking

9. Simple Arithmetic Check each correct answer.
4+7=__11__ 17+5=__22__ 48/4=__12__ 23-6=__17__ 13 x 3=__39__ 6 x 9=__54__
The score is the sum of all correct answers, plus 2 (Total+2)………...……………... Score:___/8

10. Proverb Interpretation Check the most appropriate answer.
Don't Cry Over Spilt Milk-
Don't be upset over problems in the past/Don't let past mistakes bother you..   4 Points __
Little things don't matter/Don't worry about the past/What's done is done....   2 Points __
Concrete Answers: It spilled, forget it/Clean it up and go on.........................   0 Points __
Irrelevant Answers: Don't worry, be happy/You win some, you lose some....   0 Points __

Rome Wasn't Built in a Day-
It takes time to achieve something great/Great things take time.......................   4 Points __
Don't do things too fast/Have patience/Great things need special attention.....   2 Points __
Concrete Answers: You can't do some things in a day/It takes too much time   0 Points __
Irrelevant Answers: In Rome, do as the Romans do/Haste makes waste.........   0 Points __

The score is the sum of all points..……...................... Score:___/8

11. Set Analysis Check if the patient's answer is correct.
Truth and Justice-
Score: Something can be true but not just/Something can be just but not true...............   3 Points __
Poverty and Misery-
Score: You can be poor but not miserable/You can be miserable but not poor.............   3 Points __
Daisy and Flower-
Score: A daisy is a type of flower/All daisies are flowers, not all flowers are daisies....   2 Points __

The score is the sum of all points..……........................ Score:___/8

12. The Greek Cross
To score, measure each of the twelve lines in the patient's drawing with a ruler.
Score one error for each line that is ¼ inch longer or ¼ inch shorter than the original.
Also, score one error if the circle is drawn anywhere other than to the lower right of the
copied Greek Cross, or if the circle is omitted.
The score is 8 minus the number of errors—the lowest score is 0. (8-Errors)................... Score:___/8

13. Judgment
Scoring (arranged by level of public responsibility):
Find someone in authority and tell her there is a fire, then leave quietly.........   8 Points __
Call 911 and then tell the people around me to file out quietly.......................   7 Points __
Call 911 OR find a telephone and call the fire department..............................   6 Points __
Make a calm announcement that there is a fire so everyone can get out..........   3 Points __
Scream fire as loud as you can, then run out...   2 Points __
Run out real fast/Find the nearest door and save myself, etc............................   0 Points __
The score is the number of points......................…..….. Score:___/8

14. Insight
Scoring: assign points for the answer closest to the example (arranged by type of values).
Global/Cultural: We all live together/For harmony/For civilization to work....   8 Points __
Personal: For self-respect/Because I'm not a liar/To be a good person............   7 Points __
Interpersonal: To earn respect/So I won't be called a liar/So others trust me....   7 Points __
External Rules and Punishment: To stay out of trouble/You're supposed to....   5 Points __
No answer, doesn't know, or answer is irrelevant..   0 Points __
The score is the number of points......................…….. Score:___/8

Tests of Sequential Thinking (Executive Function)

15. Serial Sevens

Check patient's answers. After an error, next correct answer is 7 minus the prior answer.

100 – 7 = 93   ___86   ___79   ___72   ___65   ___58   ___51   ___44   ___37

The score is the sum of correct answers………………......………................................. Score:___/8

16. Arithmetic Story Problem Check the patient's answer.

If the patient answers "55," check……………………..	8 Points ___
If the patient gives any number between 50-60 other than 55, check...............	4 Points ___
If the patient gives any other number that is not between 50-60, check...........	2 Points ___
If the patient cannot answer, check…………………………..	0 Points ___

The score is the number of points...…………...……………...……….….....................…...... Score:___/8

Tests of Delayed Memory

(Transfer the scores for Questions 17 and 18 to the Memory section)

17. Uncued Delayed Memory (transfer score to the Memory section)

Check if correct: ___ Watch   ___ Pen   ___ Shoe

The score is the sum of all correct answers times 2, plus 2 [(Totalx2)+2]…....................... Score:___/8

18. Cued Delayed Memory (transfer score to the Memory section)

Check if correct: ___ RED   ___ BALL   ___ BLUE   ___ CAR   ___ CITY   ___ CHICAGO

The score is the sum of all correct answers, plus 2 (Total+2)………..…........................ Score:___/8

TOTAL SCORE

The TOTAL SCORE is the sum of all points: ………………………….…..................... TOTAL SCORE ____/144

AVERAGE SCORE

The AVERAGE SCORE is the TOTAL SCORE, divided by the number of tests given (18).

TOTAL SCORE / 18=…..………….......................…………..….............................. AVERAGE SCORE ___/8

APPENDIX VI
THE NONVERBAL TESTS OF ABSTRACT THINKING
© *Wes Burgess, M.D., Mental Status Examination, 2011*

For each question, circle the shape does not belong with the others.

1. Circle the shape that does not belong: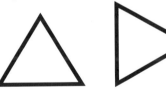

2. Circle the shape that does not belong: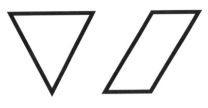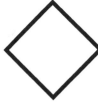

3. Circle the shape that does not belong: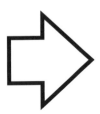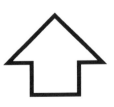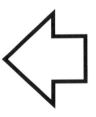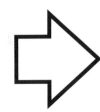

4. Circle the shape that does not belong: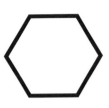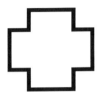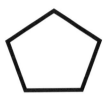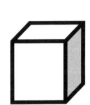

Abstraction Score____

NONVERBAL TESTS OF SEQUENTIAL THINKING

After each question, draw a new shape that should come next in the sequence.

1. Draw the shape that comes next:

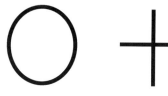 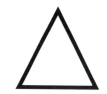

2. Draw the shape that comes next:

3. Draw the shape that comes next:

4. Draw the shape that comes next:

Sequential Score _____

Total Score _____

APPENDIX VII
THE LURIA FIGURE DRAWING TEST

© Wes Burgess, M.D., Mental Status Examination

This is an exercise in copying figures. Copy each figure below into the space next to it.
Try to make each of your drawings as similar as possible to the original.

DRAW YOUR COPY HERE:

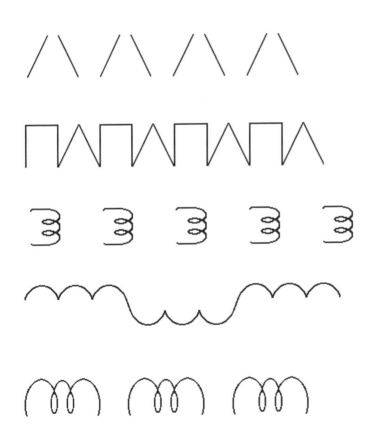

Score _____

THE AUTHOR

Wes Burgess, M.D., Ph.D. is a Los Angeles psychiatrist who trained at Stanford University and has taught at Stanford Medical School, UCLA Medical School, and the University of California, Davis, Department of Psychology. He is the author of *Mental Status Examination for Personality Disorders*, a companion book that focuses on the evaluation and diagnosis of personality disorders, plus *Calm Your Mind* and other books on relaxation techniques for your clients. Dr. Burgess has also written books on Bipolar Disorder and Major Depression. He is a winner of the Purdue Literary Award, the Mead Johnson Award for Excellence in Writing, and the Southern California Psychiatric Association Award for his monthly column on diagnosis. Dr. Burgess has served as a consultant for the Los Angeles Superior Courts and the California Bar Association as well as appearing as a psychiatric expert on National Public Radio, television, and films.

FROM THIS AUTHOR

Mental Status Examination. Volume 1 of the Mental Status Examination Series. CreateSpace, 2011.

Mental Status Examination for Personality Disorders. Volume 2 of the Mental Status Examination Series. CreateSpace, 2013.

Calm Your Mind: Exercises to Reduce Stress, Improve Focus, and Control Anxiety, Anger, and Depression. CreateSpace, 2011.

The Tao Te Ching by Lao Tse. CreateSpace, 2012.

The Gateless Gate of Zen. CreateSpace, 2012.

Transtorno Bipolar. Editora Gaia, São Paulo, Brazil, 2010. (Portuguese)

The Depression Answer Book. Sourcebooks, 2009.

The Bipolar Handbook for Children, Teens, and Families. Avery/Penguin, 2008.

Guia del Bipolar. Ediciones Robinbook, Barcelona, Spain, 2007. (Spanish)

The Bipolar Handbook. Avery/Penguin Press, 2006.

DISCLAIMER

Each of these stories is a teaching example made up of a compilation of experiences with many patients. No symptom, action, or event mentioned in the text refers to any single person. In all cases, names, ages, genders and all personal details are made up for the purpose of writing the book. Symptom lists and diagnostic charts are adapted from the Personality Inventory Scales (1991) and *Mental Status Examination* (2011), with additional support from the American Psychiatric Association's *Diagnostic and Statistical Manual of Mental Disorders* and the World Health Organization's *International Statistical Classification of Diseases and Related Health Problems, 10th Revision*. For the complete wording, consult the original texts referenced in Chapter 8.

Medical treatment information is given here solely for the purpose of illustration and education for clinical students and professionals. Some medications discussed are not licensed for the indications described. Only a licensed clinician can evaluate the unique presentation and needs of an individual patient—this book is not a substitute for a doctor's personal assessment and care. If you are a clinician seeing a patient, always use your own best clinical judgment, and if you are unsure, consult with specialists and utilize professional references and resources. If you are a patient, seek the recommendation of a licensed, credentialed, and experienced clinical professional. Please recognize that the success of any treatment is dependent on a strong, healthy, collaborative relationship between clinician and patient.

Made in the USA
Lexington, KY
16 October 2013